I0886921

Global Perspectives on Health Communication in the Age of Social Media

Seif Sekalala
Kean University, USA

Brandon C. Niezgoda
Drexel University, USA

A volume in the Advances in Healthcare Information Systems and Administration (AHISA) Book Series

IGI Global
DISSEMINATOR OF KNOWLEDGE

Published in the United States of America by
IGI Global
Medical Information Science Reference (an imprint of IGI Global)
701 E. Chocolate Avenue
Hershey PA, USA 17033
Tel: 717-533-8845
Fax: 717-533-8661
E-mail: cust@igi-global.com
Web site: http://www.igi-global.com

Copyright © 2018 by IGI Global. All rights reserved. No part of this publication may be reproduced, stored or distributed in any form or by any means, electronic or mechanical, including photocopying, without written permission from the publisher.
Product or company names used in this set are for identification purposes only. Inclusion of the names of the products or companies does not indicate a claim of ownership by IGI Global of the trademark or registered trademark.

Library of Congress Cataloging-in-Publication Data

Names: Sekalala, Seif, 1985- editor. | Niezgoda, Brandon C., 1988- editor.
Title: Global perspectives on health communication in the age of social media / Seif Sekalala and Brandon C. Niezgoda, editors.
Description: Hershey PA : Medical Information Science Reference, [2018] | Includes bibliographical references.
Identifiers: LCCN 2017020878| ISBN 9781522537168 (hardcover) | ISBN 9781522537175 (ebook)
Subjects: | MESH: Health Communication | Self-Help Groups | Social Media
Classification: LCC RA423.2 | NLM WA 590 | DDC 362.101/4--dc23 LC record available at https://lccn.loc.gov/2017020878

This book is published in the IGI Global book series Advances in Healthcare Information Systems and Administration (AHISA) (ISSN: 2328-1243; eISSN: 2328-126X)

British Cataloguing in Publication Data
A Cataloguing in Publication record for this book is available from the British Library.

All work contributed to this book is new, previously-unpublished material.
The views expressed in this book are those of the authors, but not necessarily of the publisher.

For electronic access to this publication, please contact: eresources@igi-global.com.

Advances in Healthcare Information Systems and Administration (AHISA) Book Series

ISSN:2328-1243
EISSN:2328-126X

Editor-in-Chief: Anastasius Moumtzoglou, Hellenic Society for Quality & Safety in Healthcare and P. & A. Kyriakou Children's Hospital, Greece

MISSION

The **Advances in Healthcare Information Systems and Administration (AHISA) Book Series** aims to provide a channel for international researchers to progress the field of study on technology and its implications on healthcare and health information systems. With the growing focus on healthcare and the importance of enhancing this industry to tend to the expanding population, the book series seeks to accelerate the awareness of technological advancements of health information systems and expand awareness and implementation.

Driven by advancing technologies and their clinical applications, the emerging field of health information systems and informatics is still searching for coherent directing frameworks to advance health care and clinical practices and research. Conducting research in these areas is both promising and challenging due to a host of factors, including rapidly evolving technologies and their application complexity. At the same time, organizational issues, including technology adoption, diffusion and acceptance as well as cost benefits and cost effectiveness of advancing health information systems and informatics applications as innovative forms of investment in healthcare are gaining attention as well. **AHISA** addresses these concepts and critical issues.

COVERAGE

- Role of informatics specialists
- IT Applications in Physical Therapeutic Treatments
- Telemedicine
- Virtual health technologies
- Measurements and Impact of HISA on Public and Social Policy
- Clinical Decision Support Design, Development and Implementation
- Pharmaceutical and Home Healthcare Informatics
- E-Health and M-Health
- Medical informatics
- IS in Healthcare

IGI Global is currently accepting manuscripts for publication within this series. To submit a proposal for a volume in this series, please contact our Acquisition Editors at Acquisitions@igi-global.com or visit: http://www.igi-global.com/publish/.

The Advances in Healthcare Information Systems and Administration (AHISA) Book Series (ISSN 2328-1243) is published by IGI Global, 701 E. Chocolate Avenue, Hershey, PA 17033-1240, USA, www.igi-global.com. This series is composed of titles available for purchase individually; each title is edited to be contextually exclusive from any other title within the series. For pricing and ordering information please visit http://www.igi-global.com/book-series/advances-healthcare-information-systems-administration/37156. Postmaster: Send all address changes to above address. ©© 2018 IGI Global. All rights, including translation in other languages reserved by the publisher. No part of this series may be reproduced or used in any form or by any means – graphics, electronic, or mechanical, including photocopying, recording, taping, or information and retrieval systems – without written permission from the publisher, except for non commercial, educational use, including classroom teaching purposes. The views expressed in this series are those of the authors, but not necessarily of IGI Global.

Titles in this Series

For a list of additional titles in this series, please visit:
https://www.igi-global.com/book-series/advances-healthcare-information-systems-administration/37156

Handbook of Research on Data Science for Effective Healthcare Practice and Administration
Elham Akhond Zadeh Noughabi (University of Calgary, Canada) Bijan Raahemi (University of Ottawa, Canada) Amir Albadvi (Tarbiat Modares University, Iran) and Behrouz H. Far (University of Calgary Canada)
Medical Information Science Reference • ©2017 • 545pp • H/C (ISBN: 9781522525158) • US $255.00

Patent Law and Intellectual Property in the Medcal Field
Rashmi Aggarwal (Institute of Management Technology Ghaziabad, India) and Rajinder Kaur (Panjab University, India)
Medical Information Science Reference • ©2017 • 257pp • H/C (ISBN: 9781522524144) • US $200.00

Design, Development, and Integration of Reliable Electronic Healthcare Platforms
Anastasius Moumtzoglou (P&A Kyriakou Children's Hospital, Greece)
Medical Information Science Reference • ©2017 • 357pp • H/C (ISBN: 9781522517245) • US $205.00

Cloud Computing Systems and Applications in Healthcare
Chintan M. Bhatt (Charotar University of Science & Technology, India) and S. K. Peddoju (Indian Institute of Technology Roorkee, India)
Medical Information Science Reference • ©2017 • 282pp • H/C (ISBN: 9781522510024) • US $205.00

Handbook of Research on Healthcare Administration and Management
Nilmini Wickramasinghe (Epworth HealthCare, Australia & Deakin University, Australia)
Medical Information Science Reference • ©2017 • 825pp • H/C (ISBN: 9781522509202) • US $345.00

For an enitre list of titles in this series, please visit:
https://www.igi-global.com/book-series/advances-healthcare-information-systems-administration/37156

IGI Global
DISSEMINATOR OF KNOWLEDGE

701 East Chocolate Avenue, Hershey, PA 17033, USA
Tel: 717-533-8845 x100 • Fax: 717-533-8661
E-Mail: cust@igi-global.com • www.igi-global.com

Editorial Advisory Board

Aslıhan Ardıç Çobaner, *Mersin University, Turkey*
Mine Gencel Bek, *University of Siegen, Germany*
Kristin Maki, *University at Buffalo (SUNY), USA*
Sarah Parsloe, *Ohio University, USA*
Matthew Pittman, *University of Oregon, USA*

Table of Contents

Preface xiii

Acknowledgment xxiii

Section 1
Introduction: A Theoretical and Empirical Overview of Contemporary Online Health Communities

Chapter 1
Online Social Support Groups/Communities: Implications of Theoretical and Empirical Findings for Individuals Coping With Health Concerns 1
Liza Ngenye, George Mason University, USA
Kevin Wright, George Mason University, USA

Section 2
International Perspectives: Four Case Studies Showcasing International Communities of Practice Online

Chapter 2
Cyber-Moms Facing Motherhood: Holding Functions and Regressive Movements in Parenting Websites 29
Valentina Boursier, University of Naples Federico II, Italy
Valentina Manna, Association for Social Promotion Roots in Action, Italy
Francesca Gioia, University of Naples Federico II, Italy
Federica Coppola, University of Naples Federico II, Italy
Noemi Venosa, University of Naples Federico II, Italy

Chapter 3
Analyzing Online Social Support Within the Type 1 Diabetes Community 59
Kristin G. Maki, University at Buffalo (SUNY), USA
Aisha K. O'Mally, University at Buffalo (SUNY), USA

Chapter 4
Social Support Through Digital Media? Breast Cancer Groups at Facebook 85
Aslıhan Ardıç Çobaner, Mersin University, Turkey
Mine Gencel Bek, University of Siegen, Germany

Chapter 5
Insight Into Sub-Saharan African Discussions of Anxiety and Depression Online.......107
Seif Sekalala, Drexel University, USA
Kristin G. Maki, University at Buffalo (SUNY), USA

Section 3
Rethinking the Current Paradigm: Analyzing Individual/Collective Agency in a Technologically Mediated Society

Chapter 6
Lonely Typers at Midnight: Investigating the Quandaries of Millennial Illness Through Digital Ethnography of Reddit.......162
Brandon Niezgoda, Drexel University, USA

Chapter 7
Sharing Your Personal Medical Experience Online: Is It an Irresponsible Act or Patient Empowerment?.......185
Claudia Lisa Moeller, Istituto Alti Studi Strategici e Politici (IASSP), Italy

Chapter 8
Social Media for Mental Health Initiatives.......210
Gemma Richardson, Humber College, Canada

Related References....... 225

Compilation of References....... 273

About the Contributors....... 344

Index....... 347

Detailed Table of Contents

Preface xiii

Acknowledgment xxiii

Section 1
Introduction: A Theoretical and Empirical Overview of Contemporary Online Health Communities

Chapter 1
Online Social Support Groups/Communities: Implications of Theoretical and Empirical Findings for Individuals Coping With Health Concerns 1
Liza Ngenye, George Mason University, USA
Kevin Wright, George Mason University, USA

Numerous studies over the past two decades suggest that people with a variety of health concerns are increasingly turning to online networks for social support. This has led to the rise of online support groups/communities for people facing health concerns. Researchers have found that these groups/communities provide patients, disease survivors, and caregivers a number of advantages and disadvantages in terms of mobilizing social support for their health-related concerns. This chapter will examine these issues in greater detail as well as the theoretical and practical implications of this body of research for patients who use online support communities to help cope with and manage a variety of health issues. It will provide an overview of online social support and health outcomes, discuss key processes and theoretical explanations for the efficacy of online support communities for people facing health concerns, and the limitations of this body of research as well as an agenda for future communication research on health-related online support groups/communities.

Section 2
International Perspectives: Four Case Studies Showcasing International Communities of Practice Online

Chapter 2
Cyber-Moms Facing Motherhood: Holding Functions and Regressive Movements in Parenting Websites 29
Valentina Boursier, University of Naples Federico II, Italy
Valentina Manna, Association for Social Promotion Roots in Action, Italy
Francesca Gioia, University of Naples Federico II, Italy
Federica Coppola, University of Naples Federico II, Italy
Noemi Venosa, University of Naples Federico II, Italy

Mothers and mothers-to-be often become e-health users because of their need for sharing emotional and practical parental experiences. In this sense, web forums seem to positively contribute to parenting skills and transition to motherhood. This study aims at exploring how 379 Italian mothers use two Italian forums, the manifest and latent contents of their interactions, and the emotional connections between their own maternal experiences and the e-group dynamics. The qualitative analysis of 7433 comments pointed out five main themes, describing how mothers make sense of their experiences through the online dimension: the group; I am; personal experience; perspective knowhow; tech-moms. This study confirms that parenting experience represents a big challenge for rising mothers. Moreover, it shows that the e-groups can alternatively reproduce a peer group functioning and a feeding breast, a reassuring container with holding functions, or a "toilet breast", encouraging progressive as well as regressive movements.

Chapter 3
Analyzing Online Social Support Within the Type 1 Diabetes Community 59
Kristin G. Maki, University at Buffalo (SUNY), USA
Aisha K. O'Mally, University at Buffalo (SUNY), USA

Social support has been linked with many health outcomes, ranging from heart disease to depression. Although its importance has been recognized, less is known about how individuals with chronic illnesses may use social media to provide and seek social support. This chapter's focus is on the way in which people with Type 1 diabetes (T1D) use social media to provide and solicit social support. A mixed-methods approach is utilized. First, posts from two social media platforms were qualitatively content analyzed. Second, the data were quantitatively analyzed to provide a finer-grained understanding of the messages. The results show informational support as the most prevalent on both sites, although there are some differences in content and use. This chapter's implications highlight the importance of social media as a conduit for social support among caregivers and individuals affected by T1D.

Chapter 4
Social Support Through Digital Media? Breast Cancer Groups at Facebook 85
Aslıhan Ardıç Çobaner, Mersin University, Turkey
Mine Gencel Bek, University of Siegen, Germany

This chapter aims to analyze the use of online support groups for breast cancer in Turkey. After describing the general characteristics of such groups, the authors closely analyze the two Facebook groups on breast cancer. The analysis focuses on how the patients read the illness and their struggle to cope with the illness; how social support mechanisms are used; and which aims and motivations are foregrounded. Both quantitative and qualitative techniques are used in the research. Informed by the international research literature, the chapter also tries to underline the similarities and differences of online social media in the Turkish context. Although the main purpose of the groups is to share information, emotional empathy and shared personal experience are also obvious.

Chapter 5
Insight Into Sub-Saharan African Discussions of Anxiety and Depression Online.....107
Seif Sekalala, Drexel University, USA
Kristin G. Maki, University at Buffalo (SUNY), USA

This chapter presents a brief review of past studies on the topics of stigma towards clinical anxiety and depression among populations of African descent in the US and Sub-Saharan Africa, as well as the efficacy of online searches for assistance and moral support. It also reports the findings of a study of nine African patients or survivors of clinical anxiety and depression who share their stories two online platforms, i.e., the website of the South African Depression and Anxiety Group (SADAG), and the www.depression-understood.org forum.

Section 3
Rethinking the Current Paradigm: Analyzing Individual/Collective Agency in a Technologically Mediated Society

Chapter 6
Lonely Typers at Midnight: Investigating the Quandaries of Millennial Illness Through Digital Ethnography of Reddit 162
Brandon Niezgoda, Drexel University, USA

Also known as Generation Y, Millennials—an American construct to classify those born from the early 1980 to mid-1990s—have been targeted by mainstream media as narcissistic, and internet obsessed. But gross generalizations of the American cohort's vanity may only contain nuggets of truth. If millennials are in fact narcissistic and technologically oriented, this research attempts to understand whether this psychological assessment is innate, or deterministic. Contemporary online platforms allow users to voice their opinions and insight regarding predominant frames constructed by once exclusive media domains. Analysis of Reddit discussions through digital ethnography has worked to better understand modes of agency, or lack thereof, as this demographic navigates health problems in a technologically mediated society; providing insight for practitioners, patients, and family members in how to properly conceptualize illness to best help them, and the social order.

Chapter 7
Sharing Your Personal Medical Experience Online: Is It an Irresponsible Act or Patient Empowerment? 185
Claudia Lisa Moeller, Istituto Alti Studi Strategici e Politici (IASSP), Italy

What happened between Mrs. Kardashian West and the FDA in 2015 is very interesting to all of us. She praised and suggested a prescribed drug against morning sickness. The FDA claimed it was a commercial and sent a warning letter to the company, which produced the drug. Kim Kardashian West changed her post and admitted it was a commercial. Was it true? Mrs. Kardashian West just expressed her personal opinion and wanted to share with her followers a piece of advice. She share her personal story, like many other Internet users, and her patient experience should have been respected. Her story shows what patient empowerment is and how the Net is a precious resource for patients to share their stories that might help other patients. For this reason, doctors should not be afraid of the Net and its potentiality.

Chapter 8
Social Media for Mental Health Initiatives 210
Gemma Richardson, Humber College, Canada

Social media has added a new dynamic for those living with mental illness. There are several benefits to using social media to obtain information and support for mental health issues, but there are also new challenges and drawbacks. This chapter explores social media for mental health initiatives, with a focus on two case studies: Facebook's suicide prevention tools and the Bell Let's Talk campaign. These case studies highlight the unique ways that social media can be harnessed to raise awareness and provide support and resources to vulnerable populations, while also providing insights into the challenges of utilizing these platforms.

Related References 225

Compilation of References 273

About the Contributors 344

Index 347

Preface

GENERAL ACADEMIC AND SEMI-AUTOETHNOGRAPHIC BACKGROUND OF RESEARCH

The origins of this volume can be traced to the Spring of 2013 when Seif Sekalala, one of the two co-editors (and co-author of this preface), was enrolled in a Narrative Analysis seminar class in the Drexel University Culture, Communication and Media Ph.D. program. In that class, students were tasked with a term project in which a substantive narrative analysis would have to be carried out on one or more short biographical story/ies.

Incidentally, Sekalala had struck up a friendship with Brandon Niezgoda—the other co-editor of this volume—since their first year in the program, and the former had shared with the latter the traumatic story of his pancreatic cancer ordeal. Seeing as a narrative analysis tends to yield more interesting data if it contains what Labov (2006) calls a dramatic "reportable event" (p. 5), it made sense to use his story.

Sekalala thus held an audio-recorded interview with Niezgoda, prompting him to share his cancer survival story for the record, this time for the specific purpose of a research project. Sekalala also proceeded to gather as much relevant literature as he could find on the topics of illness narratives, and he discovered that in fact, numerous studies have been carried out about illness narratives over the past few decades (e.g., Chatwin, 2006; Delbene, 2011; Vevea & Miller, 2010). Overall, the resultant paper was received enthusiastically by Dr. Barbara Hoekje, the instructor of that seminar, and by numerous participants at two conferences where we presented the findings of the study.

But in the course of writing that paper—which was later revised and co-authored by both Niezgoda and Sekalala, we realized that various websites have a sizable number of stories similar to Brandon's. Such stories are divulged mostly in written testimonies, but are also told using video and audio file media (e.g., on YouTube). And yet, within the aforementioned plethora of relevant past illness narrative research, there was a dearth of studies reporting and analyzing these testimonies, both quantitatively and qualitatively, as they diffuse in online space.

Thus, this book is the consequence of that realization. In the first chapter, readers are given a basic contextualization of the topic. This is followed by relevant research studies in the next seven chapters which analyze the virtual interaction dynamics of various patient and well-wisher support groups and communities across the globe, as encountered on various websites and online social media platforms.

IMPLICATIONS, CAVEATS, QUESTIONS, AND ANSWERS FOR A NEW PARADIGM OF SOCIAL SUPPORT IN HEALTH COMMUNICATION

For indeed, beyond the basic illness narrative on a website or online forum, in the past two decades, diverse interactions on an ever-growing set of internet-based social media platforms have revolutionized the ways in which various populations of afflicted and vulnerable individuals experience, discuss, and make meaning of physical, psychological, and other forms of illness. These platforms, or communities of practice, range from the larger online support group forums (for various specific afflictions) which proliferated in the late 1990s, through today's discussion threads on sites/platforms such as Reddit and Facebook between burgeoning groups of friends, and possible enemies.

When citizens can get and share information freely online about health topics—e.g. using Wikipedia, WebMD, the CDC website etc., and when they can and do share their personal health and illness experiences on various social media platforms, old paradigms of how health-related advice is received (accepted or rejected) and used, are necessarily displaced (Blease, 2016; Breathnach & Kelly, 2016; Kuper & Mustanski, 2014).

Such information and advice includes disease prevention and treatment, coping mechanisms, and tips for caretakers, etc. Thus clearly, healthcare practitioners and policy-makers—among other parties—have to be informed through current scholarship vis-à-vis the trends of the topic of health communication in the age of social media.

And yet, challenges to this research abound, and have to be duly acknowledged in any such endeavor. Arguably, foremost among these—especially given the current dizzying rate of proliferation and unpredictability of social media platforms—is the fact it is quite challenging if not impossible to keep track of a sufficient majority of online health support groups in any given study (of notable size or other worthy consequence). And as Turkle (2012) and others (e.g., Boyd, 2015; Carr, 2011; Rushkoff, 2013[1]) have pointed out, the general public and techno-enthusiasts often overlook various dangers of social media.

Still, scholars can reasonably pose questions with which we can execute actionable research, including: 1) (for any proposed and current study or set of studies,) how can this research improve our understanding of health communication and support in the age of online social media, and 2) why was the particular (set of) online community(/ies) analyzed in this study started, what has it accomplished, and what are its implications for the future vis-à-vis health communication and support via online social media? In the remaining section of this preface below, we briefly summarize and discuss the answers to the above questions from each of this book's eight chapters.

SECTION 1: INTRODUCTION

Chapter 1: Brief Literature Review and Theoretical Framework

In a nutshell, Chapter 1 by Liza Ngenye discusses the history of the existence and evolution, as well as the academic study of the advantages and disadvantages of health communication online by patients, illness survivors, and caretakers. Foundational concepts such as the direct effects and buffering models of social support are briefly recapped, as well as a synthesis of computer-mediated vs. face-to-face communication benefits in the specific context of health communication. Finally, Ngenye utilizes a total of four Communication Studies theories to hypothesize the deeper "*whys*" and "*hows*" of the dynamics of health communication and support via online social media.

SECTION 2: INTERNATIONAL PERSPECTIVES

Topic 1: Across Chapters 2-5 – International Comparisons

These four chapters—(co-)authored respectively by Valentina Boursier et al.; Kristin Maki and Aisha O'Mally; Aslihan Adiç Çobaner and Mine Gencel Bek; and Seif Sekalala and Kristin Maki—offer a varied set of answers to the concerns highlighted in the preceding summary of the literature review chapter, as well as the questions posed further above, that is: 1) how can this work improve our understanding of health communication and support in the age of online social media, and/or 2) why was the online community analyzed in this chapter started, what has it accomplished, and what are its implications for the future? In the comparative context of these four chapters, one of the most remarkable features about Chapter 3 (i.e., compared to the other three chapters) is the fact that it deals with data gathered mostly—apparently—

from the United States, whereas the other three chapters (2, 4, 5) discuss research findings from countries in Europe and Sub-Saharan Africa (Chapters 6-8 also discuss findings from the US and Canada).

Overall, viewed from the prism of the overarching theoretical hypotheses of Chapter 1, one can argue that these chapters tend to demonstrate identical advantages and challenges vis-à-vis online health communication and social support. However, the dearth of relevant data in the research study of Chapter 5 necessarily suggests underlying structural economic and other disadvantages faced by sub-Saharan African populations, which hamper access to helpful online communication and support resources. While future research and advocacy can help in the filling of the relevant knowledge gaps in that regard, readers of these four chapters might gain valuable insights via any notable/consequential specific cross-cultural commonalities and/or differences vis-à-vis health communication and support between the US vs. Europe (i.e., Italy and Turkey) and Sub-Saharan Africa (i.e., South Africa).

Topic 2: Across Chapters 2-5 – Preview of Findings

Each of these chapters focuses on a unique community or (sets of) group(s) of individuals, namely 1) mothers-to-be and new mothers, type-1 diabetics, breast cancer support groups, and individuals dealing with clinical anxiety and depression. And yet, regardless of their specific population, the studies of each of these groups highlight two basic facts, namely 1) individuals dealing with illnesses or other similar challenges actively *seek* social support online. Perhaps they do so after failing to get the type of help they need via face-to-face interactions, or in an attempt to supplement it. 2) There are individuals on among these groups that actively *provide* social support online. Readers should keep in mind the fact that not all individuals who are members or regular visitors to these groups' pages on the various social media platforms are both seekers and providers. On the contrary, platform/site members or visitors are often "lurkers" or passive consumers. Thus, in these chapters, readers will encounter the authors' specific syntheses and analyses of the discussion themes and other features of these groups' online interaction dynamics, and the implications thereof.

In addition to the above commonalities between the analyses of the communities or groups in these chapters, it should be noted that most of the interactions analyzed in these chapters are of a mutual bi- or multi-directional nature between the groups of fellow illness (or other health condition) sufferers or survivors. Granted, Chapter 3 highlights an apparently minimal participation by various organizations, both for- and non-profit, and Chapter 5's data includes that from a non-profit advocacy organization in South Africa.

Still, having noted these chapters' bi-/multi-directional message structure, readers might benefit from an active comparison between their analyses, versus those of Chapters 7-8, which explicitly analyze findings from studies that focus on unidirectional messages, that is messages to the general public from large for- and/ or non-profit organizations, and from a single individual—albeit a celebrity, that is, Ms. Kim Kardashian West.

Overall, these four chapters demonstrate a number of specific benefits and challenges experienced by the group members or visitors of the four sites or platforms analyzed, namely a number of support group groups on Facebook, a forum site, and messages on Twitter. The benefits and challenges discussed include the specific types, quantities, and qualities of practical pieces of advice and resources—for example, how to practice better breastfeeding techniques; where to seek treatment for breast cancer; and how to avoid or manage type-1 diabetes, as well as moral support—for example, exhortations to stay positive in the face of doubts and anxiety during pregnancy, and/or the struggle with cancer, diabetes, and clinical anxiety and depression. Moreso, the chapters advocate for increased understanding in the specific historical and cultural discourses that are perpetuated around an illness, and how they are in play online (i.e., the lack of men found in Turkish Breast Cancer online groups marking a long-lasting cultural construct that the ailment is the women's responsibility, or the continued stigma in African that depression is not openly communicated).

SECTION 3: RETHINKING THE CURRENT PARADIGM – CHAPTERS 6-8

The final three chapters of the volume work as a conclusion: addressing some of the implications of the still malleable paradigm. As has been proclaimed, this is a new dimension of healthcare (Moorhead, Hazlett, Harrison, & Carrol, 2013).

Through virtual ethnography, in Chapter 6, "Lonely Typers at Midnight," Brandon Niezgoda establishes predominant specters of contemporary online virtual communities. With Web 2.0 technology, media frames may now be openly debated. For those who are willing to listen, and spend some time, the millennial demographic is not all how it is perceived by some derogatory mainstream media reports. More to the point, in their discursive practices many have shown a resilience to share knowledge, and help others. While true, just as some groups have been able to create a positive-community, these platforms can just as easily become venues of despair, and group-think, creating further isolation.

This can be exacerbated when coupled with parallel contemporary facets of modernization, where upstart web based media platforms can confirm one's insidious beliefs (e.g., Infowars), or the reforming Pharmaceutical industry can infiltrate web space just as had been done with television. With widespread disapproval of the almost passed American Health Care Act (July 2017) it is imperative for demographics to see how they are similar, and importantly, for these sub-communities of medical anomie to communicate with each other. This is important not only for more communication, and integration between subreddits, but more communication in real life (between patients and doctors, between generation x and generation y). Increased research is necessary to understand just how these groups enact physical change, with formed protests, with decisions to support only specific types of medical practices, and, on the other side of the spectrum, with medical practitioners addressing of these spaces and how traditional institutions (FDA, Mainstream Media) react to these spaces and associated practices that are not just used by the "digital natives."

As Claudia Moeller situates in Chapter 7, "Sharing Online Your Personal Medical Experience: Is It an Irresponsible Act or a Patient Empowerment," there are vast philosophical components to every communicative act on these online spaces. Rhetorically analyzing an Instagram post by Kim Kardashian West, and the subsequent response from the FDA, Moeller sees this current paradigm as riddled with ethical implications. At the core of her study, and this book, is someone simply trying to share information and enter a discourse with their "community." But, one must ask, who owns this virtual space, what is our obligation to each other, what is an advertisement in contemporary society, and, in particular when it comes to medical issues, what if we break the fundamental medical ethic: do no harm? But as the author makes clear, these institutions have never been perfect, and plenty of harm has been done continuously in modern society. Internet space have provided us an opportunity to rethink our roles, and our agency, in the medical field.

In her chapter, Moeller has questioned the ethical implications of contemporary online practices from various stakeholders. She looks from the perspective of a follower, or lurker, searching online for information. She analyzes the state of affairs from the role of a celebrity the trying to make sense of the same medical ailment countless women before have gone through, only now marked by a new type of contemporary career gauged by personal marketability. Moeller too analyzes the changing and shifting landscape from the position of an overworked doctor, whose field of practice, and the rules and regulation that guide his or her actions, have been complicated by not only new technology, but shifts in political economy, and continued poverty/hardships/illnesses. It is, in this philosophical and phenomenological sense, important in this new paradigm for each person to rethink their role and position in contemporary society, and their role, in both online medical communities and contemporary society as a whole.

But, beyond human perspectives, Moeller thinks from the position of the technology itself. She identifies the internet as having two characteristics that doctors do not have: the ability to be available anytime and anywhere, and the possibility to provide anonymous help. Still, these technological affordances and riddled with paradoxes and risks (Speed, Davison, & Gunnell, 2016).

As more research and data is compiled to better understand the communicative actions of Web 2.0, and more books are written about how and why people use the internet, more problems may occur. In Chapter 8, "Social Media for Mental Health Initiatives," Gemma Richardson speaks of a posed future where more understanding, and more data, only seems to systematically break humans down into algorithmic communicative data and phrases. As the first section of this book has situated, our online practices are discursively complicated. The majority of humans that comprise these communities as desperate for hope, change, and empathy. On the contrary, the possibilities of "bot" based analysis of comments may be more dehumanizing. For those dealing with depression to have their words broken down to a base level sense of suicidal tendencies in order to provide "proactive" general communication is condescending and belittling. This is especially when many of these subjects have turned to online spaces because traditional outlets have been inadequate.

Further, predominant debates about network-neutrality pose lingering problems for these online spaces. The Bell Let's Talk Campaign, as highlighted by Richardson, may be meritorious, but is a commercialized online landscape. Her discussion deconstructs some of the more utopian ideals seen in the new landscape. Internet space can be commercially co-opted, and in the process, deconstruct perceived benefits. What is the role of medical practitioners in shaping the internet to make it a space of mutual trust, while facing long lasting bureaucratic battles within the healthcare system outside of virtual space? The difference in social media use between medical students and medical physicians (Von Muhlen & Ohno-Machado, 2012) poses ongoing questions as the doctors rethink their own phenomenological positions and how they are constructed (Karnieli-Miller, Vu, Holtman, Clyman, & Inui, 2010).

Detailed analysis is provided of The Samaritans, a British suicide prevention group. Their 2014 application to alert users when someone they followed was posting troubling comments verbiage would only last one week. In analyzing the actual technical affordances, the developers realized that while the application may have positive externalities, it in turn could be used to mine data on vulnerable people for future targeting (which in the best-case scenario can be a drug that can help them cope, but in the worst-case scenario can be someone to diminish the significance of their pain). There will be persistent problems as web-developers continue to come to terms with the specific user-affordances their websites engender. In these virtual spaces for communicative acts, particular modes of agency have been granted, or lack thereof, by the already existing social and technological structures. This becomes even more complicated when taking into proper consideration, the historical and cultural intricacies of illness and place.

Stressed in each of these chapters is that activism and change must work both ways. The practices online dealing with medical experience come to shape the external world (i.e., breast cancer groups refusing to give their money to predatory private hospitals), but in turn, the outside spaces will continue to shape these virtual spaces (Guggenheim, Jang, Bae, & Neuman, 2015). For reddit community members, the more the external world has chosen to shun, mislabel, and enframe them (Heidegger, 1954), the more people may turn to online spaces. But similarly stressed by each of the authors, within actor networks these online outlets should never be conceptualized as self-contained solutions, and instead, as either symptoms or microcosms to ongoing social and cultural issues.

Research must be geared towards understanding, primarily, the motives of individuals, and the social and technical practices that can help engender change. As Garden (2015) situated in her article: "Who Speaks for Whom? Health Humanities and the Ethics of Representation":

The media or health humanities are in essence a form of advocacy, a means of addressing a problem of under representation. They focus on suffering, rather than pathology, and on sociocultural understandings of illness and disability, rather than a narrow biomedical perspective. The health humanities thus analyze and attempt to recalibrate the power imbalance in healthcare. (p. 77)

It has been our purpose in this book to contribute, further, to this growing body of Health Humanities research. This book has been written to provide a shared sense of knowledge built upon the experiences of a multitude of patients, practitioners, and family members—of which this book is dedicated to—in order to better understand their online practices, and what they mean for both the past, and future, across the globe.

REFERENCES

Blease, C. (2016). In defense of utility: The medical humanities and medical education. *Medical Humanities*, *42*(2), 103–108. doi:10.1136/medhum-2015-010827 PMID:26842744

Boyd, D. (2015). *It's complicated: The social lives of networked teens*. Yale University Press.

Carr, N. G. (2011). *The shallows: What the Internet is doing to our brains*. New York, NY: Norton.

Chatwin, J. (2006). Patient narratives: A micro-interactional analysis. *Communication & Medicine*, *3*(2), 113–123.

Delbene, R. (2011, January 01). Patients' narratives of chronic illnesses and the notion of biographical disruption. *Communication & Medicine*, *8*(1), 17–27. doi:10.1558/cam.v8i1.17 PMID:22616353

Garden, R. (2015). Who speaks for whom? Health humanities and the ethics of representation. *Medical Humanities*. PMID:25795700

Guggenheim, L., Jang, S. M., Bae, S. Y., & Neuman, W. R. (2015). The dynamics of issue frame competition in traditional and social media. *The Annals of the American Academy of Political and Social Science*, *659*(1), 207–224. doi:10.1177/0002716215570549

Karnieli-Miller, O., Vu, T. R., Holtman, M. C., Clyman, S. G., & Inui, T. S. (2010). Medical students' professionalism narratives: A window on the informal and hidden curriculum. *Academic Medicine*, *85*(1), 124–133. doi:10.1097/ACM.0b013e3181c42896 PMID:20042838

Labove, W. (n.d.). *Oral Narratives of Personal Experience*. Retrieved August 27, 2017, from http://www.ling.upenn.edu/~wlabov/Papers/FebOralNarPE.pdf

Rushkoff, D. (2014). *Present shock: When everything happens now*. New York: Current.

Speed, E., Davison, C., & Gunnell, C. (2016). The anonymity paradox in patient engagement: Reputation, risk and web-based public feedback. *Medical Humanities*, *42*(2), 135–140. doi:10.1136/medhum-2015-010823 PMID:26879526

Turkle, S. (2011). *Alone together: Why we expect more from technology and less from each other*. Academic Press.

Vevea, N., & Miller, A. (2010). Patient Narratives: Exploring the Fit of Uncertainty-Management Models of Health Care. *Review of Communication*, *10*(4), 276–289. doi:10.1080/15358593.2010.501907

Von Muhlen, M., & Ohno-Machado, L. (2012). Reviewing social media use b clinicians. *Journal of the American Medical Informatics Association*, *19*(5), 777–781. doi:10.1136/amiajnl-2012-000990 PMID:22759618

ENDNOTE

1 Special thanks to Matthew Pittman for pointing us in the right direction with this sub-topic.

Acknowledgment

The editors of this volume would like to earnestly thank all the authors who have contributed chapters to it. Thank you for your hard work and patience throughout the pre-publication process. We also wish to solemnly thank all the members of the editorial advisory board, both internal (i.e., members who are also authors) and external, namely Aslıhan Ardıç Çobaner, Mine Gencel Bek, and Kristin Maki (internal), as well as Matthew Pittman and Sarah Parsloe (external). Last but certainly not least, we would like to thank Ms. Jordan Tepper, our development editor at IGI Global, who has gone above and beyond to help bring this volume to fruition.

Section 1

Introduction:

A Theoretical and Empirical Overview of Contemporary Online Health Communities

Chapter 1
Online Social Support Groups/Communities:
Implications of Theoretical and Empirical Findings for Individuals Coping With Health Concerns

Liza Ngenye
George Mason University, USA

Kevin Wright
George Mason University, USA

ABSTRACT

Numerous studies over the past two decades suggest that people with a variety of health concerns are increasingly turning to online networks for social support. This has led to the rise of online support groups/communities for people facing health concerns. Researchers have found that these groups/communities provide patients, disease survivors, and caregivers a number of advantages and disadvantages in terms of mobilizing social support for their health-related concerns. This chapter will examine these issues in greater detail as well as the theoretical and practical implications of this body of research for patients who use online support communities to help cope with and manage a variety of health issues. It will provide an overview of online social support and health outcomes, discuss key processes and theoretical explanations for the efficacy of online support communities for people facing health concerns, and the limitations of this body of research as well as an agenda for future communication research on health-related online support groups/communities.

DOI: 10.4018/978-1-5225-3716-8.ch001

Copyright © 2018, IGI Global. Copying or distributing in print or electronic forms without written permission of IGI Global is prohibited.

INTRODUCTION

Numerous studies over the past two decades suggest that people with a variety of health concerns are increasingly turning to online networks for social support. This has led to the rise of online support groups/communities for people facing health concerns, growing from several thousand support groups/communities in the late 1990's to hundreds of thousands of groups/communities by 2012 (Chou, Hunt, Beckjord, Moser, & Hesse, 2009; Fox, 2011; National Cancer Institute, 2013; Wright & Bell, 2003). A survey conducted by the National Cancer Institute (2012) indicated that almost 5% of all adult American Internet users—approximately 7.5 million people—visited a health-related online support community during 2012. Another study found that 18% of people had used the Internet in the last year to find information from a peer with similar health concerns (Fox &Duggan, 2013).

Researchers have found that these groups/communities provide patients, disease survivors, and caregivers a number of advantages (and some disadvantages) in terms of mobilizing social support for their health-related concerns. Online health-related support groups/communities are frequently used by individuals with rare health conditions/issues that are not well understood by physicians, conditions/issues that are difficult for health care providers to explain in layperson terms, or if members of one's primary social network (i.e. friends and family members) have limited knowledge of a person's health condition (Campbell-Grossman et al., 2009; Tanis, 2008; Tong et al., 2013). Due to these issues, many individuals report that they receive inadequate informational support from their traditional social networks and health care providers; and they appear to perceive online support groups/communities as a better alternative for receiving health information (Wicks et al., 2010).

Moreover, research in this area has found that online community members enjoy the ability to draw upon the collective experience of other online participants who are dealing with a similar health issue in ways that are not possible in the face-to-face world. For example, the Internet allows people to access and interact with others in health-related online communities that cross geographical and temporal boundaries (Rains & Wright, 2016). In addition, other participants within these online communities appear to replace or extend traditional offline support networks in terms of providing greater access to different forms of social support. Accessing support providers online has the added benefit of finding people who are available in a larger, easier to maintain, network of (often) geographically separated individuals compared to face-to-face sources of social support (Ellison et al., 2007; Kim & Lee, 2011; Walther & Boyd, 2002). Online support groups/communities can also help individuals facing health concerns during times of stress and transition to access new networks of support, such as providing connections to others facing the same or similar transitions and stressors (such as if a person moves to a small town where the likelihood of meeting others living with a similar health condition is low).

In addition to convenience, online sources of social support can help individuals with health problems overcome accessibility barriers and high service fees associated with other (more traditional) sources of information and support, such as therapy (Barrera, 2000). The asynchronous and mediated nature of online communication helps alleviate time and space barriers that exist for support settings that require the simultaneous presence of conversational partners (Turner, Grube, & Meyers, 2001). Online support groups/communities often offer people who are coping with health problems higher quality health information and support for health behavior change than is available among traditional, face-to-face sources of support (Wright & Miller, 2010).

This chapter will examine each of these issues in greater detail as well as the theoretical and practical implications of this body of research for patients who use online support communities to help cope with and manage a variety of health issues. Specifically, it will review current literature on communication issues related to social support within online support groups/communities for individuals facing health concerns published within the health communication literature. Toward that end, it will provide an overview of online social support and health outcomes, and it will discuss key processes and theoretical explanations for the efficacy of online support communities for people facing health concerns. Finally, the chapter provides an overview of some of the limitations of this body of research as well as an agenda for future communication research on health-related online support groups/communities.

ONLINE SOCIAL SUPPORT AND HEALTH OUTCOMES

Social support refers to the emotional (e.g., empathy and encouragement), informational (e.g., advice), or instrumental (e.g., financial and physical) resources provided by one's social networks that help her or him to cope with stressful events (Cohen, 2004). Studies across a number of disciplines have reported the benefits of peer-to-peer social support groups (both in groups led by peers and supervised by professionals) where individuals can interact with others who are experiencing the same disease or similar health condition (Ussher, Kirsten, Butow, & Sandoval, 2006). Supportive communication with peers who share common health-related experiences may decrease feelings of isolation and increase a sense of belonging (Cohen, Underwood, & Gottlieb, 2000; Ussher et al., 2006). Based on a shared identity and perceived similarity among peers, individuals in peer support groups (both face-to-face and online) tend to perceive information provided by peers as more credible (Campbell & Wright, 2002; Petosa & Smith, 2014) and participants are more likely to engage in empathic communication (Helgeson & Gottlieb, 2000) than in other contexts.

Social support plays an important role in one's ability to cope with a range of stressors from mundane everyday stressful situations to significant life events (Goldsmith, 2004; Uchino, 2004). Two general explanations have been offered for the effects of social support on well-being. First, the *direct-effects model* posits that simply being involved in interpersonal relationships can lead to physical and psychological benefits (Aneshensel & Stone, 1982; Thoits, 2011), even in the absence of a specific stressor. Ties between individuals influence human health positively if they satisfy the need to be socially and emotionally connected with others (Sorkin, Rook, & Lu, 2002). Second, the *buffering model* suggests that social support serves to directly shield a person from a stressor or positively alter one's appraisal of the stressor. For example, an individual may receive advice to help him or her solve a problem or feedback to change his or her perceptions of its severity. Researchers have linked the buffering model to positive health outcomes in terms of morbidity and mortality (Berkman & Syme, 1979).

Studies have found that social support in online support communities buffers the harmful physiological consequences of stress from breast cancer (Barak, Boniel-Nissim, & Suler, 2008). For example, depressive symptoms such as feelings of isolation, hopelessness, anxiety, and a lack of interest were found to be decreased in patients who received emotional support, such as empathy and encouragement, from peers in a number of online support communities (Batenburg & Das, 2015). Individuals using health-related online support communities report higher quality of life after participating in online communities (Lieberman & Goldstein, 2006). Moreover, the information that is exchanged within online support communities appears to contribute to an improvement in information competence (Han et al., 2012) and knowledge of disease and its treatment among patients (Høybye et al., 2005; Owen et al., 2004), leading them to feel more in control of their health situation.

The amount of time spent using online support communities has been shown to be associated with users' size and satisfaction with their online support network (Wright, 2000) as well as decreased rates of depression over the course of a year among depression community members (Houston, Cooper, & Ford, 2002; Wright et al., 2010). Participating in health-related online support groups/communities has also been linked to other positive mental health outcomes such as self-efficacy and optimism (Mo & Coulson, 2013). Online support is associated with online support group participants' perceived coping abilities (Seçkin, 2013). In general, studies have shown a positive association between members' well-being and support received from using online groups/communities (Mo & Coulson, 2013; Oh, Ozkaya, & LaRose, 2014; Rains & Keating, 2011).

Researchers have also investigated the impact that online support groups/communities have on how people cope with critical or chronic diseases (Eichhorn, 2008; Guo & Goh, 2014; Johnston, Worrell, Di Gangi, & Wasko, 2013; Rodgers & Chen, 2005), how often people use the online health communities looking for health information (Kummervold et al., 2008), which sources of information are used in online health communities (Rodgers & Chen, 2005), which factors contribute or obstruct the use of the online health communities when searching for health information (Lemire, Paré, Sicotte, & Harvey, 2008), and how social support is requested and offered on these sites (Mazzoni & Cicognani, 2014).

BENEFITS AND PROBLEMS ASSOCIATED WITH SEEKING SUPPORT WITHIN ONLINE SUPPORT GROUPS/COMMUNITIES

A growing number of studies have investigated the benefits of online support groups/communities for people facing a variety of health concerns (See Green-Hamann, Campbell Eichhorn, & Sherblom, 2011; Malik & Coulson, 2008; Rains, Peterson, & Wright, 2015; Rains & Young, 2009; Wright & Bell, 2003). In terms of benefits, online support communities allow individuals to discuss health-related topics with others who have been through similar experiences, to support one another and talk about the unique difficulties associated with illness (Attard & Coulson, 2012; Coulson, 2005). Online communities provide flexible access to social support at any time of the day or night (Malik & Coulson, 2008), making it easy to fit support needs around work, family, study or other commitments. However, the lack of physical proximity can make it difficult to develop meaningful relationships and offer physical comfort, which may leave some members feeling isolated in real life. Research examining computer-mediated communication (CMC) support has largely focused on explaining why people choose to use CMC for exchanging support (Tanis, 2008; Walther & Boyd, 2002; Wright, 2002) and identifying the types of support messages shared online (Rains, Peterson, & Wright, 2015). Although less plentiful, there is also evidence to suggest that support received or available in computer-mediated contexts can be a valuable coping resource (Rains & Keating, 2011; Wright, 2000).

The sense of community an online support group creates for its members provides similar health benefits to traditionally shared face-to-face social support in terms of important outcomes like reduced stress and depression, faster recovery times, etc. (Rains & Young, 2009), but online support offers the affordances of being able to transcend geography and temporality as well as offer people greater ease in terms of communicating with a large network of potential support providers (Bambina, 2007; Wright & Bell, 2003). Several studies have found that participation in online support groups/communities is influenced by perceptions of the convenience, flexibility, and relative anonymity of computer-mediated communication associated with these groups. Online support groups/communities typically include greater accessibility (e.g., lack of time and travel constraints), anonymity, and the ability to obtain information without having to personally interact with others (Eichhorn, 2008; Green-Hamann, Campbell Eichhorn, & Sherblom, 2011; Wright & Bell, 2003) compared to face-to-face forms of social support. Unlike face-to-face support groups, online support venues offer participants access via computer and other Internet accessible devices 24 hours a day and access to potential support providers all over the world (Tanis, 2008; Wright & Bell, 2003). In addition, the anonymity of online groups/communities appears to influence increased self-disclosure of one's health issues to other group/community members (Wright & Bell, 2003).

However, online support group members can also face a variety of challenges (van Uden-Kraan et al., 2008), such as the quality and validity of information exchanged (Finn, 1999; Wright, 2002) and potential exposure to negative or self-destructive postings that may undermine the health benefits of online support (Campbell & Wright, 2002; Wright & Bell, 2003). Moreover, researchers have identified other negative aspects of online support communities that may influence health outcomes, including flaming and delayed feedback in computer-mediated interactions, short-term participation, and negative social comparisons (Wright, 2000; Wright & Bell, 2003). More recent studies have identified online communities that actually support and encourage unhealthy behaviors, such as anorexia, and substance abuse, and other health behaviors (Custers & Van den Bulck, 2009; Davey, Schifano, Corazza, & Deluca, 2012).

THEORETICAL EXPLANATIONS OF ONLINE SUPPORT COMMUNITY COMMUNICATION PROCESSES AND HEALTH BENEFITS FOR PARTICIPANTS

Similarity/Social Comparisons

Similarities between participants in online support groups/ communities appear to increase the persuasiveness and influence of the messages that are exchanged. For example, Wang, Walther, Pingree, and Hawkins (2008) showed that perceived similarity of support group members influenced perceptions of their credibility and, in turn, the evaluation of health information they provided. In addition, Wright (2000) and Campbell and Wright (2002) found that similarity was a key perception that was associated with social support satisfaction with support providers within health-related online support groups (which may be a motivation to participate). Campbell et al. (2004), for example, claimed that "those who have survived the disease have an understanding and first-hand experience of the disease and its treatment that facilitates shared experiences" (p. 4). Similarly, Meyer, Coroiu, and Korner (2015) found that patients can be ideal support providers because they have "authentic knowledge of what it is like to live with the disease, and they are able to bring a unique perspective to the support process. Moreover, disease survivors generally present better physical functioning and emotional well-being than newly diagnosed patients (Baker, Denniston, Haffer, & Liberatos, 2009). Survivors and long-term online community members may possess more resources to provide informational and emotional support to other participants who are newly diagnosed or in the early stages of a health problem (Cameron, Ashbury, & Iverson, 1997; Wright, 2000). More experienced online community members can take a leading role in offering social support by providing information and their experiences of coping (Meier, Lyons, Frydman, Forlenza, & Rimer, 2007; Wright & Bell, 2003).

Social comparison theory (Festinger, 1954) proposes that people use either upward or downward comparison to cope with stressful events. Upward comparison includes seeking affiliation with and information from those who are in a better condition, whereas downward comparison refers to self-evaluation against others in a worse situation (Taylor & Lobel, 1989). Buunk, Collins, Taylor, VanYperen, and Dakof (1990) later distinguished positive upward comparison, in which individuals become optimistic to see others in a better situation (i.e., upward identification), from negative upward comparison by which people become pessimistic to see others in a better situation (i.e., upward contrast).

Studies have found that participants often glean information about the status of their health issues through social comparisons that take place within supportive interactions in online support groups/communities (Batenburg & Das, 2015; Vilhauer, 2009; Wright & Bell, 2003). Such social comparison processes do not even require actual participation in the online group; rather, individuals may engage in these practices passively by reading the posted group discussions. A few studies have shown that (positive) upward comparison is related to the self-improvement of cancer patients, such as developing coping strategies, finding hope, and learning useful information (Taylor & Lobel, 1989). Furthermore, women with breast cancer tend to have a greater desire for upward comparison, thereby seeking information and emotional support from better-adjusted patients versus poorly adjusted patients (Stanton et al., 1999). Although the previous literature on social comparison in cancer care has not specified the role of cancer survivors, given a better understanding of cancer treatment and psychological adjustment of survivors (Baker et al., 2009; Meyer et al., 2015), positive upward comparison may occur when newly diagnosed patients receive social support from survivors, which in turn contributes to the psychological adjustment of new patients. However, there are also several significant limitations of support community participation from a social comparison perspective. The most common involves stress resulting from hearing about difficulties experienced by other community members (Holbrey & Coulson, 2013; Malik & Coulson, 2008). Other drawbacks include social comparisons with others who are improving (Malik & Coulson, 2008) and becoming negatively focused on one's illness (Holbrey & Coulson, 2013).

Strength of Weak Ties

Online support groups/communities are generally considered networks of largely weak-tie relationships (Wright & Bell, 2003). Online groups can be beneficial by offering connections to relevant peers (Scharer, 2005) and expanding access to resources and social capital by gaining access to others' online networks via the online support community (Walther & Boyd, 2002; Wright & Miller, 2010). However, weak-tie networks can also come with costs because members of online groups lack control over the quality, content, and validity of presented information (Finn, 1999; Klemm et al., 2003; Wright, 2002). According to Colineau and Paris (2010), people choose weak tie networks because of the members' ability to understand their experience and because of the emotional distance afforded by the online communication. Another advantage of weak ties is that they tend to be more plentiful than strong ties, and they are more likely to be different from the receiver and from one another. This means there is a greater likelihood of being able to find an expert in a particular area in weak tie rather than strong tie sources.

Members of weak tie networks may be more willing to talk about illness since these individuals tend to be less emotionally attached to a person (Adelman, & Albretcht, 1987). Weak tie network members are often able to provide more objective feedback about a problem since they are less emotionally attached to a person with health problems than family and friends. According to Goldsmith and Albrecht (2011), weaker ties tend to be perceived as helpful when a person is coping with an issue that requires new information or skills (that may be limited within a close-knit family or friendship social network). These features of weak ties can be beneficial to people who are coping with health concerns that may be difficult to ameliorate in strong ties due to lack of information and relational problems in close relationships (Winefield, 2006; Wright & Miller, 2010).

Several researchers have found weak tie network theory to be applicable to explaining why some individuals prefer to obtain social support online (including online support groups/communities) versus via traditional offline networks (Green-Hamman & Sherblom, 2014; Wright & Rains, 2013; Wright, Rains, & Banas, 2010; Wright & Miller, 2010). When members of traditional offline social networks have limited knowledge about a stressful situation, there is evidence that individuals often turn to online sources of information and social support (Wright & Miller,

2010) despite the fact that they may feel less close relationally to the people with whom they interact online. Additionally, when online sources are able to offer specialized information about a problem and/or may be in a better position to offer desired types of social support (such as increased empathy and less judgment due to sharing similar problems).

Reduced Stigma

Another important theoretical explanation for why online support groups/community participation is associated with positive health outcomes is the group's ability to help individuals cope with the stigma that the larger culture attaches to many diseases and health conditions (Ballantine & Stephenson, 2011; Faith, Thorburn, & Sinky, 2016; Lewis, Thomas, Blood, Castle, Hyde, & Komesaroff, 2011; Rains, 2014; Wright & Rains, 2014). Health-related stigma is a significant problem that many individuals facing health concerns have to deal with on a daily basis (Herek & Glunt, 1988). It has been linked to reductions in the size of individuals' support networks, problems discussing concerns with others, dissatisfaction with one's support network, reduced compliance with treatment recommendations, and increased health problems (Vanable, Carey, Blair, & Littlewood, 2006). Stigmatized health issues have been linked to increased stress and depression (Wolitski, Pals, Kidder, Courtenay-Quirk, & Holtgrave, 2008), substance abuse, anxiety, and increased physical health problems (Duncan, Hart, Scoular, & Bigrigg, 2001). Health-related stigma is also associated with reduced levels of self-esteem and self-efficacy (Herek & Glunt, 1988). Researchers have found that people with stigmatized health problems are drawn to online support groups/ communities because these groups/communities help them to manage the stigma, leading them to feel less isolated and less judged by others (Lewis et al., 2011; Rains, 2014; Wright & Miller, 2010; Wright & Rains, 2014).

Reduced Cues/Social Information Processing Theory

One variable that makes computer-mediated communication (CMC) unique is the reduction in social cues relative to face-to-face interaction (Caplan & Turner, 2007; Rains & Young, 2009; Tanis, 2008; Walther & Parks, 2002; Wright & Bell, 2003). This reduction in social cues is particularly important given the setting in which several popular forms of CMC are used for support. Although it is possible to routinely communicate with well-known others (e.g., Turner et al., 2001), one-time interactions often take place in online health-related communities and blogs among individuals who have never met and will not interact in the future. Informal social support communities, for example, typically have open membership in which an unlimited number of individuals can come and go as they please (Rains & Young, 2009).

Computer-mediated communication (CMC) can be unique from face-to-face interaction in several important ways (See Caplan & Turner, 2007; Tanis, 2008; Wright & Bell, 2003). For example, many of the social cues available in face-to-face interaction (e.g., eye contact, paralinguistic cues, etc.) are reduced or absent in online interaction. Walther and Parks (2002) referred to the reduction in social cues as one of two structural aspects of social support that are fundamentally altered by CMC. Even as communication technologies continue to evolve, the reduction in social cues is likely to remain an important variable across different CMC modes. The hyperpersonal communication model (Walther, 1996) is a popular theoretical framework that has been applied to the context of online supportive communication (Caplan & Turner, 2007; Walther & Boyd, 2002; Wright & Bell, 2003). This model outlines a process resulting in communication that is "more socially desirable than we tend to experience in parallel [face-to-face] interactions'' (Walther, 1996, p. 17). Two aspects of the hyperpersonal model are important in terms of explaining the influence of using CMC on the outcomes of supportive interaction. The reduced social cues associated with CMC create opportunities for selective self-presentation that may serve to mitigate self-presentation concerns and allow individuals to give greater attention to message construction (Walther & Boyd, 2002; Wright & Bell, 2003).

Support seekers report feeling less self-conscious and more comfortable sharing supportive messages since health-related online communities are typically perceived as comfortable and non-threatening environments in terms of forming and maintaining interpersonal relationships (Caplan & Turner, 2007). This more comfortable communication environment appears to facilitate individuals' efforts to cope with their stressor and allow them to better manage their uncertainty as well as feel less worry and greater self-efficacy relative to a face-to-face interaction. Features of computer-mediated communication within online support communities may also lead support seekers to construct idealized perceptions of support providers (Walther & Boyd, 2002; Wright & Bell, 2003).

Idealized perceptions can be explained by the hyperpersonal model. According to Walther (1996), the reduced number of available nonverbal cues in CMC increases message-editing capabilities, and the temporal features of CMC allow communicators to be more selective and strategic in their self-presentation, and engage in more intimate exchanges than people in face-to-face situations. These features of computer-mediated communication appear to offer people more interactional control over face-to-face communication, and they appear to influence perceptions of the attractiveness of online relational partners. Walther, Slovacek, and Tidwell (2001) found that individuals rated online interaction partners as more socially attractive and affectionate when a photo was not present compared to those who did view a photo of the interaction partner. In addition, dyads in computer-mediated settings also appear to self-disclose more than face-to-face dyads (Tidwell & Walther, 2002). Given the nature of supportive interactions in which support providers are attempting to be empathetic and offering encouragement and advice, receivers may develop inflated perceptions of the degree to which providers are caring or knowledgeable. The reduced social cues associated with CMC may ultimately result in receivers developing an exaggerated sense of being supported by providers (Wright & Bell, 2003).

Similar to social information processing theory, the dual-process theory of supportive message outcomes (Bodie & Burleson, 2008; Burleson, 2010) has been used to help understand the implications of the reduced social cues in CMC during supportive interactions. An important way that the reduced social cues in CMC may impact support processes is by increasing support recipients' attentional resources. Because they have less responsibility for managing nonverbal behavior (e.g., eye contact) relative to face-to-face interaction, individuals using CMC may pay greater attention to articulating their thoughts and feelings as well as the messages received from a communication partner. This appears to allow for the construction of more thoughtful and competent supportive messages.

However, the reduced social cues in computer-mediated interaction have the potential to undermine the benefits of supportive interactions. The cues-filtered-out perspective (Culnan & Markus, 1987) is grounded in the idea that the reduction in social cues stemming from CMC inhibits socio-emotional messages and the development of personal relationships (Kiesler, Siegel, & McGuire, 1984). In the context of social support, the cues-filtered-out perspective suggests that the reduction in social cues could serve to encourage more impersonal interactions (White & Dorman, 2001) and make the process of exchanging support more difficult (Lewandowski, Rosenberg, Parks, Siegel, 2011; Wright & Bell, 2003).

In terms of the influence of reduced cues in CMC and self-disclosure to others in online support groups/communities, Wright (2000) found that older adults using SeniorNet (an early online community for older adults) reported disclosing information about their health to anonymous members of the online community that they were reluctant to discuss with family members and friends in face-to-face settings. Anonymity led seniors using the community to feel safer disclosing health information within the online group. Walther and Boyd (2002) found that hyperpersonal interaction within online support groups/communities enhanced the attractiveness of seeking support within this context. In particular, these researchers found that perceived social distance from other participants facilitated perceptions of reduced risk in terms of disclosing sensitive or stigmatized issues (including health concerns). Eysenbach (2003) drew upon social information processing theory, and found that anonymity of virtual support communities was particularly helpful in terms of facilitating the participation of men living with health concerns to interact with others within these groups. Eysenbach (2003) argued that the reduced cues in this environment were particularly helpful for men to obtain online support for health concerns since they tend to be culturally and socially conditioned not to ask for help and support.

AGENDA FOR FUTURE RESEARCH IN THE AREA OF ONLINE SUPPORT GROUPS/COMMUNITIES

Since online support groups/communities will likely continue to flourish and change in the coming years, as newer technologies will likely transform the ways in which people with health concerns connect and garner support from others online, it is important to examine some of the limitations of the current literature in this area of research as well as opportunities to better understand online support groups/communities, supportive communication processes within them, and their relationship to important psychological and physical health outcomes. This section presents a brief agenda for scholars who are interested in conducting research in this area.

Theories and methods in future research in this area need to take into account a more comprehensive perspective of the influence of both types of social support on health outcomes, including the main effects and interaction effects of online and offline sources of social support, additional predictors of engaging in online support, mediated variables (i.e., the influence of different computer-mediated channels and contexts), and key demographic and environmental variables on health outcomes. There are many limitations of the existing research in this area that need to be addressed in future work. While a number of theoretical frameworks have been utilized in the study of online support and health outcomes, this area would benefit from the development of new theories that shed light on features of online support that are unique from offline supportive contexts. This section discusses some of the key limitations to the existing research as well as fruitful areas of research and theory development within this area.

One of the first limitations of previous studies concerns the need to account for the influence of overlapping sources of social support on key outcome variables, such as stress and depression. For example, according to Haythornthwaite (2002), both online and off-line supportive exchanges influence health outcomes. In short, it becomes difficult to separate online supportive influences from off-line influences. Most individuals typically mix face-to-face contact with e-mail, or searching the Internet for health information and then discussing it with people in their face-to-face social network. Future research should assess the interaction of both online and face-to-face support networks on key outcome variables such as satisfaction, well-being, stress, depression, and physical health outcomes while also comparing differences between support from these two networks in terms of how they uniquely contribute to these outcomes. Future research in this area would benefit from the development of theories and methods that take into account a more comprehensive perspective of the influence of social support on health outcomes, including the main effects and interaction effects of online and off-line sources of social support, additional predictors of engaging in online support, mediated variables (i.e., the influence of different computer-mediated channels, contexts), and key demographic and environmental variables on health outcomes.

Research is also needed to examine interaction(s) between face-to-face and online social support networks as well as how new communication technologies are facilitating the intersection of virtual and face-to-face interactions through media convergence (e.g., GPS chips and applications that allow you to find key people in your support network in the face-to-face world). For example, although research has examined the influence of mobile games on physical activity levels (Fanning, Mullen, McAuley, 2012), few studies have specifically focused on the role of social support on health outcomes within this context. More research is needed to better understand a wider variety of health issues and the influence of multimodal communication (e.g., online communication combined with face-to-face interaction) and mobile/online social support processes on key health outcomes, such as stress, depression, and physical health.

As research studies on social support networks/relationships and health continue to develop, more meta-analyses and meta-analytic reviews will be needed to assess the impact of social networks/relationships on health across similar studies. Meta-analytic reviews have contributed greatly to our understanding of newer areas, such as online support group network, influences on health. For example, Rains and Young (2009) conducted a meta-analysis of 28 published online support group studies dealing with people coping with health concerns and found that greater participation in their online support groups was related to increased perceived support, reduced depression, increased quality of life, and increased self-efficacy in terms of managing health problems. Meta-analytic can also help researchers identify key mechanisms that help to explain or moderate the influence of online support networks on health outcomes.

More studies are needed to better understand complex cultural differences in how social support networks influence is conceptualized, how social support communication processes may differ, and cultural influences on health outcomes across a wide variety of cultural contexts. In addition, more research is needed in the area of cross-cultural and international comparisons in terms assessing the relationship between social network and interpersonal dyadic support on important health outcomes (including regionally specific health issues) (Goldsmith & Albrecht, 2011). In addition, more research is need to better understand how online social support is used by older adults and the challenges they may face in terms of accessing and using newer communication technologies. While researchers have examined online support and health-related technology for older adults (Wright, 2000; LeRouge et al., 2014), more research and interventions are needed to design online support platforms and technologies for older adult populations. Relatively little is known about how minority groups and other populations facing health disparities use computer-mediated support groups. However, it appears that members of minority groups engage in a variety of online social support activities, and individuals within these groups may benefit from online support group/community interventions (Hong, Pena-Purcell, & Ory, 2012). For example, Fogel, Albert, Schnabel, Ann Ditkoff, and Neugut (2003) found that while African Americans, Hispanics, and Asian Americans tend to use the Internet less than whites, their Internet use was associated with greater ability to talk with someone about problems and to obtain other types of social support. Weinert and Hill (2005) found that rural women (including a high percentage of minorities) using an online support group intervention had lower levels of depression and higher self-reported management of day-to-day chronic illness symptoms than a control group of similar rural women living with chronic illness. Qualitative research and quantitative studies can both make important contributions to the study of cultural influences on social support network and health outcome processes (as well as to the larger area of social support and health research). While quite a bit research in the area of social support groups/communities and health outcomes has been conducted in a variety of countries around the world, most of the research has been conducted in a relatively small number of countries in Europe and Asia (mainly China) (Deng et al., 2010; Rao et al, 2012; Van Tilburg, 1998).

In recent years, smartphones have become the primary way people gain access to the Internet and social media. New mobile applications have taken advantage of the media convergence potential of smartphone (e.g., GPS combined with wireless Internet, video, etc.). At the same time, we have witnessed the emergence of wearable electronic devices that track physical activity (e.g., Fitbit). Both innovations have led to the burgeoning field of MHealth (Boulos et al., 2014; Luxton et al., 2011). While much of this research has examined the impact of smartphones on provider-patient communication, a number of researchers have examined the social support potential of smartphones (Boulos et al., 2014). Although diet and exercise applications and devices are currently the most widely used health-related features of smartphones (Boulos et al., 2014), other applications are available for a variety of health issues, including alcohol addiction recovery support, smoking cessation support, and support for mental health issues (Luxton et al., 2011; Alvarez-Jimenez et al., 2014). These types of MHealth applications can allow researchers to access available data from smartphones, including activity levels and diet information, which can be used as important health outcome measures. Moreover, these applications also provide the names/online contacts of online social network members with whom an individual shares his or her health information *via* these applications.

CONCLUSION

The findings from the reviewed literature provide support for the idea that online support groups/communities have health benefits for a variety of people facing health concerns. As online support among members of these populations will likely continue in the future, researchers need to continue gaining a better understanding of the nature of online support group/ community processes and outcomes. While scholars have identified a number of theoretical frameworks that help to explain key processes of online support groups/communities and their relationship to health outcomes, new theoretical perspectives are needed to capture the complexity of this phenomenon. Scholars should work on integrating overlapping concepts from the major theories discussed in this article, and they should take into account the unique influences that computer-mediated communication has on supportive relationships within these groups/communities.

REFERENCES

Adelman, M. B., & Albrecht, T. L. (1987). *Communicating social support*. Sage Publications.

Alvarez-Jimenez, M., Alcazar-Corcoles, M. A., González-Blanch, C., Bendall, S., McGorry, P. D., & Gleeson, J. F. (2014). Online, social media and mobile technologies for psychosis treatment: A systematic review on novel user-led interventions. *Schizophrenia Research*, *156*(1), 96–106. doi:10.1016/j.schres.2014.03.021 PMID:24746468

Aneshensel, C. S., & Stone, J. D. (1982). Stress and depression: A test of the buffering model of social support. *Archives of General Psychiatry*, *39*(12), 1392–1396. doi:10.1001/archpsyc.1982.04290120028005 PMID:7149899

Attard, A., & Coulson, N. S. (2012). A thematic analysis of patient communication in Parkinson's disease online support group discussion forums. *Computers in Human Behavior*, *28*(2), 500–506. doi:10.1016/j.chb.2011.10.022

Baker, F., Denniston, M., Haffer, S. C., & Liberatos, P. (2009). Change in health-related quality of life of newly diagnosed cancer patients, cancer survivors, and controls. *Cancer, 115*(13), 3024–3033. doi:10.1002/cncr.24330 PMID:19402049

Ballantine, P. W., & Stephenson, R. J. (2011). Help me, I'm fat! Social support in online weight loss networks. *Journal of Consumer Behaviour, 10*(6), 332–337. doi:10.1002/cb.374

Bambina, A. (2007). *Online social support: the interplay of social networks and computer-mediated communication*. Cambria Press.

Barak, A., Boniel-Nissim, M., & Suler, J. (2008). Fostering empowerment in online support groups. *Computers in Human Behavior, 24*(5), 1867–1883. doi:10.1016/j.chb.2008.02.004

Barrera, M. (2000). Social support research in community psychology. In J. Rappaport & E. Seidman (Eds.), *Handbook of Community Psychology* (pp. 215–245). New York: Kluwer Academic/Plenum. doi:10.1007/978-1-4615-4193-6_10

Batenburg, A., & Das, E. (2015). Virtual Support Communities and Psychological Well-Being: The Role of Optimistic and Pessimistic Social Comparison Strategies. *Journal of Computer-Mediated Communication, 20*(6), 585–600. doi:10.1111/jcc4.12131

Berkman, L. F., & Syme, S. L. (1979). Social networks, host resistance, and mortality: A nine-year follow-up study of Alameda County residents. *American Journal of Epidemiology, 109*(2), 186–204. doi:10.1093/oxfordjournals.aje.a112674 PMID:425958

Bodie, G. D., & Burleson, B. R. (2008). Explaining variations in the effects of supportive messages a dual-process framework. *Annals of the International Communication Association, 32*(1), 355–398. doi:10.1080/23808985.2008.11679082

Boulos, M. N. K., Brewer, A. C., Karimkhani, C., Buller, D. B., & Dellavalle, R. P. (2014). Mobile medical and health apps: State of the art, concerns, regulatory control and certification. *Online Journal of Public Health Informatics, 5*(3). PMID:24683442

Burleson, B. R. (2010). Explaining recipient responses to supportive messages. *New directions in interpersonal communication research*, 159-179.

Buunk, B. P., Collins, R. L., Taylor, S. E., VanYperen, N. W., & Dakof, G. A. (1990). The affective consequences of social comparison: Either direction has its ups and downs. *Journal of Personality and Social Psychology, 59*(6), 1238–1249. doi:10.1037/0022-3514.59.6.1238 PMID:2283590

Cameron, C., Ashbury, F. D., & Iverson, D. C. (1997). Perspectives on Reach to Recovery and CanSurmount: informing the evaluation model. Cancer prevention & control: CPC= Prevention & controle en cancerologie. *PCC, 1*(2), 102–107. PMID:9765731

Campbell, H. S., Phaneuf, M. R., & Deane, K. (2004). Cancer peer support programs—do they work? *Patient Education and Counseling, 55*(1), 3–15. doi:10.1016/j.pec.2003.10.001 PMID:15476984

Campbell, K., & Wright, K. B. (2002). Online support groups: An investigation of relationships among source credibility, dimensions of relational communication, and perceptions of emotional support. *Communication Research Reports, 19*(2), 183–193. doi:10.1080/08824090209384846

Campbell-Grossman, C. K., Hudson, D. B., Keating-Lefler, R., & Heusinkvelt, S. (2009). New mothers network the provision of social support to single, low-income, African American mothers via e-mail messages. *Journal of Family Nursing, 15*(2), 220–236. doi:10.1177/1074840708323048 PMID:19211545

Caplan, S. E., & Turner, J. S. (2007). Bringing theory to research on computer-mediated comforting communication. *Computers in Human Behavior, 23*(2), 985–998. doi:10.1016/j.chb.2005.08.003

Chou, W. Y., Hunt, Y. M., Beckjord, E. B., Moser, R. P., & Hesse, B. W. (2009). Social Media Use in the United States: Implications for Health Communication. *Journal of Medical Internet Research, 11*(4), e48. doi:10.2196/jmir.1249 PMID:19945947

Colineau, N., & Paris, C. (2010). Talking about your health to strangers: Understanding the use of online social networks by patients. *New Review of Hypermedia and Multimedia, 16*(1-2), 141–160. doi:10.1080/13614568.2010.496131

Coulson, N., & Knibb, R. (2007). Coping with food allergy: Exploring the role of the online support group. *Cyberpsychology & Behavior, 10*(1), 145–148. doi:10.1089/cpb.2006.9978 PMID:17305463

Coulson, N. S. (2005). Receiving social support online: An analysis of a computer-mediated support group for individuals living with irritable bowel syndrome. *Cyberpsychology & Behavior, 8*(6), 580–584. doi:10.1089/cpb.2005.8.580 PMID:16332169

Coulson, N. S., Buchanan, H., & Aubeeluck, A. (2007). Social support in cyberspace: A content analysis of communication within a Huntington's disease online support group. *Patient Education and Counseling, 68*(2), 173–178. doi:10.1016/j.pec.2007.06.002 PMID:17629440

Culnan, M. J., & Markus, M. L. (1987). Information technologies. Handbook of organizational communication: An interdisciplinary perspective, 420-443.

Custers, K., & Van den Bulck, J. (2009). Viewership of pro-anorexia websites in seventh, ninth and eleventh graders. *European Eating Disorders Review*, *17*(3), 214–219. doi:10.1002/erv.910 PMID:19142974

Davey, Z., Schifano, F., Corazza, O., & Deluca, P. (2012). e-Psychonauts: Conducting research in online drug forum communities. *Journal of Mental Health (Abingdon, England)*, *21*(4), 386–394. doi:10.3109/09638237.2012.682265 PMID:22823094

Deng, J., Hu, J., Wu, W., Dong, B., & Wu, H. (2010). Subjective well-being, social support, and age-related functioning among the very old in China. *International Journal of Geriatric Psychiatry*, *25*(7), 697–703. doi:10.1002/gps.2410 PMID:20033902

Duncan, B., Hart, G., Scoular, A., & Bigrigg, A. (2001). Qualitative analysis of psychosocial impact of diagnosis of Chlamydia trachomatis: Implications for screening. *BMJ (Clinical Research Ed.)*, *322*(7280), 195–199. doi:10.1136/bmj.322.7280.195 PMID:11159612

Eichhorn, K. C. (2008). Soliciting and providing support over the Internet: An investigation of online eating disorder groups. *Journal of Computer-Mediated Communication*, *14*(1), 67–78. doi:10.1111/j.1083-6101.2008.01431.x

Ellison, N. B., Steinfield, C., & Lampe, C. (2007). The benefits of Facebook "friends": Social capital and college students' use of online social network sites. *Journal of Computer-Mediated Communication*, *12*(4), 1143–1168. doi:10.1111/j.1083-6101.2007.00367.x

Eysenbach, G. (2003). The impact of the Internet on cancer outcomes. *CA: a Cancer Journal for Clinicians*, *53*(6), 356–371. doi:10.3322/canjclin.53.6.356 PMID:15224975

Faith, J., Thorburn, S., & Sinky, T. H. (2016). Exploring healthcare experiences among online interactive weight loss forum users. *Computers in Human Behavior*, *57*, 326–333. doi:10.1016/j.chb.2015.12.048

Fanning, J., Mullen, S. P., & McAuley, E. (2012). Increasing physical activity with mobile devices: A meta-analysis. *Journal of Medical Internet Research*, *14*(6), e161. doi:10.2196/jmir.2171 PMID:23171838

Festinger, L. (1954). A theory of social comparison processes. *Human Relations*, *7*(2), 117–140. doi:10.1177/001872675400700202

Finn, J. (1999). An exploration of helping processes in an online self-help group focusing on issues of disability. *Health & Social Work*, *24*(3), 220–231. doi:10.1093/hsw/24.3.220 PMID:10505283

Fogel, J., Albert, S. M., Schnabel, F., Ann Ditkoff, B., & Neugut, A. I. (2003). Racial/ethnic differences and potential psychological benefits in use of the internet by women with breast cancer. *Psycho-Oncology*, *12*(2), 107–117. doi:10.1002/pon.617 PMID:12619143

Fox, S. (2011). *Pew Internet & American Life Project: Health Topics*. Retrieved March 11, 2011 from http://www.perwinternet.org/Reports/2011/HealthTopics.aspx

Fox, S., & Duggan, M. (2013). *Health online 2013*. Washington, DC: Pew Internet & American Life Project.

Frost, J. H., & Massagli, M. H. (2008). Social uses of personal health information within PatientsLikeMe, an online patient community: What can happen when patients have access to one another's data. *Journal of Medical Internet Research*, *10*(3), e15. doi:10.2196/jmir.1053 PMID:18504244

Goldsmith, D. J. (2004). *Communicating social support*. Cambridge University Press. doi:10.1017/CBO9780511606984

Goldsmith, D. J., & Albrecht, T. L. (2011). Social support, social networks, and health. The Routledge handbook of health communication, 335-348.

Granovetter, M. S. (1973). The strength of weak ties. *American Journal of Sociology*, *78*(6), 1360–1380. doi:10.1086/225469

Green-Hamann, S., Campbell Eichhorn, K., & Sherblom, J. C. (2011). An exploration of why people participate in Second Life social support groups. *Journal of Computer-Mediated Communication*, *16*(4), 465–491. doi:10.1111/j.1083-6101.2011.01543.x

Green-Hamann, S., & Sherblom, J. C. (2014). *The influences of optimal matching and social capital on communicating support. Journal of Health Communication*. doi:10.1080/10810730.2013.864734

Guo, Y., & Goh, D. H. L. (2014). "I Have AIDS": Content analysis of postings in HIV/AIDS support group on a Chinese microblog. *Computers in Human Behavior*, *34*, 219–226. doi:10.1016/j.chb.2014.02.003

Han, J. Y., Kim, J. H., Yoon, H. J., Shim, M., McTavish, F. M., & Gustafson, D. H. (2012). Social and psychological determinants of levels of engagement with an online breast cancer support group: Posters, lurkers, and nonusers. *Journal of Health Communication*, *17*(3), 356–371. doi:10.1080/10810730.2011.585696 PMID:22085215

Helgeson, V. S., & Gottlieb, B. H. (2000). Support groups. *Social support measurement and intervention: A guide for health and social scientists*, 221-245.

Herek, G., & Glunt, E. K. (1988). An epidemic of stigma: Public reactions to AIDS. *The American Psychologist*, *43*(11), 886–891. doi:10.1037/0003-066X.43.11.886 PMID:3063145

Hlebec, V., Manfreda, K. L., & Vehovar, V. (2006). The social support networks of internet users. *New Media & Society*, *8*(1), 9–32. doi:10.1177/1461444806058166

Holbrey, S., & Coulson, N. S. (2013). A qualitative investigation of the impact of peer to peer online support for women living with polycystic ovary syndrome. *BMC Women's Health*, *13*(1), 51. doi:10.1186/1472-6874-13-51 PMID:24341398

Hong, Y., Pena-Purcell, N. C., & Ory, M. G. (2012). Outcomes of online support and resources for cancer survivors: A systematic literature review. *Patient Education and Counseling*, *86*(3), 288–296. doi:10.1016/j.pec.2011.06.014 PMID:21798685

Houston, T. K., Cooper, L. A., & Ford, D. E. (2002). Internet support groups for depression: A 1-year prospective cohort study. *The American Journal of Psychiatry*, *159*(12), 2062–2068. doi:10.1176/appi.ajp.159.12.2062 PMID:12450957

Høybye, M. T., Johansen, C., & Tjørnhøj-Thomsen, T. (2005). Online interaction. Effects of storytelling in an internet breast cancer support group. *Psycho-Oncology*, *14*(3), 211–220. doi:10.1002/pon.837 PMID:15386774

Johnston, A. C., Worrell, J. L., Di Gangi, P. M., & Wasko, M. (2013). Online health communities: An assessment of the influence of participation on patient empowerment outcomes. *Information Technology & People*, *26*(2), 213–235. doi:10.1108/ITP-02-2013-0040

Kiesler, S., Siegel, J., & McGuire, T. W. (1984). Social psychological aspects of computer-mediated communication. *The American Psychologist*, *39*(10), 1123–1134. doi:10.1037/0003-066X.39.10.1123

Kim, J., & Lee, J. E. (2011). The Facebook paths to happiness: Effects of the number of Facebook friends and self-presentation on subjective well-being. *Cyberpsychology, Behavior, and Social Networking*, *6*(6), 359–364. doi:10.1089/cyber.2010.0374 PMID:21117983

Klemm, P., Bunnell, D., Cullen, M., Soneji, R., Gibbons, P., & Holecek, A. (2003). Online cancer support groups: a review of the research literature. CIN: Computers, Informatics. *Nursing*, *21*(3), 136–142. PMID:12792194

Kummervold, P., Chronaki, C., Lausen, B., Prokosch, H. U., Rasmussen, J., Santana, S., & Wangberg, S. et al. (2008). eHealth trends in Europe 2005-2007: A population-based survey. *Journal of Medical Internet Research, 10*(4), e42. doi:10.2196/jmir.1023 PMID:19017584

Lemire, M., Paré, G., Sicotte, C., & Harvey, C. (2008). Determinants of Internet use as a preferred source of information on personal health. *International Journal of Medical Informatics, 77*(11), 723–734. doi:10.1016/j.ijmedinf.2008.03.002 PMID:18434246

LeRouge, C., Van Slyke, C., Seale, D., & Wright, K. (2014). Baby boomers' adoption of consumer health technologies: Survey on readiness and barriers. *Journal of Medical Internet Research, 16*(9), e200. doi:10.2196/jmir.3049 PMID:25199475

Lewandowski, J., Rosenberg, B. D., Parks, M. J., & Siegel, J. T. (2011). The effect of informal social support: Face-to-face versus computer-mediated communication. *Computers in Human Behavior, 27*(5), 1806–1814. doi:10.1016/j.chb.2011.03.008

Lewis, S., Thomas, S. L., Blood, R. W., Castle, D., Hyde, J., & Komesaroff, P. A. (2011). 'I'm searching for solutions': Why are obese individuals turning to the Internet for help and support with 'being fat'? *Health Expectations, 14*(4), 339–350. doi:10.1111/j.1369-7625.2010.00644.x PMID:21199200

Lieberman, M. A., & Goldstein, B. A. (2006). Not all negative emotions are equal: The role of emotional expression in online support groups for women with breast cancer. *Psycho-Oncology, 15*(2), 160–168. doi:10.1002/pon.932 PMID:15880627

Luxton, D. D., McCann, R. A., Bush, N. E., Mishkind, M. C., & Reger, G. M. (2011). mHealth for mental health: Integrating smartphone technology in behavioral healthcare. *Professional Psychology, Research and Practice, 42*(6), 505–512. doi:10.1037/a0024485

Malik, S. H., & Coulson, N. S. (2008). Computer-mediated infertility support groups: An exploratory study of online experiences. *Patient Education and Counseling, 73*(1), 105–113. doi:10.1016/j.pec.2008.05.024 PMID:18639409

Mazzoni, D., & Cicognani, E. (2014). Sharing experiences and social support requests in an Internet forum for patients with systemic lupus erythematosus. *Journal of Health Psychology, 19*(5), 689–696. doi:10.1177/1359105313477674 PMID:23479300

Meier, A., Lyons, E. J., Frydman, G., Forlenza, M., Rimer, B. K., & Winefield, H. (2007). How cancer survivors provide support on cancer-related Internet mailing lists. *Journal of Medical Internet Research, 9*(2), e12. doi:10.2196/jmir.9.2.e12 PMID:17513283

Meyer, A., Coroiu, A., & Korner, A. (2015). One-to-one peer support in cancer care: A review of scholarship published between 2007 and 2014. *European Journal of Cancer Care*, *24*(3), 299–312. doi:10.1111/ecc.12273 PMID:25512107

Mo, P. K., & Coulson, N. S. (2013). Online support group use and psychological health for individuals living with HIV/AIDS. *Patient Education and Counseling*, *93*(3), 426–432. doi:10.1016/j.pec.2013.04.004 PMID:23669152

Mo, P. K. H., Malik, S. H., & Coulson, N. S. (2009). Gender differences in computer-mediated communication: A systematic literature review of online health-related support groups. *Patient Education and Counseling*, *75*(1), 16–24. doi:10.1016/j.pec.2008.08.029 PMID:19233586

National Cancer Institute. (2013). *Health Information National Trends Survey*. Retrieved from http://hints.cancer.gov

Oh, H. J., Ozkaya, E., & LaRose, R. (2014). How does online social networking enhance life satisfaction? The relationships among online supportive interaction, affect, perceived social support, sense of community, and life satisfaction. *Computers in Human Behavior*, *30*, 69–78. doi:10.1016/j.chb.2013.07.053

Owen, J. E., Klapow, J. C., Roth, D. L., Nabell, L., & Tucker, D. C. (2004). Improving the effectiveness of adjuvant psychological treatment for women with breast cancer: The feasibility of providing online support. *Psycho-Oncology*, *13*(4), 281–292. doi:10.1002/pon.733 PMID:15054732

Petosa, R. L., & Smith, L. H. (2014). Peer mentoring for health behavior change: A systematic review. *American Journal of Health Education*, *45*(6), 351–357. doi:10.1080/19325037.2014.945670

Rains, S. A. (2014). The implications of stigma and anonymity for self-disclosure in health blogs. *Health Communication*, *29*(1), 23–31. doi:10.1080/10410236.2012.714861 PMID:23356432

Rains, S. A., & Keating, D. M. (2011). The social dimension of blogging about health: Health blogging, social support, and well-being. *Communication Monographs*, *78*(4), 511–534. doi:10.1080/03637751.2011.618142

Rains, S. A., Peterson, E. B., & Wright, K. B. (2015). Communicating social support in computer-mediated contexts: A meta-analytic review of content analyses examining support messages shared online among individuals coping with illness. *Communication Monographs*, *82*(4), 403–430. doi:10.1080/03637751.2015.1019530

Rains, S. A., & Young, V. (2009). A meta-analysis of research on formal computer-mediated support groups: Examining group characteristics and health outcomes. *Human Communication Research*, *35*(3), 309–336. doi:10.1111/j.1468-2958.2009.01353.x

Rao, D., Chen, W. T., Pearson, C. R., Simoni, J. M., Fredriksen-Goldsen, K., Nelson, K., & Zhang, F. et al. (2012). Social support mediates the relationship between HIV stigma and depression/quality of life among people living with HIV in Beijing, China. *International Journal of STD & AIDS*, *23*(7), 481–484. doi:10.1258/ijsa.2009.009428 PMID:22844001

Rodgers, S., & Chen, Q. (2005). Internet community group participation: Psychosocial benefits for women with breast cancer. *Journal of Computer-Mediated Communication, 10*(4).

Scharer, K. (2005). Internet social support for parents: The state of science. *Journal of Child and Adolescent Psychiatric Nursing*, *18*(1), 26–35. doi:10.1111/j.1744-6171.2005.00007.x PMID:15701096

Seçkin, G. (2013). Satisfaction with health status among cyber patients: Testing a mediation model of electronic coping support. *Behaviour & Information Technology*, *32*(1), 91–101. doi:10.1080/0144929X.2011.603359

Sorkin, D., Rook, K. S., & Lu, J. L. (2002). Loneliness, lack of emotional support, lack of companionship, and the likelihood of having a heart condition in an elderly sample. *Annals of Behavioral Medicine*, *24*(4), 290–298. doi:10.1207/S15324796ABM2404_05 PMID:12434940

Stanton, A. L., Danoff-burg, S., & Huggins, M. E. (2002). The first year after breast cancer diagnosis: Hope and coping strategies as predictors of adjustment. *Psycho-Oncology*, *11*(2), 93–102. doi:10.1002/pon.574 PMID:11921325

Tanis, M. (2008). Health-related online forums: What's the big attraction. *Journal of Health Communication*, *13*(7), 698–714. doi:10.1080/10810730802415316 PMID:18958781

Taylor, S. E., & Lobel, M. (1989). Social comparison activity under threat: Downward evaluation and upward contacts. *Psychological Review*, *96*(4), 569–575. doi:10.1037/0033-295X.96.4.569 PMID:2678204

Thoits, P. A. (2011). Mechanisms linking social ties and support to physical and mental health. *Journal of Health and Social Behavior*, *52*(2), 145–161. doi:10.1177/0022146510395592 PMID:21673143

Tidwell, L. C., & Walther, J. B. (2002). Computer-mediated communication effects on disclosure, impression, and interpersonal evaluations: Getting to know one another a bit at a time. *Human Communication Research, 28*(3), 317–348. doi:10.1111/j.1468-2958.2002.tb00811.x

Tong, S. T., Heinmann-LaFave, D., Jeon, J., Kolodziej-Smith, R., & Warshay, N. (2013). The use of pro-ana blogs for online social support. *Eating Disorders, 21*(5), 408–422. doi:10.1080/10640266.2013.827538 PMID:24044597

Turner, J. W., Grube, J. A., & Meyers, J. (2001). Developing an optimal match within online communities: An exploration of CMC support communities and traditional support. *Journal of Communication, 51*(2), 231–251. doi:10.1111/j.1460-2466.2001.tb02879.x

Uchino, B. N. (2004). *Social support and physical health: Understanding the health consequences of relationships*. Yale University Press. doi:10.12987/yale/9780300102185.001.0001

Ussher, J., Kirsten, L., Butow, P., & Sandoval, M. (2006). What do cancer support groups provide which other supportive relationships do not? The experience of peer support groups for people with cancer. *Social Science & Medicine, 62*(10), 2565–2576. doi:10.1016/j.socscimed.2005.10.034 PMID:16303220

Van Tilburg, T. (1998). Losing and gaining in old age: Changes in personal network size and social support in a four-year longitudinal study. *The Journals of Gerontology. Series B, Psychological Sciences and Social Sciences, 53*(6), S313–S323. doi:10.1093/geronb/53B.6.S313 PMID:9826973

van Uden-Kraan, C. F., Drossaert, C. H., Taal, E., Shaw, B. R., Seydel, E. R., & van de Laar, M. A. (2008). Empowering processes and outcomes of participation in online support groups for patients with breast cancer, arthritis, or fibromyalgia. *Qualitative Health Research, 18*(3), 405–417. doi:10.1177/1049732307313429 PMID:18235163

Vanable, P. A., Carey, M. P., Blair, D. C., & Littlewood, R. A. (2006). Impact of HIV-related stigma on health behaviors and psychological adjustment among HIV-positive men and women. *AIDS and Behavior, 10*(5), 473–482. doi:10.1007/s10461-006-9099-1 PMID:16604295

Vilhauer, R. P. (2009). Perceived benefits of online support groups for women with metastatic breast cancer. *Women & Health, 49*(5), 381–404. doi:10.1080/03630240903238719 PMID:19851944

Walther, J. B. (1992). Interpersonal effects in computer-mediated interaction: A relational perspective. *Communication Research*, *19*(1), 52–90. doi:10.1177/009365092019001003

Walther, J. B. (1996). Computer-mediated communication: Impersonal, interpersonal, and hyperpersonal interaction. *Communication Research*, *23*(1), 3–43. doi:10.1177/009365096023001001

Walther, J. B. (2007). Selective self-presentation in computer-mediated communication: Hyperpersonal dimensions of technology, language, and cognition. *Computers in Human Behavior*, *23*(5), 2538–2557. doi:10.1016/j.chb.2006.05.002

Walther, J. B., & Boyd, S. (2002). Attraction to computer-mediated social support. In C. A. Lin & D. Atkin (Eds.), *Communication technology and society: Audience adoption and uses* (pp. 153–188). Cresskill, NJ: Hampton Press.

Walther, J. B., & Parks, M. R. (2002). Cues filtered out, cues filtered in. Handbook of interpersonal communication, 3, 529-563.

Walther, J. B., Slovacek, C., & Tidwell, L. C. (2001). Is a picture worth a thousand words? Photographic images in long term and short term virtual teams. *Communication Research*, *28*(1), 105–134. doi:10.1177/009365001028001004

Wang, Z., Walther, J. B., Pingree, S., & Hawkins, R. P. (2008). Health information, credibility, homophily, and influence via the Internet: Web sites versus discussion groups. *Health Communication*, *23*(4), 358–368. doi:10.1080/10410230802229738 PMID:18702000

Weinert, C., & Hill, W. G. (2005). Rural women with chronic illness: Computer use and skill acquisition. *Women's Health Issues*, *15*(5), 230–236. doi:10.1016/j.whi.2005.06.002 PMID:16165009

White, M., & Dorman, S. M. (2001). Receiving social support online: Implications for health education. *Health Education Research*, *16*(6), 693–707. doi:10.1093/her/16.6.693 PMID:11780708

Winefield, H. R. (2006). Support provision and emotional work in an Internet support group for cancer patients. *Patient Education and Counseling*, *62*(2), 193–197. doi:10.1016/j.pec.2005.07.002 PMID:16139466

Wolitski, R. J., Pals, S. L., Kidder, D. P., Courtenay-Quick, C., & Holtgrave, D. R. (2008). The effects of HIV stigma on health, disclosure of HIV status, and risk behavior of homeless and unstably housed persons living with HIV. *AIDS and Behavior*, *13*(6), 1222–1232. doi:10.1007/s10461-008-9455-4 PMID:18770023

Wright, K. B. (1999). Computer-mediated support groups: An examination of relationships among social support, perceived stress, and coping strategies. *Communication Quarterly*, *47*(4), 402–414. doi:10.1080/01463379909385570

Wright, K. B. (2000). Perceptions of online support providers: An examination of perceived homophily, source credibility, communication and social support within online support groups. *Communication Quarterly*, *48*(1), 44–59. doi:10.1080/01463370009385579

Wright, K. B. (2002). Social support within an online cancer community: An assessment of emotional support, perceptions of advantages and disadvantages, and motives for using the community. *Journal of Applied Communication Research*, *30*, 195–209. doi:10.1080/00909880216586

Wright, K. B. (2005). Researching Internet-based popu0lations: Advantages and disadvantages of online survey research, online questionnaire authoring software packages, and web survey services. *Journal of Computer-Mediated Communication*, *10*(3), article 11. Available: http://jcmc.indiana.edu/vol10/issue3/wright.html

Wright, K. B. (2012). Emotional support and perceived stress among college students using Facebook.com: An exploration of the relationship between source perceptions and emotional support. *Communication Research Reports*, *29*(3), 1–10. doi:10.1080/08824096.2012.695957

Wright, K. B., Bell, S. B., Wright, K. B., & Bell, S. B. (2003). Health-related support groups on the Internet: Linking empirical findings to social support and computer-mediated communication theory. *Journal of Health Psychology*, *8*(1), 37–52. doi:10.1177/1359105303008001429 PMID:22113899

Wright, K. B., Johnson, A. J., Bernard, D. R., & Averbeck, J. (2011). Computer-mediated social support: Promises and pitfalls for individuals coping with health concerns. In T. L. Thompson, R. Parrott, & J. F. Nussbaum (Eds.), *The Routledge handbook of health communication* (2nd ed.; pp. 349–362). New York: Routledge.

Wright, K. B., & Miller, C. H. (2010). A measure of weak tie/strong tie support network preference. *Communication Monographs*, *77*(4), 502–520. doi:10.1080/03637751.2010.502538

Wright, K. B., Rains, S., & Banas, J. (2010). Weak tie support network preference and perceived life stress among participants in health-related, computer-mediated support groups. *Journal of Computer-Mediated Communication*, *15*(4), 606–624. doi:10.1111/j.1083-6101.2009.01505.x

Wright, K. B., & Rains, S. A. (2014). Weak tie support preference and preferred coping styles as predictors of perceived credibility within health-related computer-mediated support groups. *Health Communication*, *29*(3), 281–287. doi:10.1080/10410236.2012.751084 PMID:23790220

Wright, K. B., Rosenberg, J., Egbert, N., Ploeger, N., Bernard, D. R., & King, S. (2013). Communication competence, social support, and depression among college students. A model of Facebook and face-to-face support network influence. *Journal of Health Communication*, *18*(1), 41–47. doi:10.1080/10810730.2012.688250 PMID:23030518

KEY TERMS AND DEFINITIONS

Asynchronous/ Computer Mediated Communication/CMC: Information sent and received through computer, internet or other forms of media.

Emotional Support: The sharing of emotions to assist one during health-related challenges, such as empathy and encouragement.

Informational Support: The sharing of information to assist one during health-related challenges, such as advice and referrals.

Instrumental Support/Resources: The sharing of financial or physical resources to assist one during health-related challenges, such as transportation or donations.

Online Community/Network: Social networks that primarily engage through online platforms such as social media.

Online Support Community/Network: Social networks that engage to provide informational and emotional support for various health-related challenges.

Social Network: Members of one's primary social environment such as friends and family.

Social Support: The emotional, informational, or instrumental resources provided by one's social networks that help one to cope with stressful events.

Section 2

International Perspectives:

Four Case Studies Showcasing International Communities of Practice Online

Chapter 2
Cyber-Moms Facing Motherhood:
Holding Functions and Regressive Movements in Parenting Websites

Valentina Boursier
University of Naples Federico II, Italy

Valentina Manna
Association for Social Promotion Roots in Action, Italy

Francesca Gioia
University of Naples Federico II, Italy

Federica Coppola
University of Naples Federico II, Italy

Noemi Venosa
University of Naples Federico II, Italy

ABSTRACT

Mothers and mothers-to-be often become e-health users because of their need for sharing emotional and practical parental experiences. In this sense, web forums seem to positively contribute to parenting skills and transition to motherhood. This study aims at exploring how 379 Italian mothers use two Italian forums, the manifest and latent contents of their interactions, and the emotional connections between their own maternal experiences and the e-group dynamics. The qualitative analysis of 7433 comments pointed out five main themes, describing how mothers make sense of their experiences through the online dimension: the group; I am; personal experience; perspective knowhow; tech-moms. This study confirms that

DOI: 10.4018/978-1-5225-3716-8.ch002

Copyright © 2018, IGI Global. Copying or distributing in print or electronic forms without written permission of IGI Global is prohibited.

parenting experience represents a big challenge for rising mothers. Moreover, it shows that the e-groups can alternatively reproduce a peer group functioning and a feeding breast, a reassuring container with holding functions, or a "toilet breast", encouraging progressive as well as regressive movements.

INTRODUCTION

Pregnancy and the transition to parenthood represent some of the biggest life challenges, which need support. As Albrecht and Adelman (1984) highlighted, social support allows people to manage the uncertainty related to the stress and improve the sense of personal control or efficacy over their environments. Web communities offer a great opportunity to create online groups and receive necessary and appropriate experiences of social support and comparison. Probably, for this reason, parents and parents-to-be represent a large category of *e-health* users, as they can express and satisfy online their need for sharing emotional and practical experiences. For example, a recent multicenter Italian cross-sectional study (Bert et al., 2013) revealed that around 20% of pregnant women use online forums to share information and to experience support from other pregnant women. It has been demonstrated that pregnant women frequently use the internet to search for pregnancy-related information (Scaioli et al., 2005).

Furthermore, the increasing role of the Internet in everyday life has changed the meaning of what a community is. Indeed, on the Web, parents can create communities based on shared interests (Kirk & Milnes, 2015), setting up groups composed of different individuals who offer different perspectives, experiences, opinions and sources of information (Brady & Guerin, 2010), and, lastly, to receive Internet-based peer support, despite the geographical distance or time constraints (Niela-Vilén et al., 2014). Thus, what the parents and parents-to-be are searching for on the *e*-communities? How and why they are using them? The reason for participating in e-parents' groups should be investigated, taking into account the underlying meanings and psychological dynamics which possibly characterize an identity and role transition.

Background

Overall, future parents have to face changes with a number of adaptive and transformative tasks (Stern & Bruschweiler-Stern, 1998) to successfully transit from the couple dyad to the family triad (Montigny, Lacharité, & Amyot, 2006), crossing an important adulthood crisis (Cadei & Simeone. 2011). Moreover, they are required to transform their roles and identities, integrating new parental functions

(Deave, Johnson, & Ingram, 2008; Slade, Cohen, Sadler, & Miller, 2009; Widarsson, Kerstis, Sundquist, Engström, & Sarkadi, 2012; Spinelli et al., 2016). Particularly, the psychodynamic literature strongly highlighted how much these challenges influence in a specific way the mothers rather than the fathers, due to the cultural stereotype of the "perfect mother", socially established and internalized by women, thus becoming a kind of phantasy (Chodorow & Contratto, 1989), not present in the same vein among fathers. Indeed, during pregnancy women undergo a physical and psychological transformation in preparing to become a mother. From a psychodynamic perspective, the *birth of a mother* (Stern & Bruschweiler-Stern, 1998) involves a reorganization of the woman's inner world and the creation of a mental space to host both the ideas of the child and herself as a parent (Bibring, 1959; Ambrosini & Stanghellini, 2012). Moreover, assuming that motherhood is both a site of social and identity change (Thomson, 2011), the process of becoming a mother includes a deep psychological *re-negotiation* of several aspects of the woman's life and identity as a woman, partner, daughter, and mother. On the one hand, internal conflicts and ambivalence (in a psychodynamic sense, i.e. the coexistence of disparate feelings at the same time), also fostered by prior movements of identification and parental representations above mentioned, need solution and integration (Slade et al, 2009), passing through an interpersonal and a transgenerational[1] dimension (Grienenberger & Slade, 2002; Kelly, Slade, & Grienengerger, 2005). On the other hand, these movements have now increased due to modifications of maternal involvement in the society: the maternal identity and role construction cover a difficult *self-balancing*, for example involving work and family issues as the Work-Family Conflict perspective profusely argues (Hammer & Thompson, 2003). All these topics basically represent mothering tasks, thus the ways mothers respond to the inner role and identity conflicts affect parenting styles (Greenberger, O'neil, & Nagel, 1994; Repetti & Wood, 1997; Crouter & Bumpus, 2001; Costigan, Cox, & Cauce, 2003; Anderson 2007), revealing peculiarities of the mother-child functioning or the adoption of a specific model of what being a mother means to that woman. Indeed, following Brown's reasoning (2010), the modern female identity is a social phenomenon which stems from the relationship that mothers entertain with the social institution of motherhood, and with the social expectations of the maternal role. For example, according to Blair-Loy (2003) and Ridgeway and Correll (2004), the cultural normative of idealized sacrificial motherhood (McCormick, 2010), consistent with the ideology of intensive mothering (Hays, 1996), usually requires an exclusive attentive focus on child rearing in order to be an excellent mother (Stuart, 2007). Consequently, working women often feel guilty because they are not conforming to the societal standard of what a good mother is deemed to be (Guendouzi, 2006), facing the truth that they cannot be both a good worker and a good mother at the same time (Williams & Segal,

2003). Thus, ambivalence about motherhood, choices, and time frequently appears (Chodorow, 2003; Hewlett, 2002).

The informal and professional support and the family's encouragement appear extremely important for mothers and mothers-to-be, helping them to face stressful events like the transition to parenthood (Montigny et al., 2006), the body changes, the baby birth, and their life with a newborn or a growing child.

MAIN FOCUS OF THE CHAPTER

Issues, Controversies, Problems

As Parks (2011) explained, there are two conceptualizations of the term "community": one usually restrict it to groups of people who share physical space, are relatively self-sufficient within that space, and who are linked by ties that include kinship. The second one had lost the geographical trait, becoming stands for culture, a set of ideas and interpersonal sentiments rather than as a physical place (Bender, 1978; Calhoun, 1980). Within this framework, a virtual community is a social group that has the psychological and cultural qualities of a strong community without physical proximity (Willson, 2006). Every group, also virtual, can be defined a community if it acts collectively, thinks of itself as a community and the members identify with the community, sharing and exchanging information and exhibiting attachments to one another and to the community more generally (Willson, 2006; Parks, 2011). Thus, web communities offer a great opportunity to create online groups and receive necessary and appropriate experiences of social support and comparison (Gibson & Hanson, 2013; Niela-Vilén, Axelin, Salanterä, & Menelnder, 2014), as an alternative to face-to-face ones. Due to the increased geographical mobility of people and families, also according to work and career plans, parents, especially mothers, feel more isolated and they are losing daily support from their own family networks (Litt, 2000; Plantin & Daneback, 2009; Gibson & Hanson, 2013). Moreover, grandparents' experiences result in more "out of date" than in the past (they become grandparents at older age than before), thus new parents' requirements are mainly directed to the experience-based source of information, i.e. other "modern" parents in similar situations (Litt, 2000; Niela-Vilén et al., 2014). For example, during postpartum hospital recovery *strangers* become *confidants* because hospitalized new mothers share similar parenting doubts (Oakley & Roberts, 1981), and the parental website offers the opportunity to recreate the hospital scenario (Madge & O'Connor, 2004). Thus, new parents and parents-to-be represent a large category of users (Bartholomew, Schoppe-Sullivan, Glassman, Kamp Dush, & Sullivan, 2012; Morris, 2014), and the *e-health* communities have some advantages for them, especially mothers (Mo,

Malik, & Coulson, 2009; Moorhead et al., 2013), in particular when they are socially and geographically isolated.

Sundstrom (2016) underlined how social attachments in online communities may facilitate associations despite the anonymity of members. Several studies describe the reasons for and benefits of the online support group participation (i.e. emotional and instrumental support, community connections and protection, anonymity which allow to express itself candidly) (Drentea & Moren-Cross, 2005; Hall & Irvine, 2009; Brady & Guerin, 2010; Jang, Dworkin, & Connell, 2012; Palmén, Korpela, & Saranto, 2012).

New mothers use the Internet for sharing their baby stories by posting photos or text messages, and reporting special events in their family life (Jomhari, Gonzalez, & Kurniawan, 2009); moreover, they enjoy social communities satisfying their desire of social interactions (Gibson & Hanson, 2013). Indeed, online communities can be considered an important medium in the communication process, serving the function of personal influence and promoting direct interpersonal connection through forum and blogs (Sundstrom, 2016). Particularly, it seems that blogs and forums' participation increase the well-being of mothers, as they receive support in return, more than on the social networks sites (McDaniel, Coyne, & Holmes, 2012). Furthermore, future mothers using online forums declare to be more likely to change their own behavior (for example, concerning the breastfeeding and childcare) according to their online findings. Overall, the time spent on motherhood specific sites seem to have a greater impact on maternal intentions and behaviors despite normative pressures (McKeever & McKeever, 2017).

According to Rogers (2003), interpersonal communication channels can lead the social change more than mass media and, as Tangherlini et al. (2016) highlighted, the persuasive nature of a personal storytelling can catalyze the decision-making process. Additionally, the internet anonymity allows personal disclosure (Suler, 2004; Quian & Scott, 2007; Jordan, 2010) through a direct or an indirect participation in the conversation (Kraut et al., 2004): it reduces inhibitions, and facilitates the users to be honest about their own opinions and feelings (O'Connor & Madge, 2001). As Ley (2007) showed, sites' design influences members' commitment (including loyalty, obligation, attachment, respect, encouragement), developing a sense of security and safety regarding the site because of their evolving and active nature based on shared cultural values, practices, and collective identity that improve support and trust within the online group's boundaries. As Sundstrom (2016) demonstrate, mothers prefer texting as form of communication because of flexibility that text messages offer, because of their easy access, and the possibility to delete it either save it as a future reference or forward it. Thus, writing or replying to posts on the Internet, mothers can create virtual relations through an open and interactive writing; moreover, they can share personal thoughts and feelings, disclosing parental concerns (McDaniel et al., 2012), and experiencing ways of self-expression (Gibson & Hanson, 2013; Morris, 2014), which can or cannot reveal something about the author's identity (Cadei & Simeone. 2011).

At a personal level, people in cyberspace seem to be influenced by the online disinhibition effect, which involves six factors: dissociative anonymity, invisibility, solipsistic introjections, dissociative imagination, and minimization of status and authority. It is not a mere representation of a "true self" but a complex process of "working through" as a shift among deeper aspects of intrapsychic structure (Suler, 2002, 2004). At a relational level, as highlighted by Walther (2007), in a hyperpersonal perspective the computer mediated communication can facilitate desired relationships: the users' self-presentation takes advantage of the written interface and the extra time to edit and re–write the messages before sending them. In this way, this communication channel contributes to greater intimacy and desirability. Thus, from a psychodynamic perspective, *e*-parents may become a protective community and a source of emotional, formal, informal and instrumental support (Drentea & Moren-Cross, 2005), performing a "holding" function[2], and normalising mothers' *in*experience (Madge & O'Connor, 2004; Brady & Guerin, 2010). In this sense, they may provide a safe space for mothers who need to escape from a romanticized motherhood model (Mungham & Lazard, 2011), space where they can admit that they are not "perfect". Moreover, these communities allow parents to transition from being passive containers of information towards actively searching for different perspectives, experiences, and information (Brady & Guerin, 2010; Jang et al., 2012). Indeed, the online peer support groups represent an endless source of medical data and social assistance (Plantin & Daneback, 2009), characterized by instant responses and low costs (Madge & O'Connor, 2004), even though they cannot constitute an alternative to high-quality professional websites (Reichow et al., 2012) because of the risk of sharing inaccurate information (Madge & O'Connor, 2004; Jordan, 2010).

Furthermore, despite the geographical distances or time constraints (Niela-Vilén et al., 2014), online peer support groups are a rich source of comparison and practical advice. They make a positive contribution to parents and parenting (Nieuwboer, Fukkink, & Hermanns, 2013), for example: satisfying mothers' needs when they suffer from postpartum depression (Dennis et al., 2009; Dennis, 2010); helping new mothers to feel more connected with others through the Internet (McDaniel et al., 2012); and committing mothers practically to online activities, thus helping them to be awake during the night while feeding (Gibson & Hanson, 2013). Thus, e-groups seem to make a positive contribution to parenting skills and transition to motherhood. Recently, an Italian study on families of patients with rare diseases (Tozzi et al., 2013) showed that 66% of parents participate in an online forum on health and demonstrated that Italian parents of children with rare diseases are active Internet users (searching for information and/or joining online communities), confirming that the information management is an important component of coping with illness and illness-related uncertainties (Brashers, Goldsmith, & Hsieh, 2002). What about parents not specifically involved with child's diseases? And what about mothers-to-be? The Italian context is lack of studies on this issue, i.e. on if, how and why mothers and mothers-to-be use the web communities. Two Italian studies (Bert et al., 2013; Scaioli et al., 2015) carried out a multicentre survey to assess the sociodemographic and geographic differences existing in a sample of pregnant women searching for information on the web. These studies also explored the factors influencing the choices of childbirth after the Internet consultation and investigated potential differences between primiparous and multiparous women in the Internet use. Moreover, Tozzi et al. (2013) conducted an online survey among Italian parents of patients with rare diseases to describe their Internet user profile and to explore how Internet use affects their health decisions. Nevertheless, there is a lack of Italian studies about the use of web forums dedicated to mothering and about motivations for its use by mothers, *mothers-to-be*, and women trying to have a baby.

SOLUTIONS AND RECOMMENDATIONS

Aims

From a psychodynamic perspective, the aim of the present study is to explore the Italian e-mothers context -specifically focusing on the rising maternity- questioning *whether*, *why*, and *how* they use specific online forums. The analysis of the manifest and latent contents of the mothers' interactions and of the emotional connections between their own maternal experiences and their online group belonging represents a specific task.

Methods

Data Collection

According to Kraut et al. (2004), although conducting online research can potentially affect data quality, researchers' actions, and human subjects, it does not involve more risks than traditional research. Rather, it changes the nature of the risks and investigators' ability is required to evaluate them. First, the online research entails serious sampling problems, especially for traditional quantitative studies. Indeed, recruiting a random or representative sample and verifying the identity of online participants is not possible (Madge & O'Connor, 2002). Moreover, possible risks to subjects participating in internet-based interviews and surveys regard their direct participation, for example, emotional reactions or experimental manipulations, and harm resulting from a breach of confidentiality (Kraut et al., 2004). The issues relating to anonymity, informed consent, boundaries, and the difference between public and private behaviors have still not been clarified and the debate is far from over.

However, internet-based methodologies offer new and many opportunities. They allow researchers to interact with participants in innovative ways, to use different sampling strategies, to conduct qualitative research (Mann & Stewart, 2000; Madge & O'Connor, 2002; Hooley, Wellens, & Marriott, 2011), to explore the online and offline experience in everyday life, and to involve marginalized populations (Sparks, Collins, & Kearns, 2016). Moreover, as Kraut et al. (2004) explained, the use of the Internet in psychological research allows researchers to recognize psychological phenomena that would be much more difficult to identify in traditional settings. It is very difficult to chase the evolution of groups because of the difficulties and costs of tracking many individuals for a long time. In this regard, the Internet represents a valuable tool for long-term research on groups.

Data for this study were extracted on the Internet by searching for Italian websites with forums about maternity. Forums were searched on Google search engine using few representative Italian keywords, descriptive of this study interest: forum, mothers, children. Two forums specifically directed to mothering and raising maternity, with mothers coming from all over Italy, were selected because of their users' daily activity and the variety of themes discussed. From these two forums, 231 relevant threads were extracted. They have been written in a time frame of three years (2013-2016).

After a first summary reading of posts and personal users' account, threads were selected using following criteria:

- written or active from January 1, 2013, to December 31, 2016;
- written by mothers-to-be and mothers of young children (0-3 years).

The data collection focused on women who were having their first child as the study focused on the maternity process, assuming that pregnant women and mothers experiencing maternity with very young children could specifically face with similar topics (different from mothers of adolescents for example). Moreover, it was not possible to select only a specific target of mothers, as mothers of young children often participate in forum discussions about pregnancy, presenting their quite close experience. On the contrary, it was improbable to find a mother of an adolescent.

Finally, a total number of 7433 comments were collected. Each thread was extracted by copying and printed into a document for a pencil on paper analysis.

To protect forum members' real identity (Kraut et al., 2004), all the identifying data in the text were omitted, such as the Internet forum name, names or pseudonyms of the writers, or references to places. Also, the usernames or URLs for any specific threads were omitted. Therefore, it is not possible to identify any single forum user in our final results.

Sample

In the collected data, 379 Italian writers were included: mothers of young children and 57 declared mothers-to-be. The gender and the geographical origin of users were explicitly declared on their personal forum profile. Being a mother, pregnant or trying to have a baby were determined by information explicitly provided by the authors (i.e., in profiles) or inferred from the content of comments (for example, “my baby is 20 months old”, “I and my husband are trying to have a baby”). On the personal forum profile, nobody had explicitly declared her age.

Data Analysis

According to the guidelines described by Braun and Clarke (2006), a Latent Thematic Analysis was realized to identify, analyze, and report themes from a qualitative source of data. Taking into account the psychodynamic epistemological authors’ background, an inductive data-driven (not theory-driven) analysis was conducted through an analytic process, which moves from the data description to the interpretation. Indeed, thematic analysis entails research across the data set to find repeated patterns of meaning, mainly in the latent thematic analysis the development of the themes themselves involves an interpretative work. Specifically, a line by line thematic analysis at a latent level “goes beyond the semantic content of the data, and starts to identify or examine the *underlying* ideas, assumptions, and conceptualizations” (Braun & Clarke, 2006, p. 13).

According to Braun and Clarke (2006), the Latent Thematic Analysis is not a linear process from one phase to the next. Rather, it is a recursive process and consists of different phases, where the researcher move back and forth as needed, throughout them (Table 1). First, two researchers independently and simultaneously read all the material to familiarize with the data corpus, and after a “repeated reading” of the data in an active way, searching for meanings, patterns and so on, they wrote notes on the margins to record interesting contents. The codes could refer to semantic or latent contents that appear interesting to the analysts. Gradually, from these contents, they created a preliminary list of codes, writing notes in the text, using highlighters or colored pens to indicate potential patterns or to identify segments of data. Later, the researchers started to analyze the codes matching them up with data extracts, consider how different codes may combine to form an overarching theme, and think about the relationship between codes, between themes, and between different levels

Table 1. Phases of thematic analysis (Braun & Clarke, 2006)

Phase	Description of the Process
1. Familiarising yourself with your data:	Transcribing data (if necessary), reading and re-reading the data, noting down initial ideas.
2. Generating initial codes:	Coding interesting features of the data in a systematic fashion across the entire data set, collating data relevant to each code.
3. Searching for themes:	Collating codes into potential themes, gathering all data relevant to each potential theme.
4. Reviewing themes:	Checking in the themes work in relation to the coded extracts (Level 1) and the entire data set (Level 2), generating a thematic 'map' of the analysis.
5. Defining and naming themes:	Ongoing analysis to refine the specifics of each theme, and the overall story the analysis tells; generating clear definitions and names for each theme.
6. Producing the report:	The final opportunity for analysis. Selection of vivid, compelling extract examples, final analysis of selected extracts, relating back of the analysis to the research question and literature, producing a scholarly report of the analysis (eventually including a thematic map).

of themes. Following Braun and Clarke (2006), they discussed the findings searching for the meanings beyond the surface, unraveling the reality. Through the comparison among the researchers, a critical revision of proposed themes was conducted to guarantee internal homogeneity and external heterogeneity (data within themes should cohere together meaningfully, while there should be clear and identifiable distinctions between themes). Finally, searching for themes that work in relation to the coded extracts and the entire data set, five main themes emerged and it was possible to determine which features of data was captured by each theme, generating clear definitions and names for each of them and a "thematic map" of the analysis. In this way, it was possible to make sense of patterns of meaning (Braun & Clarke, 2013).

RESULTS

Five main themes emerged from the thematic analysis, resulting from the final identification of 41 codes and 12 subthemes. These 5 themes and their connections describe the complexity of the relations among the e-mothers and (a) their on-going parental experience, (b) their identities under construction, (c) their worries and fantasies, and (d) the online group. In our interpretation, all these topics shape how mothers make sense of their experiences through the online dimension. (Figure 1)

Figure 1. The map of themes connected to the categories and related codes

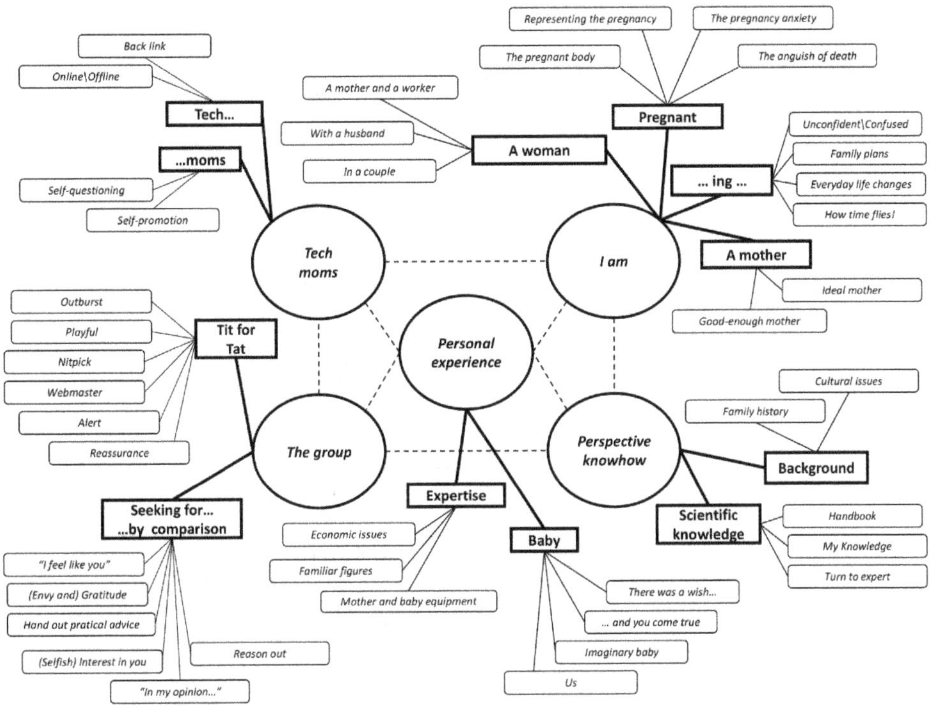

Themes were so called: *the group* (53.06%); *I am* (17.93%); *personal experience* (14.82%); *perspective knowhow* (8.92%); *tech-moms* (5.27%) (Table 2).

On the total frequency of the codes, it has been calculated the percentage of the sub-themes and, consequently, the percentage of the themes. The first theme is the biggest one, including a little more than half of the entire corpus of data. Even though Latent Thematic Analysis does not take care of statistics and invites researchers to consider the emotional value it can be captured beyond the data description (Braun & Clarke, 2006), this amount should be considered as it refers to "the weight" the online group dynamics and functioning have in this context.

The Group

This theme seems to well describe the group functioning, how and why the members use the community. On these parenting websites, mothers can share personal experiences and knowledge with people interested in the same issue, receiving information and practical advice. The e-group interactions, as the face-to-face group, are often characterized by a *tit for tat* functioning, a back and forth communication.

Table 2. Codes frequency on 7433 messages; subthemes % on total codes frequency and related themes %

<table>
<tr><th>THEMES
(% On Total Sub Themes)</th><th>SUB THEMES
(% On Total Frequency)</th><th>CODES
(Frequency)</th></tr>
<tr><td rowspan="2">THE GROUP
(53.06)</td><td>Tit for tat
(20.61)</td><td>Playful (2260)
Nitpick (1023)
Reassurance (843)
Alert (265)
Outburst (227)
Webmaster and censorship (155)</td></tr>
<tr><td>Seeking for… By comparison
(32.45)</td><td>"In my opinion" (2605)
"I feel like you" (2239)
Hand out practical advice (1233)
(Selfish) Interest in you (925)
(Envy and) Gratitude (389)
Reason out (131)</td></tr>
<tr><td rowspan="4">I AM
(17.93)</td><td>A mother
(5.65)</td><td>Ideal mother (734)
Good enough mother (575)</td></tr>
<tr><td>A woman
(3.9)</td><td>In a couple (442)
A mother and a worker (250)
With a husband (211)</td></tr>
<tr><td>Pregnant
(5)</td><td>The anguish of death (445)
The pregnant body (377)
Representing the pregnancy (171)
The pregnancy anxiety (165)</td></tr>
<tr><td>… ing …
(3.38)</td><td>Unconfident/Confused (471)
Everyday life changes (158)
Family plans (98)
How time flies! (58)</td></tr>
<tr><td rowspan="2">PERSONAL EXPERIENCE
(14.82)</td><td>Baby
(11.78)</td><td>… And you come true (1667)
There was a wish … (847)
Imaginary baby (191)
Us (23)</td></tr>
<tr><td>Expertise
(3.04)</td><td>Mother and baby equipment (372)
Familiar figures(192)
Economic issues (138)</td></tr>
<tr><td rowspan="2">PERSPECTIVE KNOWHOW
(8.92)</td><td>Background
(1.21)</td><td>Cultural issues (226)
Family history (54)</td></tr>
<tr><td>Scientific knowledge
(7.71)</td><td>Turn to expert (1027)
My knowledge (720)
Handbook (40)</td></tr>
<tr><td rowspan="2">TECH-MOMS
(5.27)</td><td>Tech …
(1.29)</td><td>Back link (263)
Online/Offline (35)</td></tr>
<tr><td>… Moms
(3.98)</td><td>Self-promotion (608)
Self-questioning (314)</td></tr>
</table>

Moreover, as in a typical face-to-face group, both the *nitpicks* (i.e. conflicts and arguments) and *playful* moments (i.e. jokes and complicity) are unavoidable and seem to reinforce cohesion and intimacy among members. For example:

Your nickname is awesome… So funny!!!!! (Playful)

There are topics full of venom against your mothers. Has anybody ever told you to shut up?!

Seriously, what kind of speeches are these? (Nitpicks)

Maybe... the first childbirth was too hard for your husband, and maybe HE doesn't want to repeat that experience!!!!!!!!!!!! (Nitpicks)

However, in the specific online context, a *webmaster* mediates the members' exchanges.

I covered the bad word you used with asterisks… Just be careful, please!!!

Through their interactions, sometimes *e*-mothers seem to verbalize their worries, anxiety, and the *alert* they undergo about their first experiences with children and/or pregnancy, transmitting it to the other members and evacuating it in the group that can contain these feelings. Thus, the e-group seems the place in which concerns and *Outbursts* (releases of negative and strong emotions) are permitted, accepted and held back by *Reassurances*. For example:

I am so irate, I know I could be egoistic, but I'm tired and I was very patience! I am very irritated! (Outburst)

Girls, thank you so much for your reassuring words, but I am so worried. Even if he is growing, the pediatrician told me that growth parameters are not good... I am so worried... The chow time is a fight, he cries and doesn't open his mouth. It's become too much for me… I need a solution! (Reassurance and Outburst)

Furthermore, the sub-theme named *comparison* includes comparative experiences reported by mothers with someone who feels the same feelings (*"I feel like you"*), *hands out practical advice*, offers a personal opinion (*"In my opinion…"*), and expresses attention and interest in other people (*Interest in you*), helping grateful mothers (*Gratitude*) to make decisions (*Reason out*).

Thank you very much for your valuable suggestion... I will take your advice! (Gratitude and Reason out)

I like so much these threads! When someone asks a question, each of us answers based on personal experiences, therefore we have a number of completely different replies. So, there are no well-specific guidelines with regard to children, only common sense (In my opinion... and Interest in you)

Indeed, the group is also the virtual place in which *selfish*ness and *envy* can be expressed, for example towards who is living actual maternity experience or pregnancy, caring their baby, while other women are trying to get pregnant.

Girls, I don't know if it's the same for you, but every day pregnant friends pop up around me. Obviously, I am happy for them, but I wish the same to me, possibly getting over the first trimester.

Sometimes it seems an obstacle course of enthusiasms and falls, often with the unpleasant feeling of seeing so many women who make it, while we keep running, falling and rising up after all this trouble, may we will be in good shape mothers.

Last year, when I started to try, all the women around me caught the stork, everyone but me. I brought good luck to many women, but now, I really would want some fortune!

I Am

The "I am" dimension involves transformations in the feminine identity the woman is experiencing. Forums about maternity seem to include hints and variations of women's identity, according to how the on-going maternity implicates a revolution in women's sense of be-*ing*: they are constantly in changing, their new lives and identities are in progress, and these transformations connect past to present and future, involving *everyday life changes, family plans*, and *unconfident* feelings. The personal identity, as *a woman* and as *a mother,* needs to become gradually and deeply integrated and balanced.

Hello, moms! This morning, drinking my coffee, I enjoyed the sunrise and the silence... Amazing! I was thinking about the need to have our own space, despite the family, where we could seek shelter from everyday life routine and problems. Have you a place to find your thoughts and yourself again? Have you a place to collect your thoughts and to process your problems and feelings?

We are first of all women, as well as mothers... Delicate souls subjected to a lot of sacrifices and continuous trials... No one of us is better than others: we are amazing women that are trying to best manage our own lives.

Mothers need to resolve a difficult mix: the job's responsibilities (as *a mother and a worker)* need to match with the woman *in a couple*, and with the mothering that implies children's requests and maternal duty; such as the idealized image of maternity (*the ideal mother*) needs to encounter reality boundaries (*the good enough mother).*

I lasted two months... I hardly saw her because of my office hours.

In the morning I took her to the nest, during the lunch break I brought back her at home where my mother was waiting for us. I went back to work, and then I returned at home no earlier than 8 p.m., when she was already asleep. I asked for the part-time, but it was denied me. So I decided to fire me. After a while, my husband and I tried to have another child. I came back at work when my second baby was 3 years old and the first daughter started primary school

Despite my breast pain, I fed my daughter until 14 months, but I want, to be honest... I'm not sure what my strong motivation was, whether it was the love for my baby or the fear of being accused of being a bad mother

She would be labeled as a bad mother because that's how it works. In sorrow shall thou bring forth children»; you will feed them and you will forget yourself!!!

Nobody will ever tell you how you can be a parent. Being a parent means to learn from the children, reviewing themselves and the relationship with own parents.

There is no right or wrong: the important thing is the harmony you establish with your child.

All these aspects discuss an identity under construction and evolution, as it refers to the first years of the child life and to the *mother-to-be* dimension when the woman faces *body* transformations:

Your body is preparing for the event, and your mind should do the same.

How long after the childbirth can I dress in my old jeans again? I mean, how long will it take to get back in shape? I miss my favorite jeans...

... inner fantasies, and fears as the pregnancy anxiety, and the anguish of death.

I use the Angel Care, a sensor that you put under the mattress of the child, which sounds in case of absence of breath.

Today I had some slight blood losses... Hey, you [the baby] please settle at the right place!

When you are pregnant you have a thousand thoughts, even about trivial things. So you are troubled by so many doubts: « This will hurt him? Can I use, eat, do such a thing?»

Personal Experience

Digital writers often share with the *e*-group an event occurred in their everyday life. Moreover, the baby's birth implies the constitution of an "*us*" dimension that activates emotional and practical issues.

I haven't been apart from her since we checked out of the hospital... We are always together! I know that moment will come, but for now, she is so tiny!!!

Mothers narrate their experiences with the *baby*: the *imaginary* one...

I am not afraid that he might be disabled.

...the desired one *(there was a wish ...)*...

I simply felt that this was the right moment for me to realize the desire of having a child.

Just remember: you are a mother now and forever. You are a mother for this angel who lived for a too short time inside of you, bringing a lot of happiness. You will be a mother for your future babies. When the desire of a baby touch a woman's heart she is already a mother: a mother in the making.

...and the real one (... *and you come true)*. However, mothers also provide for the construction of a personal *expertise* focusing on the *mother and baby equipment,* the *familiar figures'* support and the *economic issues*. For example:

I found a great offer on e-bay, I paid 9€, it was great, wasn't it?

We bought: two baby bottles, thermos, diapers, napkins, dummy, clothes, towels, beach chair, toys, and stroller. is there something missing? What kind of ointment have I to use when I will change his diaper? Have I to buy physiological saline for his nose?

Sharing personal experiences seems to reinforce women's belonging to a new on-going dimension, facing fantasies and reality. Emotional and practical issues proceed simultaneously like two dimensions which sometimes cover and discover each other.

Perspective Knowhow

Parenting challenges and desires encourage mothers to work hard improving their own capabilities as a caregiver. The experiences they had as children basically imprint their own parental style. Indeed, a personal and cultural *background* transmitted across generations *(family history, cultural issues)* give the mothers a first direction equipping them deeply and a guide to an initial approach to mothering. This cultural background is often discussed and criticized by mothers in the *e*-group especially about themes as breastfeeding, job and gender role.

All women in my family have fed the children. For me, there can be no other kind

In my family, everybody has breastfed, maybe I didn't want to be outdone...it influenced my decision of course...

S*cientific knowledge* certainly can solve parenting doubts and dull pain, representing an important task for mothers. By reading *handbook*s or (positively or negatively) referring *to the experts*, mothers can build a personal portfolio *(my knowledge)* they can share with the other e-parents and proudly show them.

In my opinion, some good reading is necessary ... You cannot start the parental adventure without adequate training!

I was so scared before of the childbirth! But I remember a paper about this and how to get over it. It was very useful to me.

My pediatrician wrote to me the feed schedule...

Unfortunately, most pediatricians do not consider the newborns' pain as a relevant issue to be faced.

But I would like to know... why the pediatricians have to psychologically terrorize the parents?

I beg to tell you that the 10-minute-feed method is greatly exceeded: scientific studies highlighted that the first milk is lighter and more thirst-quenching than the second one. The second milk is fatter and more filling: it allows to your child to grow up. Feeding your baby 10 minutes for breast, she sucks just the first, lighter and digestible milk, so she will be hungry sooner.

Anguishes can decrease through the knowledge. Although online forums do not always represent high-quality sources of information, the Internet and the social networks offer a great opportunity to an instant access to scientific information to learn, and experiences to compare with the personal one. Sometimes this immediacy becomes more successful than the experience transmitted through generations by other family members which, on the contrary, often feed anguishes and ideals, not always useful for an identity under construction.

Tech-Moms

This theme refers to the relation between mothers and the technological medium: mothers seem to use the *e*-groups to express their style of motherhood and improve their technology-related capabilities. Within and through the safe online forum, the mothers have the opportunity to share and discuss common experiences. Moreover, moms' competencies are conveyed in the forum group as *self-promotion* (a tendency to give value to their maternal roles, experiences, and decisions) or as *self-questioning* (due to the uncertainty linked to their new roles, experiences, and decisions as a mother). For examples:

I really laughed for your expensive stroller... My 3 wheels one is perfect and costs less (Self-promoting)

I don't know, they are just messy thoughts of a mother who wants to do the best and sometimes she mess up! (Self-questioning)

Have you ever heard of guilt? Sometimes you have to seriously decide (I couldn't sleep and after a long day of struggles was too hard) but you don't know if you are right: you are tortured by self-doubt and fear, especially about your baby (Self-questioning)

The *e-group* allows promoting and improving mother's *tech*-skills: knowledge and experiences can be easier transmitted online through the *back link* or supporting them through photos or video records.

I sent you the link!

Please, share the video with us

What kind of stroller do you suggest? [Two links]

Often, thanks to the online medium, relations among mothers also become a bridge to an offline meeting and an occasion to build a close friendship, connecting the *online* to the *offline* dimensions.

Wow, where do you live exactly? I think we are very close!

I read you live in Milan, if you need the stroller, please contact me

FUTURE RESEARCH

This study confirms that parenting experience represents a big challenge for new mothers and mothers-to-be. Turning to online forums and e-groups, mothers express their need for communication, sharing emotional and practical support. Learning through shared experiences seems to have a key role in the e-group functioning.

Naturally, this qualitative and explorative study presents some limits that could direct future research: exploring how other digital device work or focusing on possible differences between mothers and fathers in regards to how they use online groups, and analyzing their subjective experiences also taking care of gender and role differences. It was not possible to delineate the specificity of the primiparous vs multiparous women through the forum's threads, but it could be very interesting to analyze whether and how experiencing e-groups diverges. Furthermore, it would be very interesting to compare these e-parents outcomes with other countries and cultures, and with other e-communities of parents facing different developmental diseases, i.e. adolescence for example, or parents facing their children special needs. Future research could provide answers to these curiosities.

CONCLUSION

The group, the *I am* dimension, *personal experience, perspective knowhow* and *tech-moms* represent the emotional core issues of the e-mothers whose forum's participation has been analyzed. The e-group functioning and the identity dimension arising from the group's dynamics are two main aspects which need to be discussed. On the one hand, it seems that the e-group membership (*the group*) can reproduce an offline peer group functioning (Parks, 2011), allowing members to identify each other, and to reshape the personal identity (*I am*) (Suler, 2002, 2004) thanks to the comparison among *personal experience*s and knowledge (*perspective knowhow*) through the technological medium (*Tech-moms*) (Kirk & Milnes, 2015). It seems to be confirmed the greater impact of the time spent on motherhood-dedicated web sites on maternal intentions, behaviors, and decisions (Rogers, 2003; McKeever & McKeever, 2017), and mothers' self-presentation (Walther, 2007) and experiences can take advantages through the online forum medium (Sundstrom, 2016).

Thus, the e-group functioning allows members' personal growth, through essential mirroring functions the woman often need during the transitional periods of life, such as the on-going experience of maternity. Indeed, rising maternity naturally implies the re-definition of personal and relational dimensions (Stern & Bruschweiler-Stern, 1998). Internal conflicts and ambivalence can characterize this condition such as a crisis of woman's identity, and this represents a social and a psychological matter. According to literature, people in difficult stages of life and experiences, need to be sustained by a social network (Montigny et al., 2006), that increasingly means a virtual plot of relationships, able to guarantee an emotional and concrete support even though in a potential space (Bert et al., 2013; Gibson & Hanson, 2013; Niela-Vilén et al., 2014). Sharing the same experiences with peers, the mothers seem to reinforce progressively their own identity, often "under construction". On the other hand, taking into account the emotional needs the rising maternity experience elicits, the e-group virtually become a breast with feeding, holding and reassuring functioning, responding to these necessities. The online community represent a source of social personal that helps mothers to face and manage the stress (Albrecht & Adelman, 1984) related to their new lives, roles, and identities. Into the large e-group container, mothers and *mothers-to-be* seem to throw up the pain they feel and through the e-group emotional functioning they can collect pieces of experiences, memories, knowledge, identity. Sometimes a reassuring container with holding functions, or a "toilet breast" (Meltzer, 1967) for evacuated anguishes, sometimes a source of rejection which can badly raise overwhelming emotions or a source of reparation for guilty parents, the e-group can also encourage regressive movements and dependence.

Thus, regressive and progressive movements seem to characterize the e-group experience as well as the developmental experiences of life and, naturally, the individual and psychic functioning. Therefore, sharing experiences and opinions the e-group empower mothering through a kind of self-promotion and self-questioning, which sustain the women's identity and the representation of a *good-enough* mother (Winnicott, 1951), frequently against an ideal image of maternity deeply and culturally ratified. Indeed, the Italian culture confers principally to mothers the responsibility to organize children's daily activities, to integrate parenting and jobs duties (Saraceno, 2003), to face with the idealization of a role - "The Mother" - and a practice that not easily allows women to feel negative feelings toward maternity and children. Just like in face-to-face communities, also in online contexts mothers can find supportive interactions and relationships which play a major role in all aspects of people's lives, such as in physical health, emotional well-being, and work performance (Albrecht & Halsey, 1992).

A new competence seems to raise from the e-group: the tech-mom through the technological medium improves her expertise and *tech*-skills. Then, encouraging women's self-questioning and self-improvement, and new mother's proficiency, the *e*-group can alternatively increase a perfect model, this time not generated by cultural issues but by the e-identity it-self.

We are parents who wonder about their own role. We believe in the importance of sharing that makes us more aware, safer and comfortable, and overcomes stereotypes and prejudices. We propose a model of curious and informed parenting, careful above all to the needs of all children. This is a place where we can repair us as parents, by working together to become of course not perfect but simply more careful parents. (From the main forum issues)

This study tried to fill the gap about *e*-motherhood and to demonstrate that maternal identity and role constructions, with all entailed processes, are played also online, especially on peer *e*-groups. Indeed, the online forums appear to be privileged "places" for the definition of these "under construction" identities. Finally, the experts should take into account the new mothers' and mothers-to-be' needs of practical advice and comparison with peers, and not just of scientific knowledge.

REFERENCES

Albrecht, T. L., & Adelman, M. B. (1984). Social support and life stress. *Human Communication Research*, *11*(1), 3–32. doi:10.1111/j.1468-2958.1984.tb00036.x

Albrecht, T. L., & Halsey, J. (1992). Mutual support in mixed-status relationships. *Journal of Social and Personal Relationships*, *9*(2), 237–252. doi:10.1177/0265407592092005

Ambrosini, A., & Stanghellini, G. (2012). Myths of motherhood: The role of culture in the development of postpartum depression. *Annali dell'Istituto Superiore di Sanita*, *48*(3), 277–286. doi:10.4415/ANN_12_03_08 PMID:23007052

Ammaniti, M., & Trentini, C. (2009). How new knowledge about parenting reveals the neurobiological implications of intersubjectivity: A conceptual synthesis of recent research. *Psychoanalytic Dialogues*, *19*(5), 537–555. doi:10.1080/10481880903231951

Anderson, O. A. (2007). Linking work stress, parental self-efficacy, ineffective parenting, and youth problem behavior. *Journal of Family Studies*, *13*(1), 119–120.

Bartholomew, M. K., Schoppe-Sullivan, S. J., Glassman, M., Kamp Dush, C. M., & Sullivan, J. M. (2012). New parents' Facebook use at the transition to parenthood. *Family Relations*, *61*(3), 455–469. doi:10.1111/j.1741-3729.2012.00708.x PMID:23671354

Bender, T. (1978). *Community and social change in America*. New Brunswick, NJ: Rutgers University Press.

Bert, F., Gualano, M. R., Brusaferro, S., De Vito, E., De Waure, C., La Torre, G., & Torregrossa, M. V. et al. (2013). Pregnancy e-health: A multicenter Italian cross-sectional study on Internet use and decision-making among pregnant women. *Journal of Epidemiology and Community Health*, *0*, 1–6. PMID:24072743

Bibring, G. L. (1959). Some considerations of the psychological processes in pregnancy. *The Psychoanalytic Study of the Child*, *14*, 113–121.

Blair-Loy, M. (2009). *Competing devotions: Career and family among women executives*. Cambridge, MA: Harvard University Press.

Brady, E., & Guerin, S. (2010). "Not the romantic, all happy, coochy coo experience": A qualitative analysis of interactions on an Irish parenting web site. *Family Relations*, *59*(1), 14–27. doi:10.1111/j.1741-3729.2009.00582.x

Brashers, D. E., Goldsmith, D. J., & Hsieh, E. (2002). Information seeking and avoiding in health contexts. *Human Communication Research, 28*(2), 258–271. doi:10.1111/j.1468-2958.2002.tb00807.x

Braun, V., & Clarke, V. (2006). Using thematic analysis in psychology. *Qualitative Research in Psychology, 3*(2), 77–101. doi:10.1191/1478088706qp063oa

Braun, V., & Clarke, V. (2013). Successful qualitative research: A practical guide for beginners. *Sage (Atlanta, Ga.).*

Brown, I. (2010). Ambivalence of the motherhood experience. In A. O'Reilly (Ed.), *Twenty-first-century motherhood: Experience, identity, policy, agency* (pp. 121–139). New York, NY: Columbia University Press.

Cadei, L., & Simeone, D. (2011). Tra il chiaro e lo scuro. Riflessioni pedagogiche sul ruolo dell'ecografia ostetrica nel processo di transizione alla genitorialità. In E. Catarsi & J. P. Pourtois (Eds.), *Educazione familiare e servizi per l'infanzia. Education familiare et services pour l'enfance* (pp. 184–187). Firenze: University Press.

Calhoun, C. J. (1980). Community: Toward a variable conceptualization for comparative research. *Social History, 5*(1), 105–129. doi:10.1080/03071028008567472

Chodorow, N. J. (2003). "Too late": Ambivalence about motherhood, choice, and time. *Journal of the American Psychoanalytic Association, 51*(4), 1181–1198. doi:10.1177/00030651030510040701 PMID:14713010

Chodorow, N. J., & Contratto, S. (1989). The Fantasy of the Perfect Mother. In N. J. Chodorow (Ed.), *Feminism and Psychoanalytic Theory* (pp. 79–96). New Haven: Yale University Press.

Costigan, C. L., Cox, M. J., & Cauce, A. M. (2003). Work-parenting linkages among dual-earner couples at the transition to parenthood. *Journal of Family Psychology, 17*(3), 397–408. doi:10.1037/0893-3200.17.3.397 PMID:14562463

Crouter, A. C., & Bumpus, M. F. (2001). Linking parents' work stress to children's and adolescents' psychological adjustment. *Current Directions in Psychological Science, 10*(5), 156–159. doi:10.1111/1467-8721.00138

Deave, T., Johnson, D., & Ingram, J. (2008) Transition to parenthood: The needs of parents in pregnancy and early parenthood. *BioMed Central pregnancy and Childbirth, 8*(30), 1-11.

Dennis, C. L. (2010). Postpartum depression peer support: Maternal perceptions from a randomized controlled trial. *International Journal of Nursing Studies, 47*(5), 560–568. doi:10.1016/j.ijnurstu.2009.10.015 PMID:19962699

Dennis, C. L., Hodnett, E., Kenton, L., Weston, J., Zupancic, J., Stewart, D. E., & Kiss, A. (2009). Effect of peer support on prevention of postnatal depression among high risk women: Multisite randomised controlled trial. *British Medical Journal*, *338*, 280–284. PMID:19147637

Drentea, P., & Moren-Cross, J. L. (2005). Social capital and social support on the web: The case of an internet mother site. *Sociology of Health & Illness*, *27*(7), 920–943. doi:10.1111/j.1467-9566.2005.00464.x PMID:16313523

Ferraro, F., & Nunziante Cesàro, A. (1985). *Lo spazio cavo e il corpo saturato. La gravidanza come "agire" tra fusione e separazione*. Milano: Franco Angeli Editore.

Gibson, L., & Hanson, V. L. (2013). Digital motherhood: How does technology help new mothers? In J. A. Konstan, & K. Höök (Eds.), *Proceedings of the SIGCHI conference on human factors in computing systems* (pp. 313-322). ACM. doi:10.1145/2470654.2470700

Greenberger, E., O'neil, R., & Nagel, S. K. (1994). Linking workplace and homeplace: Relations between the nature of adults' work and their parenting behaviors. *Developmental Psychology*, *30*(6), 990–1002. doi:10.1037/0012-1649.30.6.990

Grienenberger, J., & Slade, A. (2002). Maternal reflective functioning, mother-infant affective communication, and infant attachment: Implications for psychodynamic treatment with children and families. *Psychologist-Psychoanalyst*, *22*(3), 1–8.

Guendouzi, J. (2006). "The guilt thing": Balancing domestic and professional roles. *Journal of Marriage and the Family*, *68*(4), 901–909. doi:10.1111/j.1741-3737.2006.00303.x

Hall, W., & Irvine, V. (2009). E-communication among mothers of infants and toddlers in a community-based cohort: A content analysis. *Journal of Advanced Nursing*, *65*(1), 175–183. doi:10.1111/j.1365-2648.2008.04856.x PMID:19016925

Hammer, L., & Thompson, C. A. (2003) Work-family role conflict. In *An encyclopedia entry for the Sloan Work and Family Research Network*. Retrieved March 18, 2017, from www.bc.edu/wfnetwork

Hays, S. (1996). *Cultural Contradictions of Motherhood*. New Haven, CT: Yale University Press.

Hewlett, S. A. (2002). *Creating a Life. Professional Women and the Quest for Children*. New York: Talk Miramax Books.

Hooley, T., Wellens, J., & Marriott, J. (2011). *What is Online research?: Using the Internet for social science research*. A&C Black.

Jang, J., Dworkin, J., & Connell, J. (2012). Babycenter. com: New parent behavior in an online community. The Forum for Family and Consumer Issues.

Jomhari, N., Gonzalez, V. M., & Kurniawan, S. H. (2009). See the apple of my eye: Baby storytelling in social space. In *Proceedings of the 23rd British HCI Group Annual Conference on People and Computers: Celebrating People and Technology* (pp. 238-243). British Computer Society.

Jordan, C. J. (2010). Evolution of autism support and understanding via the World Wide Web. *Intellectual and Developmental Disabilities*, *48*(3), 220–227. doi:10.1352/1934-9556-48.3.220 PMID:20597733

Kelly, K., Slade, A., & Grienenberger, J. F. (2005). Maternal reflective functioning, mother–infant affective communication, and infant attachment: Exploring the link between mental states and observed caregiving behavior in the intergenerational transmission of attachment. *Attachment & Human Development*, *7*(3), 299–311. doi:10.1080/14616730500245963 PMID:16210241

Kirk, S., & Milnes, L. (2015). An exploration of how young people and parents use online support in the context of living with cystic fibrosis. *Health Expectations*, *19*(2), 309–321. doi:10.1111/hex.12352 PMID:25691209

Kraut, R., Olson, J., Banaji, M., Bruckman, A., Cohen, J., & Couper, M. (2004). Psychological research online: Report of Board of Scientific Affairs' Advisory Group on the Conduct of Research on the Internet. *The American Psychologist*, *59*(2), 105–117. doi:10.1037/0003-066X.59.2.105 PMID:14992637

Ley, B. L. (2007). Vive les roses!: The architecture of commitment in an online pregnancy and mothering group. *Journal of Computer-Mediated Communication*, *12*(4), 1388–1408. doi:10.1111/j.1083-6101.2007.00378.x

Litt, J. S. (2000). *Medicalized Motherhood: Perspectives from the Lives of African-American and Jewish Women*. New Brunswick, NJ: Rutgers University Press.

Madge, C., & O'Connor, H. (2002). On-line with e-mums: Exploring the internet as a medium for research. *Area*, *34*(1), 92–102. doi:10.1111/1475-4762.00060

Madge, C., & O'Connor, H. (2004). Online methods in geography educational research. *Journal of Geography in Higher Education*, *28*(1), 143–152. doi:10.1080/0309826042000198710

Mann, C., & Stewart, F. (2000). Internet communication and qualitative research: A handbook for researching online. *Sage (Atlanta, Ga.)*.

McCormick, A. (2010). Supermothers on Film, or Maternal Melodrama in the 21st Century. In A. O'Reilly (Ed.), *Twenty-first-century motherhood: Experience, identity, policy, agency* (pp. 140–157). New York, NY: Columbia University Press.

McDaniel, B. T., Coyne, S. M., & Holmes, E. K. (2012). New mothers and media use: Associations between blogging, social networking, and maternal well-being. *Maternal and Child Health Journal, 16*(7), 1509–1517. doi:10.1007/s10995-011-0918-2 PMID:22094592

McKeever, R., & McKeever, B. W. (2017). Moms and Media: Exploring the Effects of Online Communication on Infant Feeding Practices. *Health Communication, 32*(9), 1059–1065. doi:10.1080/10410236.2016.1196638 PMID:27484216

Meltzer, D. (1967) *The Psycho-Analytical Process*. Perthshire, UK: Clunie.

Mo, P. K., Malik, S. H., & Coulson, N. S. (2009). Gender differences in computer-mediated communication: A systematic literature review of online health-related support groups. *Patient Education and Counseling, 75*(1), 16–24. doi:10.1016/j.pec.2008.08.029 PMID:19233586

Montigny, F. D., Lacharité, C., & Amyot, É. (2006). The transition to fatherhood: The role of formal and informal support structures during the post-partum period. *Texto & Contexto Enfermagem, 15*(4), 601–609. doi:10.1590/S0104-07072006000400008

Moorhead, S. A., Hazlett, D. E., Harrison, L., Carroll, J. K., Irwin, A., & Hoving, C. (2013). A new dimension of health care: Systematic review of the uses, benefits, and limitations of social media for health communication. *Journal of Medical Internet Research, 15*(4), 85–100. doi:10.2196/jmir.1933 PMID:23615206

Morris, M. R. (2014). Social networking site use by mothers of young children. In K. P. O'Hara, M. Massimi, R. Harper, S. Rubens, & J. Morris (Eds.), *Proceedings of the 17th ACM conference on Computer supported cooperative work & social computing* (pp. 1272-1282). ACM. doi:10.1145/2531602.2531603

Mungham, S., & Lazard, L. (2011). Virtually experts: Exploring constructions of mothers' advice-seeking in online parenting communities. *Radical Psychology, 9*(2).

Niela-Vilén, H., Axelin, A., Salanterä, S., & Melender, H. L. (2014). Internet-based peer support for parents: A systematic integrative review. *International Journal of Nursing Studies, 51*(11), 1524–1537. doi:10.1016/j.ijnurstu.2014.06.009 PMID:24998788

Nieuwboer, C. C., Fukkink, R. G., & Hermanns, J. M. (2013). Peer and professional parenting support on the Internet: A systematic review. *Cyberpsychology, Behavior, and Social Networking*, *16*(7), 518–528. doi:10.1089/cyber.2012.0547 PMID:23659725

O'Connor, H., & Madge, C. (2001). Cyber-mothers: Online synchronous interviewing using conferencing software. *Sociological Research Online*, *5*(4). doi:10.5153/sro.543

Oakley, A., & Roberts, H. (1981). Interviewing women: A contradiction in terms. In C. Seale (Ed.), *Social Research Methods: A reader* (pp. 261–268). London: Routledge.

Palmén, M., Korpela, M., & Saranto, K. (2012) Identifying health and wellbeing related information management activities and needs in families with young children. *Finnish Journal of eHealth and eWelfare*, *4*(3), 165-176.

Parks, M. R. (2011). Social network sites as virtual communities. In Z. Papacharissi (Ed.), *A Networked Self. Identity, community, and culture on social network sites* (pp. 105–123). New York, NY: Routledge.

Plantin, L., & Daneback, K. (2009). Parenthood, information and support on the internet. A literature review of research on parents and professionals online. *BioMed Center Family Practice*, *10*(1), 1–12. PMID:19450251

Qian, H., & Scott, C. R. (2007). Anonymity and self-disclosure on weblogs. *Journal of Computer-Mediated Communication*, *12*(4), 1428–1451. doi:10.1111/j.1083-6101.2007.00380.x

Reichow, B., Halpern, J. I., Steinhoff, T. B., Letsinger, N., Naples, A., & Volkmar, F. R. (2012). Characteristics and quality of autism websites. *Journal of Autism and Developmental Disorders*, *42*(6), 1263–1274. doi:10.1007/s10803-011-1342-6 PMID:21822761

Repetti, R. L., & Wood, J. (1997). Effects of daily stress at work on mothers' interactions with preschoolers. *Journal of Family Psychology*, *11*(1), 90–108. doi:10.1037/0893-3200.11.1.90

Ridgeway, C. L., & Correll, S. J. (2004). Motherhood as a status characteristic. *The Journal of Social Issues*, *60*(4), 683–700. doi:10.1111/j.0022-4537.2004.00380.x

Rogers, E. M. (2003). *Diffusion of innovations* (5th ed.). New York: Free Press.

Saraceno, C. (2003). La conciliazione di responsabilità familiari e attività lavorative in Italia: Paradossi ed equilibri imperfetti. *Polis*, *17*(2), 199–228.

Scaioli, G., Bert, F., Galis, V., Brusaferro, S., De Vito, E., La Torre, G., & Siliquini, R. et al. (2015). Pregnancy and internet: Sociodemographic and geographic differences in e-health practice. Results from an Italian multicenter study. *Public Health, 129*(9), 1258–1266. doi:10.1016/j.puhe.2015.06.012 PMID:26210071

Slade, A., Cohen, L. J., Sadler, L. S., & Miller, M. (2009) The psychology and psychopathology of pregnancy. Handbook of infant mental health, 3, 22-39.

Sparks, H., Collins, F. L., & Kearns, R. (2016). Reflecting on the risks and ethical dilemmas of digital research. *Geoforum*, *77*, 40–46. doi:10.1016/j.geoforum.2016.09.019

Spinelli, M., Frigerio, A., Montali, L., Fasolo, M., Spada, M. S., & Mangili, G. (2016). 'I still have difficulties feeling like a mother': The transition to motherhood of preterm infants mothers. *Psychology & Health*, *31*(2), 184–204. doi:10.1080/08870446.2015.1088015 PMID:26359768

Stern, D. N., & Bruschweiler-Stern, N. (1998). *The birth of a mother: How the motherhood experience changes you forever*. Basic Books.

Stuart, J. (2007). Work and motherhood: Preliminary report of a psychoanalytic study. *The Psychoanalytic Quarterly*, *76*(2), 439–485. doi:10.1002/j.2167-4086.2007.tb00264.x PMID:17503624

Suler, J. R. (2002). Identity management in cyberspace. *Journal of Applied Psychoanalytic Studies*, *4*(4), 455–459. doi:10.1023/A:1020392231924

Suler, J. R. (2004). The online disinhibition effect. *Cyberpsychology & Behavior*, *7*(3), 321–326. doi:10.1089/1094931041291295 PMID:15257832

Sundstrom, B. (2016). Mothers "Google It Up:" Extending communication channel behavior in diffusion of innovations theory. *Health Communication*, *31*(1), 91–101. doi:10.1080/10410236.2014.936339 PMID:26075413

Tangherlini, T. R., Roychowdhury, V., Glenn, B., Crespi, C. M., Bandari, R., Wadia, A., … Bastani, R. (2016). "Mommy Blogs" and the Vaccination Exemption Narrative: Results From A Machine-Learning Approach for Story Aggregation on Parenting Social Media Sites. *JMIR public Health and Surveillance, 2*(2).

Thomson, R. (2011). *Making modern mothers*. Policy Press. doi:10.2307/j.ctt1t898c8

Tozzi, A. E., Mingarelli, R., Gonfiantini, M., Pandolfi, E., Carloni, E., Gesualdo, F., & Dallapiccola, B. (2013). The internet user profile of Italian families of patients with rare diseases: A web survey. *Orphanet Journal of Rare Diseases*, *8*(1), 1–8. doi:10.1186/1750-1172-8-76 PMID:23680013

Walther, J. B. (2007). Selective self-presentation in computer-mediated communication: Hyperpersonal dimensions of technology, language, and cognition. *Computers in Human Behavior*, *23*(5), 2538–2557. doi:10.1016/j.chb.2006.05.002

Widarsson, M., Kerstis, B., Sundquist, K., Engström, G., & Sarkadi, A. (2012). Support needs of expectant mothers and fathers: A qualitative study. *Journal of Perinatal Education*, *21*(1), 36–44. doi:10.1891/1058-1243.21.1.36 PMID:23277729

Williams, J. C., & Segal, N. (2003). Beyond the maternal wall: Relief for family caregivers who are discriminated against on the job. *Harvard Women's Law Journal*, *26*, 77–162.

Willson, M. A. (2006). *Technically together: Rethinking community within techno-society*. New York, NY: Peter Lang.

Winnicott, D. W. (1951). Transitional Objects and Transitional Phenomena: A Study of the First Not-Me. *The International Journal of Psycho-Analysis*, *34*(2), 89–97. PMID:13061115

KEY TERMS AND DEFINITIONS

Comparison: The act of consider or estimate the similarities or dissimilarities between two things, ways or people.

Cyber: Relating to or characteristic of computers, computers network, virtual reality and Internet.

E-Group: A number of people that share virtual "place", interests, and experiences.

Motherhood: The state of being a mother; maternity.

Online Support: To help someone emotionally or in a practical way in online contexts, giving encourage, approval, comfort, or reassurance to.

Pregnancy: The state or period of being pregnant.

Tech-Moms: An e-group of mothers and mothers-to-be who use social media and technologies to share their own experiences.

Web Forum: An online meeting "place" in which discussions of issues of public interest can be conducted.

Website: A set of pages on the World Wide Web about a single topic or several closely related topics, usually published by one person or organization.

ENDNOTES

1 In psychoanalysis, the term *transgenerational* refers to the process of the unconscious transmission of inner contents (e.g. the trauma) between generations.

2. These web communities seem to provide an “environment” that is suited to parents’ needs, insulating the members from the impact of stress, supporting their emotional expression, putting themselves in the others’ place, knowing what they need.

Chapter 3
Analyzing Online Social Support Within the Type 1 Diabetes Community

Kristin G. Maki
University at Buffalo (SUNY), USA

Aisha K. O'Mally
University at Buffalo (SUNY), USA

ABSTRACT

Social support has been linked with many health outcomes, ranging from heart disease to depression. Although its importance has been recognized, less is known about how individuals with chronic illnesses may use social media to provide and seek social support. This chapter's focus is on the way in which people with Type 1 diabetes (T1D) use social media to provide and solicit social support. A mixed-methods approach is utilized. First, posts from two social media platforms were qualitatively content analyzed. Second, the data were quantitatively analyzed to provide a finer-grained understanding of the messages. The results show informational support as the most prevalent on both sites, although there are some differences in content and use. This chapter's implications highlight the importance of social media as a conduit for social support among caregivers and individuals affected by T1D.

DOI: 10.4018/978-1-5225-3716-8.ch003

Copyright © 2018, IGI Global. Copying or distributing in print or electronic forms without written permission of IGI Global is prohibited.

INTRODUCTION

Social support has been studied and defined in a number of ways. In general, social support is reflected as receiving help, comfort, or information from other people (Wallston, Alagna, DeVellis, & DeVellis, 1983). Previous research has established a link between social support and health outcomes for patients with chronic illnesses (e.g., Gallant, 2003). Sources of social support typically include family members, friends, and members of one's community. As can be expected, individuals may receive different types of social support from each source (e.g., Wallston et al., 1983). In turn, the relative importance of each source may vary across one's lifespan (e.g., Heinze, Kruger, Reischl, Cupal, & Zimmerman, 2015). For instance, in a community-based survey of adults living in Michigan, researchers found better emotional health among young adults who received social support from their family members. In contrast, support from one's community and friends was related to better emotional health for older adults (Heinze et al., 2015).

In addition to age-based differences in social support's impact, individuals with a chronic illness may reap the most benefit from disease-specific support (e.g., Aalto, Uutela, & Aro, 1997). For instance, participants who reported diabetes-specific psychosocial factors also reported better well-being in perceived health and mental health (Aalto et al., 1997). Likewise, another study examining the effects of perceived and utilized social support on diabetes control found that both were significantly related to patient outcomes. Specifically, participants who perceived and used their social support sources showed good control of their diabetes (Fukunishi, Horikawa, Yamazaki, Shirasaka, Kanno, & Akimoto, 1998). One explanation could be that patients with a chronic illness desire a community in which to discuss their illness, provide clinical information, and receive support for their treatment (Greene, Choudhry, Kibuk, & Shrank, 2010). Further, in a review of six controlled diabetes intervention studies, researchers found that receiving the right amount of social support from varied sources is important for diabetes patients (van Dam, van der Horst, Knoops, Ryck, Crebolder, & van den Borne, 2005).

The present research builds on these findings and applies it within an online setting. Specifically, this chapter discusses findings from a content analysis of two social media platforms centered on providing support and information for people with Type 1 diabetes (T1D) as well as their family members and caregivers. The messages included in the present study illustrate both action-facilitating and nurturing support, both of which are important from a communication standpoint (du Pré, 2005). This chapter's aims are three-fold: 1) provide an overview of the relevant literature and theoretical framework; 2) introduce the studies' methodology and results; and 3) discuss the contributions and future implications of this research.

BACKGROUND

Social Support

Over time, many dimensions of social support have been identified and discussed (e.g., House, 1981; House & Kahn, 1985). Using a communication scholar's lens, however, social support is built on two pillars: action-facilitating support and nurturing support (du Pré, 2005). To summarize, action-facilitating support consists of instrumental and informational support. Instrumental support refers to tangible or material support to help with specific situations or merely as an act of affirmation (Taylor, Klein, Gruenewald, Gurung, & Fernandes-Taylor, 2003). Informational support can also involve a range of interactions--varying from suggesting a new restaurant for a friend to try to making referrals for helping agencies, such as job placement firms--to other individuals as they adjust to major transitory periods of life (Chen & Choi, 2011). In contrast, nurturing support involves emotional support such as acceptance, caring, and encouragement. A sense of belonging is also incorporated with nurturing support (du Pré, 2005).

In a review of family communication behavior's effect on patients with chronic illnesses, Rosland, Heisler, and Piette (2012) found varied outcomes. For instance, attentive reactions, emphasizing self-reliance and achievement, and cohesiveness among the family were related with more positive health outcomes. In contrast, critical, controlling, distracting, and overprotective actions from family members were related to negative outcomes among the patients (Rosland et al., 2012). Similarly, parental interactions and friends' influence were associated with treatment adherence among adolescent T1D patients (Kyngäs, Hentinen, & Barlow, 1998). Specifically, treatment adherence was better for those who perceived their parents' interactions as accepting or if their friends either altered behavior to fit with diabetic treatment or diabetic treatment did not interfere with the time they spent together. In contrast, among the individuals who felt their friends had a good deal of influence, and who felt like incorporating T1D treatment did not fit with their friends' lifestyle, adherence was poorer (Kyngäs et al., 1998).

Likewise, in examining spousal influence on diabetes management among patients with Type 2 diabetes, one study found spousal undermining as a factor in poor treatment adherence (Henry, Rook, Stephens, & Franks, 2013). Specifically, undermining included temptations to eat non-allowed food, indicating disregard for the spouse's diabetic diet, and indicating lack of care whether the spouse followed his or her specified diet. Although this type of undermining was rare, occurring in only about one-third of the respondents, it was associated with higher blood glucose levels compared with those whose spouses did not undermine dietary restrictions (Henry et al., 2013).

Despite these disparate findings, social support is typically associated with positive health outcomes for patients with diabetes. For instance, in a secondary analysis of a randomized trial of a guided diabetes peer support intervention, researchers found improved hemoglobin A1c (HbA1c) levels—indicating better glycemic control for approximately three months—among patients who engaged in a greater number of peer calls. The impact was most significant for patients who had lower levels of support otherwise, or lower literacy levels (Piette, Resnicow, Choi, & Heisler, 2013).

Social Media and Health Communication

A recently published review of 348 peer-reviewed research articles examining technology in health communication showed social support as one of this interaction type's top uses (Hu, 2015). Although some disadvantages of online support groups were seen—such as short-term group membership—the findings suggest an overall positive effect (Hu, 2015). Likewise, in examining the ways that individuals use health video blogs (vlogs) as a form of social support, Huh and colleagues (2014) found users engaging in this form of communication for several reasons. Specifically, in their content analysis of 72 vlogs posted on YouTube--as well as 1,274 comments posted on the vlogs--the researchers categorized users' purposes into four categories: 1) journaling for self-reflection, documentation, or updates; 2) helping others through education, encouragement, and inspiration; 3) responding to others; and 4) entertainment. The analysis included vlogs from individuals with cancer, HIV, and diabetes. For those with diabetes, the purpose was mostly action-facilitating support as evidenced by sharing tangible tips and strategies relating to blood glucose management (Huh, Liu, Neogi, Inkpen, & Pratt, 2014). This aligns with prior research on cancer patients' uses of online social support groups. Specifically, in a review of 10 research studies' results, information seeking and giving were prominent activities within many of the groups (Klemm, Bunnell, Cullen, Soneji, Gibbons & Holecek, 2003).

Similarly, an examination of online communication between healthcare providers (HCPs) and Native American diabetes patients suggests that patients are more likely to log in to a Web portal when their HCPs send personal messages. Going a step further, the messages that are positively related to online activity among patients include informational support, emotional support, and tangible technical help (Robinson, Turner, Levine, & Tian, 2011). Finally, in examining computer-mediated social support (CMSS) among Korean diabetes patients, Oh and Lee (2012) found that higher levels of online community activity were positively related to perceived CMSS levels. Specifically, the index including duration of online community membership, time spent in the community, frequency of visiting the online community, and the number of members contacted by patients within the community (Oh & Lee, 2012).

Further, there has been an increase in online groups and pages that are specific to patients and caregivers who are dealing with a disease or chronic illness (e.g., Klemm & Wheeler, 2005; Sarasohn-Kahn, 2008; Shapiro, 2009). As suggested by Roblin (2011), Web 2.0 and related technology offer the ability to form social networks to offer support that aligns with needs outlined by the chronic care model. Specifically, the technology offered through Web 2.0 allows patients the opportunity to interact with others through sharing information, collaborating, and actively participating in communicative interactions. Moreover, the flexibility offered by Web 2.0 and similar technology interfaces may make it easier for patients with a chronic illness to receive support for their self-care (Roblin, 2011).

Importantly, social support that is offered online empowers patients and caregivers to seek and receive information and other types of support they desire (e.g., Klemm & Wheeler, 2005). One reason may be due to the ease with which participants in an online support group can exchange information about their experiences. For instance, Klemm and Wheeler (2005) note that talking about a particular problem or setback can often be met with a flood of responses from others who provided advice or comfort based on similar occurrences.

In a diabetes-specific examination of online social support, Greene and colleagues (2011) content analyzed 690 comments from wall posts and discussion topics from 15 Facebook groups with the largest following. The sample included 15 of the newest posts from the groups. It also included 15 discussion topics from the top 10 groups. The findings from Greene and colleagues' (2011) qualitative study suggest that friends, family members, and diabetes patients use Facebook to share and receive emotional support and disease-specific information. Specifically, about one-third of the posts were coded as an attempt at providing emotional support. A lower proportion of posts (13%) were responding to requests for clinical information (Greene et al., 2011). This chapter builds upon the previously detailed findings to further understanding of how patients with T1D use social media to provide and receive social support.

SOCIAL SUPPORT ENACTED THROUGH SOCIAL MEDIA

Online Social Support Relating to Chronic Illness

As previously discussed, individuals who are affected by a disease or chronic illness may benefit from online social support (e.g., Klemm & Wheeler, 2005). Although the links between social support and health have been well-established (e.g., Reblin & Uchino, 2008; Strine, Chapman, Balluz, & Mokdad, 2008; Uchino, Cacioppo, & Kiecolt-Glaser, 1996), less is known about how social support is given and received in online settings. Recently published results from a content analysis of posts on Twitter (i.e., "tweets") with the hashtag "#Stupidcancer," suggest that emotional and informational support is enacted within online communities (Myrick, Holton, Himelboim & Love, 2016). However, similar to prior research focusing on online cancer-related social support (e.g., Klemm et al., 2003), Myrick and colleagues' (2016) findings showed a majority of tweets fell into the information sharing category. Further, the study's findings showed that negative emotional expressions in the tweets were associated with few shares whereas positive emotions were linked with message sharing (Myrick et al., 2016). This finding supports prior research that connects positive emotional content with message sharing (e.g., Berger & Milkman, 2012). Despite the information gained by Myrick et al.'s (2016) findings along with other scholars' work, a void remains regarding the ways in which caregivers and T1D patients utilize social media for social support.

Another issue relating to online social support is the formation of communities. For instance, an analysis of online communities formed by breast and prostate cancer patients suggests that individuals formed relationships unlike those typically seen in a one-to-many communication setting (Himelboim & Han, 2014). More specifically, in their social networks analysis of Twitter communities surrounding breast and prostate cancer patients, Himelboim and Han (2014) found dense clusters of users who had followed a central information source.

Interestingly, although there are many accounts on Twitter that focus on health and news, these organizations did not influence the dense hubs (Himelboim & Han, 2014). Instead, the cluster of users who remained constant over time included individuals' and small websites' sources more frequently than sporadic users. Conversely, the sporadic users who mentioned breast or prostate cancer in passing relayed information from larger institutions such as the American Cancer Society (Himelboim & Han, 2014). The study also found differences based on the type of cancer. Specifically, the core community on Twitter for prostate cancer was smaller than the breast cancer community. Gender may partly explain this finding, but additional research is needed to further parse out differences in social media use based on health conditions (Himelboim & Han, 2014).

Social Media Platform Differences

Prior research has suggested personality differences may influence preferences for social media platforms. Specifically, those who possess traits such as extraversion and openness to experience may be more likely to use Facebook or other social network sites (e.g., Correa, Hinsley & De Zúñiga, 2010; Hughes, Rowe, Batey & Lee, 2012). Moreover, individual traits may influence individuals' uses of these sites. For instance, one study's findings showed that individuals who scored higher on extraversion belonged to significantly more Facebook groups than others in the study (Ross, Orr, Sisic, Arseneault, Simmering & Orr, 2009).

Similarly, Hughes and colleagues (2012) found personality differences predicted preferences for Twitter and Facebook use among individuals. Specifically, this study's findings suggest that individuals who scored higher in neuroticism were more likely to use Facebook as a channel for social contact. In contrast, informational use of Twitter was related to higher levels of need for cognition. One reason for this may be due to the utilitarianism afforded by Twitter's breadth of information without the requirement of socializing (Hughes et al., 2012). Based on the varied individual-level traits associated with social platform use as well as the sites' affordances, the present study aims to add to the literature on platform-based differences. Specifically, this chapter's discussion centers on differences seen in social support exchanges on two popular social networking sites: Facebook and Twitter.

SOLUTIONS AND RECOMMENDATIONS

In order to redress the void discussed previously, this chapter presents results from a comparative content analysis of messages from two social media platforms: 1) Twitter posts with the hashtag "T1D," and 2) posts from one of the largest public Facebook pages that focuses on T1D support and information. Based on the previously discussed literature, the present study posed four research questions.

RQ1: What kinds of social support do people affected by T1D seek and receive through social media platforms?
RQ2: Which type of social support do people affected by T1D engage in most frequently on social media platforms?
RQ3: What type of messages engage users on social media platforms focusing on T1D?
RQ4: Is there a difference in the uses of Facebook and Twitter among individuals affected by T1D?

Method

First, a sample of posts ($N = 502$) posts from a public support and information page for people who are affected with T1D on Facebook were retrieved with R's (version 3.2.5) "facebook" library. The Facebook page has a large group of followers, with more than 24,000 followers when the posts were retrieved. Because the range of users is smaller and the content more focused (e.g., Hughes et al, 2012), a sample of 500 was deemed sufficient.

Second, a sample of tweets ($N = 1{,}000$) with the "#T1D" hashtag were retrieved with R (version 3.2.5) and its "twitteR" library. The hashtag was chosen due to its specificity in differentiating T1D and T2D communities. Based on the research focus of this study, the decision to use a specific hashtag allowed the sample to center upon T1D rather than diabetes in general. The decision to retrieve 1,000 tweets was made due to the potential wide span of users (both individuals and organizations) that may utilize this hashtag as well as the known potential of spam (e.g., Yardi, Romero & Schoenebeck, 2009), as well as posts that may not be able to be analyzed due to language barriers (e.g., Ciot, Sonderegger, & Ruths, 2013) or expired content (e.g., Chang, Pimentel & Svistunov, 2011). Both samples were retrieved within 24 hours of one another and include posts from November and December 2016 in order to minimize possible time effects. This method allows a comparison to be made between T1D-related social support that was enacted on two popular social media platforms.

Procedure

To determine the specific message topics that were included in the Facebook posts, two coders began analyzing with the scheme developed by Robinson, Turner, Levine, and Tian (2011). The original use of this coding scheme was with analyzing patient-health care provider interaction on a Web-based diabetes monitoring system (Robinson et al., 2011). In its initial use, researchers developed the coding scheme to examine the types of communication and social support messages that were enacted in these Web-based exchanges between diabetes patients and their health care providers (Robinson et al., 2011). This coding scheme was selected due to its prior use and overlap with the current study.

In the present study, the two coders independently examined all responses for specific message nuances that were not captured with the scheme introduced by Robinson et al. (2011) and inductively coded for salient message topics. Next, independent lists of topics were discussed and compared to produce a final list of eight categories with thematic sub-categories. The final codebook captured the message topics as well as the essence of the participants' posts on Facebook. Throughout the process, the coders independently analyzed responses, then met after every 100 posts to discuss coding discrepancies and continue refining the codebook's rules until 100% agreement was reached. The same process was undertaken with the sample of data that were collected from Twitter. During this process, two additional coding categories emerged. Thus, a total of 10 message coding categories were implemented with the present study. The categories are described below and include:

(1) information, (2) emotion, (3) tangible, (4) request for information, (5) technical, (6) fun/humor, (7) call to action, (8) miscellaneous, (9) spam, and (10) snake oil.

Information

The first message category was information. The posts represented within this category provided information of several types about T1D. Specifically, four subcategories emerged from the data: (1) diabetes medication and/or tool-related (e.g., insulin pricing, new diabetic products); (2) diabetes-related holiday/celebration (e.g., November is National Diabetes Month); (3) facts about T1D; and (4) T1D social facts (i.e., information about the T1D community, information about individuals' T1D diagnosis, or posts that centered on experiences that are common for individuals who are affected by T1D).

Emotional

The second category was emotion, which represented posts that provided or requested some level of emotional support related to managing T1D. These posts could be written from the perspective of the person with T1D, caregiver, family members, or friends. In sum, six subcategories emerged from the data: (1) provision, (2) direct solicitation, (3) implicit solicitation, (4) description of support, (5) esteem, and (6) inspirational.

In the first subcategory, posts that offered emotional support to other individuals were coded as provision. Second, direct solicitation was seen with individuals who overtly asked for emotional support. Third, implicit solicitation was seen in messages in which an individual described a traumatic or trying situation related to diabetes. This type of post was often met with sympathetic replies or other offerings of social support, thus implicit solicitation emerged.

Fourth, messages that described support the individuals had received relating to T1D were included with this category. It is important to note that these posts could either be made by the person who has T1D or their caregiver(s), friend(s), or family members. Fifth, esteem messages centered on an individual with T1D or their caregiver(s), friend(s), and/or family member(s) describing how well they do handling T1D. This may be conceptually similar to patting oneself on the back. The sixth and final emotional subcategory, inspirational, included messages that were coded as having the intent of eliciting hope and encouragement for other people who are dealing with T1D.

Tangible

The third category of messages was described as being tangible. Much like tangible social support, these posts offer or provide physical help towards managing T1D. These messages were most frequently related to emergency situations (e.g. offering medication or diabetic tools to aid individuals with T1D in the face of a natural disaster, such as hurricanes or flooding). No subcategories emerged from the data within this category.

Request Information

The fourth category was requesting information. This type of message specifically asked others for contact or medical information related to their T1D experience (e.g., symptoms, side effects, or opinions on diabetic tools).

Technical

This category was represented by posts that requested help with maneuvering through the Facebook page. An additional function of technical messages was to remind users of the rules and protocol for posting on the page. None of the messages in the Twitter data included content that fit this category.

Fun/Humor

The sixth category was fun/humor. This category is represented by posts that utilize humor and encouraged light heartedness towards handling T1D and the daily frustrations living with a chronic illness.

Call to Action

The seventh category was call to action. This is represented by posts that make a request for others to perform a task related to T1D (e.g. wearing blue for T1D, or changing a profile picture to represent T1D). Additional topics that were included within call to action were posts that asked the audience to follow-up with some other action, such as contacting political representatives about the financial burden of T1D.

Miscellaneous

The final category was miscellaneous which represented all posts that did not fit any category. Messages that did not relate to T1D were also included in this category.

The same eight categories were used to analyze the messages included with the sample of "#T1D" tweets. However, two new categories emerged that were necessary to capture the nature of the data. These types of messages did not exist in the initial coding scheme that was honed with Facebook posts; the additional categories included with the Twitter data are described as "spam" and "snake oil."

Spam

This category is represented by the posts that resemble "junk mail." Specifically, the information in the posts coded as spam tended to lead to sites that did not directly relate to T1D. Moreover, many of the messages that were coded as spam had the intention of selling items, such as books and other products that were posted on eBay and other online marketplaces.

Snake Oil

This category is represented by posts in which the author makes claims about curing T1D through alternative methods, such as diet and exercise. Although these methods may help with T2D, they do not have similar effects on individuals diagnosed with T1D (e.g., Global Diabetes Community, 2016).

Prior to the analysis, control variables were created for the messages' content types. This was completed by creating dummy codes for the message characteristics. Specifically, four dummy variables were created in the Facebook dataset: (1) photo, (2) status, (3) video, and (4) link, with "event" serving as the comparison. There were two control variables that were included in the Twitter dataset: (1) if the post was made in reply to another user's screenname, and (2) if the post was a "retweet," which indicates that the user who posted the message was not its originator.

RESULTS

Research Question 1

First, summary statistics for all categories were conducted (see Table 1) to address RQ1, which asks what kinds of social support people who are affected by T1D seek and receive through social media platforms. The present study's findings show that most of the Facebook posts provided some level of information (72.5%) and social facts (58.4%). Emotion (29.7%) was also present within almost one-third of the Facebook posts. Additional categories outside of social support that were identified included request for information (30.7%) and call to action (15.5%).

Table 1. Correlation table for Facebook data

	1	2	3	4	5	6	7	8	9	10	11	12	13	14	15	16	17	18	19	20	21
1 Shares	1																				
2 Comment	.44**	1																			
3 Is Photo	.22**	.03	1																		
4 Is Status	-.01	.18**	-.24**	1																	
5 Is Video	-.04	-.03	-.14**	-.07	1																
6 Is Link	-.18**	-.13**	-.74**	-.37**	-.21**	1															
7 Info	.01	-.06	-.15**	-.09*	.05	.17**	1														
8 Med. Info	.09*	.05	-.15**	-.07	.00	.19**	.21**	1													
9 Month	.13**	-.07	.20**	-.03	.10*	-.22**	.15**	-.08	1												
10 T1Dinfo	.14**	-.07	.12**	-.04	.12**	-.13**	.18**	-.06	.14**	1											
11 Soc-Info	-.19**	.00	-.14**	-.04	.06	.13**	.59**	-.21**	-.08	-.18**	1										
12 Emotion	-.08	.09*	.02	.06	.01	-.07	.15**	-.18**	.00	-.12**	.24**	1									
13 Provide	-.05	-.10*	.18**	-.01	-.02	-.17**	.11*	-.01	.15**	-.05	.10*	.44**	1								
14 Solicit	-.08	.17**	.03	.03	-.04	-.03	.18**	-.16**	-.09*	-.12**	.29**	.71**	.21**	1							
15 Desc.	-.02	-.03	-.05	-.03	.26**	-.03	.05	-.03	-.02	.07	.07	.12**	-.02	-.04	1						
16. Esteem	.03	.08	.09*	.05	-.01	-.12**	-.13**	-.09	-.04	-.05	-.06	.28**	.04	-.04	-.02	1					
17. Inspire	-.03	-.08	.06	.01	.08	-.089*	-.03	-.06	-.01	-.02	.00	.26**	.10*	-.09*	-.02	.14**	1				
18. Tang.	-.03	-.07	-.05	-.05	-.03	.09	-.09*	.09	.01	-.05	-.09*	-.01	.05	-.01	-.01	-.04	-.03	1			
19. AskInfo	-.15**	-.02	-.45**	.08	-.13**	.43**	.07	-.18**	-.18**	-.21**	.26**	-.22**	-.19**	-.10*	-.05	-.15**	-.13**	-.07	1		
20. Fun	.02	.04	.32**	-.08	-.06	-.23**	-.34**	-.10*	-.06	-.07	-.09	-.11*	-.09*	-.07	-.02	-.04	-.01	-.04	-.19**	1	
21. Action	.02	-.14**	.21**	-.06	.15**	-.22**	.09*	-.02	.22**	.00	.03	.14**	.42**	.11*	-.03	-.09	.04	.09	-.26**	-.10*	1
Mean	38.19	6.71	.32	.11	.04	.73	.10	.08	.09	.58	.30	.09	.13	.06	.01	.06	.03	.02	.31	.08	.16
St. Dev.	174.15	12.78	.47	.31	.18	.45	.30	.27	.29	.49	.46	.28	.34	.25	.08	.24	.18	.15	.46	.27	.36

Note: * $p < .05$, ** $p < .01$, *** $p < .001$

Similarly, the tweets were most prominently focused on information (35.1%). Social facts (21.1%) and emotion (21.1%) were also represented equally within the sample. Spam posts were prevalent (42.4%) within the sample and excluded from further analyses. Posts that were not in English (n = 160), coded as snake oil (n = 30), or unavailable (n = 46) were also excluded from the analysis. Thus, the final sample size for the Twitter data was reduced (final n = 342). A summary of the Twitter data is included in Table 2.

Research Question 2

In order to address RQ2, which asks if the types of social support seen in social media posts for people with T1D differ in frequency, a series of chi-square tests of independence were performed. In the first, the frequencies of the two most prevalent, distinct categories (i.e., not a main category and one of its subcategories) of "information" and "emotion" were compared within the Facebook data. The relation between these variables was significant ($\chi^2(1) = 10.72, p = .001, N = 502$). Messages were more likely to be informational than emotional in content within the Facebook data.

Similarly, a chi-square test of independence was conducted with the Twitter data. Again, the two most prevalent, distinct categories within the dataset, "information" and "emotion," were included in the analysis. The relation between these variables is significant ($\chi^2(1) = 4.48, p = .03, N = 342$). Much like Facebook, messages on Twitter were more likely to contain informational rather than emotional content.

Research Question 3

To address RQ3, which asks about the types of messages that users engage with on social media surrounding T1D, a series of independent sample t-tests was conducted. Specifically, in the first, Facebook reactions (i.e., comments on the post, shares of the post, and emoji reactions that include: love, haha, wow, sad, and angry) were compared with information. There were only significant differences for two of these reactions: love (emoji), and haha (emoji).

For the first, there were more "love" emoji reactions to posts that were coded as informational ($M = 3.01, SD = 11.07$), $t(500) = 2.67, p = .008$. Second, the response of a "haha" emoji was also higher on posts that were coded as informational ($M = 0.16, SD = 1.82$), $t(500) = 3.51, p = .001$. To summarize, these results suggest that informational posts receive more reactions that involve the emoji responses of love and haha. Specifically, the present study's results indicate that when Facebook posts include informational-based content, members respond by showing a positive response.

Table 2. Correlation table for Twitter data

	1	2	3	4	5	6	7	8	9	10	11	12	13	14	15	16	17	18	19
1. Favorites	1																		
2. Retweets	.19**	1																	
3. IsReply	.00	-.08	1																
4. IsRetweet	-.26**	.52**	-.12*	1															
5. Info	-.02	-.11	-.15**	.07	1														
6. Med. Info	-.07	.03	-.08	.07	.16**	1													
7. Month	.00	.00	-.02	.02	.03	-.01	1												
8. T1D Facts	-.04	.20**	-.07	.31**	.13*	-.22**	.08	1											
9. SocialInfo	.08	-.28**	.01	-.16**	.32**	-.14*	-.14*	-.31**	1										
10. Emotion	.05	-.16**	.12*	-.14*	-.11*	-.24**	-.05	-.23**	.23**	1.									
11. Provide	-.02	-.03	-.01	.01	-.14**	-.05	-.01	-.04	-.02	.17**	1								
12. Solicit	-.03	-.06	.04	-.01	.08	-.18**	-.03	-.15**	.23**	.66**	-.02	1							
13. Describe	-.02	-.07	-.02	-.11	.03	-.07	-.01	-.06	.10	.27**	-.01	-.04	1						
14. Esteem	.08	-.09	.10	-.07	-.08	-.08	-.02	-.10	.09	.43**	.19**	.00	-.02	1					
15. Inspire	.08	-.08	.09	-.11*	-.27**	-.09	-.02	-.10	-.03	.44**	-.02	-.06	-.02	-.04	1				
16. Tangible	-.02	-.05	-.01	-.07	-.14**	-.05	-.01	-.04	-.10	-.03	-.01	-.02	-.01	-.02	-.02	1			
17. Ask-Info	-.05	-.07	-.03	-.04	-.11*	.01	-.03	.01	.10	-.07	-.02	-.07	-.03	.03	-.05	-.02	1		
18. Fun	.08	.25**	-.04	.16**	-.06	-.18**	-.03	-.15**	.17**	-.13*	-.02	-.09	-.04	-.06	-.06	-.02	-.07	1	
19. Action	-.02	.17**	-.04	.09	-.06	-.17**	.07	.23**	-.20**	-.13*	-.02	-.08	-.04	-.06	-.06	-.02	-.07	-.08	1
Mean	1.53	3.46	.02	.43	.94	.27	.01	.21	.61	.17	.01	.08	.01	.04	.04	.01	.05	.08	.08
Std. Dev.	5.07	5.34	.13	.50	.24	.44	.11	.41	.49	.37	.08	.27	.12	.18	.19	.08	.22	.27	.27

Note: * $p < .05$, ** $p < .01$, *** $p < .001$

Next, an independent sample t-test was conducted to compare Facebook reactions relating to emotion. There were significant differences in shares and the following emoji reactions: haha and sad. First, the posts that contained emotional content had a higher average number of shares than other posts ($M = 18.07$, $SD = 70.87$), $t(488.44) = 2.34$, $p = .02$. Second, posts with emotional content had a higher level of the "haha" emoji responses ($M = 0.10$, $SD = 0.68$), $t(360.49) = 3.53$, $p < .001$ than other posts.

Finally, messages that included emotional content had a lower average of the "sad" emoji responses ($M = 8.46$, $SD = 28.28$), $t(160.09) = -2.67$, p = .008 than other messages. These results suggest that emotional posts receive reactions that involve higher levels of sharing and "haha" emoji responses. Surprisingly, in contrast, emotional posts receive a lower level of "sad" emoji responses.

Due to the relatively low level of both types of solicitation (i.e., direct and indirect), a new variable was created by combining the solicitation and implicit categories to capture all requests for emotional support. Next, an independent sample t-test was conducted to compare reactions for the independent variable "Asking" in the Facebook data. There were significant differences in comments and shares. First, the average number of comments was higher in posts that requested emotional support ($M = 11.47$, $SD = 19.21$), compared to other posts $t(108.64) = -2.90$, $p = .005$. Likewise, there were more shares in the posts requesting emotional support ($M = 11.00$, $SD = 57.01$), $t(478.12) = 3.03$, $p = .003$ than other posts. These results suggest that individuals who ask for emotional support may receive responses through comments and shares. Specifically, the present study's results indicate that individuals seeking emotional support likely receive some level of this support through these reactions on Facebook.

To address RQ3 within the Twitter data, an independent sample t-test was conducted to compare the retweet count in both the information and emotion variables. There was no significant difference in the information category. However, there was a significant difference in the emotion category. Specifically, messages that contained emotional content had higher retweet counts ($M = 1.60$, $SD = 2.29$) than other messages ($t(214.92) = 4.94$, $p < .001$). Indeed, the results suggest that emotion has an effect on whether a message is retweeted. In other words, as suggested by prior research (e.g., Berger & Milkman, 2012), emotional content is related with sharing messages.

Finally, in order to address both the third and fourth research questions, four hierarchical regression models were tested. Specifically, to more fully examine which type of messages engage individuals on Twitter and Facebook, two hierarchical linear regression models were conducted for each platform. User engagement was operationalized as steps users take to further interact with one another and/or the message. There were two ways in which engagement was measured for each context, for a total of four engagement measures: (1) Facebook posts' "shares" counts; (2) Facebook posts' comments counts; (3) Twitter messages' "retweet" counts; and (4) Twitter messages' "favorite" counts.

Message engagement on Facebook was also examined with hierarchical linear regression. The first model, with shares as the dependent variable, is statistically significant ($F = 3.54_{(18, 483)}, p < .001$) and explains 12% of the variance ($R^2 = 0.12$). Messages coded as providing informational support are significantly related to retweets ($\beta = 63.25$, $p < .05$) after controlling for message type. Likewise, the model with comments as the dependent variable was also statistically significant ($F = 3.74_{(18, 483)}, p < .001$) and explains 13% of the variance ($R^2 = 0.13$). Information about medication and treatment is significantly related to the number of comments on Facebook posts ($\beta = 7.14$, $p < .001$), as is solicitation of emotional support ($\beta = 6.30$, $p < .05$). Interestingly, posts that provide emotional support ($\beta = -5.85$, $p < .05$) and that serve as a call to action ($\beta = -4.13$, $p < .05$) are negatively related to the number of comments.

The hierarchical linear regression model that examined the relationship between the message content and Twitter "retweets" was statistically significant ($F = 10.76_{(18,323)}, p < .001$) and explained more than 30% of the variance ($R^2 = 0.34$). Interestingly, of the coded content, only social information ($\beta = -2.03$, $p < .001$), fun ($\beta = 4.39$, $p < .001$), and call to action ($\beta = 2.17$, $p < .05$) are statistically significantly associated with retweets after controlling for the message type (Table 3). To examine the final engagement context, a hierarchical linear regression was conducted with favorite counts as the dependent variable. This model was also statistically significant ($F = 2.16_{(18,323)}, p < .001$), but explained less variance ($R^2 = 0.11$). Within this model, the messages that were coded as "fun" are statistically significant ($\beta = 2.42$, $p < .05$). As shown in Table 3, the other messages types are not statistically significant.

Research Question 4

The standardized regression coefficients from the Facebook (Table 3) and Twitter (Table 4) posts were examined to address RQ4, which asked if there is a difference in platform usage. This decision was made because the standardized coefficients are in standard deviation units, making them comparable across datasets (e.g., Glass & Hopkins, 1996). On Facebook, the largest significant relationship is seen between with comments on posts containing treatment and medication information (Standardized Beta = 0.17, $p < .001$). However, among tweets, the largest significant relationship is seen between posts coded as fun and retweets (Standardized Beta = 0.22, $p < .001$).

Thus, it appears as though individuals may use these platforms for different purposes. Specifically, based on the present study's results, Facebook may be used

Table 3. Regression coefficients for Facebook data

	Shares Counts					Comments Counts				
	β	SE	Std. Beta	R^2	*F*	β	SE	Std. Beta	R^2	*F*
Block 1				0.05	$6.33_{(4,497)}$				0.04	$4.90_{(4,497)}$
Constant	.00	170.56				.00	12.59			
Is Photo	92.39	171.08	.25			7.32	12.63	.27		
Is Status	32.72	172.16	.06			13.30	12.71	.32		
Is Video	.53	174.99	.00			4.68	12.91	.07		
Is Link	8.91	170.88	.03			5.19	12.61	.20		
Block 2				0.12	$3.54_{(18,483)}$				0.13	$3.74_{(18,483)}$
Information	63.25*	28.93	.16*			-2.86	2.11	-.10		
Med. Info	32.69	32.82	.06			7.14***	2.39	.17***		
Month	31.82	31.51	.05			-.05	2.29	.00		
T1D Facts	23.33	31.35	.04			-.78	2.28	-.02		
Social Info	-75.60	25.04	-.21			1.72	1.82	.07		
Emotional	14.61	35.21	.04			1.10	2.56	.04		
Provision	-61.23	34.56	-.10			-5.85*	2.51	-.13*		
Solicitation	-19.43	34.26	-.05			6.30*	2.49	.20*		
Description	-4.02	106.27	.00			-4.39	7.73	-.03		
Esteem	16.12	37.53	.02			3.30	2.73	.06		
Inspirational	-41.59	48.80	-.04			-4.38	3.55	-.06		
Info-Requests	3.85	22.31	.01			.98	1.62	.04		
Fun	-5.74	32.95	-.01			-.17	2.40	.00		
Call to Action	1.46	24.52	.00			-4.13*	1.78	-.12		

Note: * $p < .05$, ** $p < .01$, *** $p < .001$

for providing more specialized content. In contrast, Twitter may be used to share information that is less specific to the T1D community. These findings are supported by prior research examining the utilities of these platforms (e.g., Correa et al., 2010).

FUTURE RESEARCH DIRECTIONS

There are a number of contributions stemming from this chapter. As evidenced earlier, much work has been done in understanding the role of friends, family, and community members in providing social support for individuals (e.g., Gallant, 2003; Heinze et al., 2015). This is important as prior research has suggested that disease-specific support may be important for patient health outcomes (e.g., Aalto et al.,

Table 4. Regression coefficients for Twitter data

	Retweet Counts					Favorite Counts				
	β	SE	Std. Beta	R^2	F	β	SE	Std. Beta	R^2	F
Block 1				.27	$62.46_{(2,339)}$				.07	$12.72_{(2,339)}$
Constant	1.09***	.33				2.72***	.36			
Is Reply	-.75	1.90	-.02			-1.05	2.03	-.03		
Is Retweet	5.56***	.50	.52***			-2.72***	.54	-.27***		
Block 2				.34	$10.76_{(18,323)}$				.11	$2.16_{(18,323)}$
Information	-2.27	1.22	-.10			-0.16	1.38	-.01		
Med. Info	.65	.65	.05			-0.01	.74	.00		
Diabetes Month	-1.92	2.21	-.04			0.30	2.51	.01		
T1D Facts	.55	.74	.04			1.05	.84	.09		
Social Info	-2.03***	.62	-.19***			0.44	.70	.04		
Emotional	1.11	3.88	.08			2.24	4.40	.17		
Provision	-3.10	3.87	-.04			-3.33	4.39	-.05		
Soliciting	-.46	3.82	-.02			-2.61	4.34	-.14		
Description	-.58	4.32	-.01			-4.08	4.90	-.10		
Esteem	-1.64	3.60	-.06			0.28	4.09	.01		
Inspire	-2.10	4.08	-.08			-0.61	4.64	-.02		
Tangible	-3.03	3.14	-.04			-1.79	3.57	-.03		
Request Info	-.65	1.13	-.03			-1.54	1.28	-.07		
Fun	4.39***	.99	.22***			2.42*	1.13	.13*		
Call to Action	2.17*	.95	.11*			0.06	1.08	.00		

Note: * $p < .05$, ** $p < .01$, *** $p < .001$

1997). Moreover, as indicated by the findings presented above, there are discrepancies between the types of support enacted by T1D patients in an online setting. Further, as can be expected, the uses of social media platforms differs. Specifically, Facebook posts may be more analogous to a group discussion, whereas Twitter posts are more typical of a town-crier that has thrown out messages for the masses.

Understanding the instances in which social media may be the most helpful could help form interventions or information that could be shared with patients suffering a chronic illness. Moving forward, communication scholars may also examine the uses of other specialized social media sites or apps in relation to T1D management. Although some work has suggested that individuals use Snapchat to share trivial information with their close ties (e.g., Bayer, Ellison, Schoenebeck & Falk, 2016), this type of light-hearted interaction may still prove beneficial for individuals dealing with a taxing condition such as T1D. Moreover, social support may also play a role in individuals' risk for developing chronic conditions. For instance, in a review of the 2010 Danish Health and Morbidity Survey, Hempler, Ekholm, and Willaing (2013) found that people with T2D were more likely to live without a partner, see their family less than once per month, and feel less certain of being able to count on help from other people if they were ill compared to the general population. Implications from this study include the need to build additional types of social networks for patients with T2D (Hempler et al., 2013).

Building upon these findings, future research may explore ways in which patients with other chronic illnesses, such as T1D, benefit from social support that is enacted through social media and other computer-mediated sources. In other words, future research may benefit from examining ways in which other online communities may help mitigate negative effects of less desirable social support in personal networks. Importantly, the present chapter's contributions may help in guiding recommendations regarding platforms on which individuals may have the best chance of finding support to suit their needs. For instance, if individuals are looking for informational social support, both Facebook and Twitter may serve the purpose well. However, going a step further, the information messages on Facebook were more specifically focused on T1D. In other words, although both Facebook and Twitter messages provided informational support, the data suggest a stronger T1D community presence on Facebook. One reason for this finding is likely due to the centralized nature of the posts. Specifically, the data collected from Facebook originated from a public page that focuses on information and support for people affected by T1D.

In contrast, the data collected from Twitter contained the "T1D" hashtag, which marked the message as being part of the T1D conversation. However, this tag does not ensure a central location for all messages. Moreover, using a tag on Twitter does not come with the same level of monitoring as is seen on a Facebook page. The effect of this is illustrated with the data. Specifically, within the Facebook posts, the technical category of codes captured a message from a page administrator who wanted to remind the users of the guidelines for posting on the page. Conversely, the data collected from Twitter contained a high proportion of spam messages that did not contribute to the T1D conversation. Along with the inclusion of spam, a portion of the messages posted on Twitter contained critical or judgmental material that would have been flagged by an administrator.

Thus, based on these findings, individuals who are seeking consistent, constructive informational support for dealing with a chronic illness such as T1D may be best served by an online community—such as what may be found within a structured Facebook page or group. If information is desired, Twitter may be useful although users may want to be mindful of its sourcing. Despite a number of peer-reviewed, scientific articles being represented through tweets' links, there were also a number of articles and resources that lacked the same scientific rigor and credibility. Thus, caution should be utilized regarding information that is shared through social media platforms such as Twitter.

Moving forward, additional research is needed to address differences in perceived and received social support. In other words, the importance of understanding whether individuals with T1D perceive having social support available through social media is needed. One reason why the present study saw more informational posts than emotionally supportive posts could have been due to the nature of the setting. Specifically, perhaps individuals use other platforms or messaging applications—such as Instagram or Snapchat—to give and receive emotional support with close ties whereas the public Facebook page and hashtag on Twitter may be a way of receiving more diabetes-specific support from looser ties. However, as seen in prior research, the perception of having access to the desired type of social support is important for health outcomes (e.g., Gallant, 2003). Thus, further work is needed to understand whether individuals who are affected by T1D feel as though they are able to receive the types of social support they need through social media platforms. This is an area in which scholars and practitioners' work could converge to provide resources necessary for handling a chronic illness such as T1D. Additionally, the literature would benefit from further examinations of specific types of posts and the types of support they elicit. Specifically, within the present study, photo-based posts were significantly correlated with sharing ($r = 0.22, p < .01$), but not with commenting. Prior work suggests that photo-based posts on social media may be related to users' needs within a social network (e.g., Oeldorf-Hirsch & Sundar, 2016).

CONCLUSION

To summarize, this chapter adds to the literature by examining the way in which individuals affected by T1D give and receive social support on social media platforms. Its findings suggest that informational support is prevalent on both Facebook and Twitter. However, the uses of these platforms appear to differ. Specifically, on Facebook, there is a significant relationship between the number of comments and messages that contain information about treatment and medication information. Conversely, on Twitter, a significant relationship is seen between retweets and content that contains "fun" content. Thus, the two-sample study allows a comparison to be made between types of support enacted on Facebook as well as Twitter.

Despite this contribution, there are some limitations that must be addressed. First, the content was analyzed by two trained coders. Despite the coders' expertise with the topic of social support, human error is always a possibility. In order to address this limitation, the researchers decided to have coders discuss discrepancies in order to meet 100% agreement on all posts. Second, the amount of spam and other messages that were excluded from the Twitter data reduced the sample size. Although a large sample of tweets was drawn for this study in anticipation of this issue, this still presented a challenge. In further analyzing the data, it was found that nearly all of the spam messages originated from one user that appears to auto-generate tweets very frequently throughout the day, with many messages being repeated throughout the cycle. Third, the analysis included posts from one public Facebook page and one hashtag that is used widely on Twitter. Although both of these data sources are popular on their respective platforms, the researchers cannot guarantee that they are representative of the population of T1D Facebook pages and tweets. Thus, future research should include multiple sources of data from each platform.

Despite these limitations, there are a number of positive contributions stemming from the present research. Specifically, the inclusion of a mixed methods approach allowed a thorough analysis of the data to be undertaken. In other words, this chapter discusses the findings of a study in which the content of messages was qualitatively analyzed. This allowed a deeper understanding of the types of social support messages that are seen on social media platforms. Moreover, the quantitative analysis allows the results to be placed within a larger discussion. That is, this study's findings suggest that informational support is more prevalent than other types of support (or message content) on both Facebook and Twitter. This is important for scholars and practitioners as they develop future interventions and campaigns to reach individuals who are affected by T1D. In addition, the chapter's discussion of the types of content that receives user engagement suggests that information—both of the practical type (on Facebook) and for providing a lighthearted reprieve from T1D (on Twitter) is related to comments and sharing, respectively. Thus, on a conceptual level, both of these actions demonstrate individuals' interest in the topic. In other words, information and lighthearted content may be particularly valued by individuals with T1D on these platforms. Finally, on a theoretical level, the present study contributes to our knowledge of social support as it is enacted within online settings. Specifically, perhaps rather than focusing on informational support in its official format, scholars will refine its conceptualization to include informal anecdotes and personal narratives. This overlap between information exchange and emotional solicitation may become a beneficial aspect of online social support for individuals who are dealing with a chronic illness. In other words, the specificity and shared experience of this type of community—as seen with the present study's "social information" messages—may provide both helpful information as well as a sense of belonging. Thus, an overlap between information and emotion may be facilitated through social media.

REFERENCES

Aalto, A. M., Uutela, A., & Aro, A. R. (1997). Health related quality of life among insulin-dependent diabetics: Disease-related and psychosocial correlates. *Patient Education and Counseling*, *30*(3), 215–225. doi:10.1016/S0738-3991(96)00963-9 PMID:9104378

Bayer, J. B., Ellison, N. B., Schoenebeck, S. Y., & Falk, E. B. (2016). Sharing the small moments: Ephermeral social interaction on Snapchat. *Information Communication and Society*, *19*(17), 956–977. doi:10.1080/1369118X.2015.1084349

Berger, J., & Milkman, K. L. (2012). What makes online content viral? *JMR, Journal of Marketing Research*, *49*(2), 192–205. doi:10.1509/jmr.10.0353

Chang, R., Pimentel, S., & Svistunov, A. (2011). Sentiment analysis of occupy wall street tweets. In *CS 229*. Machine Learning Final Projects.

Chen, W., & Choi, A. S. K. (2011). Internet and social support among Chinese migrants in Singapore. *New Media & Society*, *13*(7), 1067–1084. doi:10.1177/1461444810396311

Ciot, M., Sonderegger, M., & Ruths, D. (2013, October). *Gender inference of Twitter users in non-English contexts*. EMNLP.

Correa, T., Hinsley, A. W., & De Zúñiga, H. G. (2010). Who interacts on the Web?: The intersection of users' personality and social media use. *Computers in Human Behavior*, *26*(2), 247–253. doi:10.1016/j.chb.2009.09.003

du Pré, A. (2005). *Communicating about health: Current issues and perspectives* (2nd ed.). New York: Oxford University Press.

Fukunishi, I., Horikawa, N., Yamazaki, T., Shirasaka, K., Kanno, K., & Akimoto, M. (1998). Perception and utilization of social support in diabetic control. *Diabetes Research and Clinical Practice*, *41*(3), 207–211. doi:10.1016/S0168-8227(98)00083-7 PMID:9829351

Gallant, M. P. (2003). The influence of social support on chronic illness self-management: A review and directions for research. *Health Education & Behavior*, *30*(2), 170–195. doi:10.1177/1090198102251030 PMID:12693522

Glass, G. V., & Hopkins, K. D. (1996). *Statistical Methods in Education and Psychology* (3rd ed.). Needham Heights, MA: Pearson.

Global Diabetes Community. (2016). *Guide to HbA1c*. Retrieved March 15, 2016, from http://www.diabetes.co.uk/what-is-hba1c.html

Greene, J. A., Choudhry, N. K., Kilabuk, E., & Shrank, W. H. (2010). Online social networking by patients with diabetes: A qualitative evaluation of communication with Facebook. *Journal of General Internal Medicine*, *26*(3), 287–292. doi:10.1007/s11606-010-1526-3 PMID:20945113

Heinze, J. E., Kruger, D. J., Reischl, T. M., Cupal, S., & Zimmerman, M. A. (2015). Relationships among disease, social support, and perceived health: A lifespan approach. *American Journal of Community Psychology*, *56*(3-4), 268–279. doi:10.1007/s10464-015-9758-3 PMID:26462808

Hempler, N. F., Ekholm, O., & Willaing, I. (2013). Differences in social relations between persons with type 2 diabetes and the general population. *Scandinavian Journal of Public Health*, *41*(4), 340–343. PMID:23554389

Henry, S. L., Rook, K. S., Stephens, M. A., & Franks, M. M. (2013). Spousal undermining of older diabetic patients' disease management. *Journal of Health Psychology*, *18*(12), 1550–1561. doi:10.1177/1359105312465913 PMID:23325381

Himelboim, I., & Han, J. Y. (2014). Cancer talk on Twitter: Community structure and information sources in breast and prostate cancer social networks. *Journal of Health Communication*, *19*(2), 210–225. doi:10.1080/10810730.2013.811321 PMID:24111482

House, J. S. (1981). *Work Stress and Social Support*. Addison-Wesley Publishing Co.

House, J. S., & Kahn, R. L. (1985). Measures and concepts of social support. In S. Cohen & L. Syme (Eds.), *Social Support and Health* (pp. 83–108). Orlando, FL: Academic Press.

Hu, Y. (2015). Health communication research in the digital age: A systematic review. *Journal of Communication in Healthcare*, *8*(4), 260–288. doi:10.1080/17538068.2015.1107308

Hughes, D. J., Rowe, M., Batey, M., & Lee, A. (2012). A tale of two sites: Twitter vs. Facebook and the personality predictors of social media usage. *Computers in Human Behavior*, *28*(2), 561–569. doi:10.1016/j.chb.2011.11.001

Huh, J., Liu, L. S., Neogi, T., Inkpen, K., & Pratt, W. (2014). Health vlogs as social support for chronic illness management. *ACM Transactions on Computer-Human Interaction*, *21*(4), 1–31. doi:10.1145/2630067 PMID:26146474

Klemm, P., Bunnell, D., Cullen, M., Soneji, R., Gibbons, P., & Holecek, A. (2003). Online cancer support groups: A review of the research literature. *CIN: Computers, Informatics. Nursing*, *21*(3), 136–142. PMID:12792194

Klemm, P., & Wheeler, E. (2005). Cancer caregivers online: Hope, emotional roller coaster, and physical/emotional/psychological responses. *CIN: Computers, Informatics. Nursing*, *23*(1), 38–45. PMID:15622203

Kyngäs, H., Hentinen, M., & Barlow, J. H. (1998). Adolescents' perceptions of physicians, nurses, parents and friends: Help or hindrance in compliance with diabetes self-care? *Journal of Advanced Nursing*, *27*(4), 760–769. doi:10.1046/j.1365-2648.1998.00608.x PMID:9578206

Myrick, J. G., Holton, A. E., Himelboim, I., & Love, B. (2016). # Stupidcancer: Exploring a typology of social support and the role of emotional expression in a social media community. *Health Communication*, *31*(5), 596–605. doi:10.1080/10410236.2014.981664 PMID:26453480

Oeldorf-Hirsch, A., & Sundar, S. S. (2016). Social and technological motivations for online photo sharing. *Journal of Broadcasting & Electronic Media*, *60*(4), 624–642. doi:10.1080/08838151.2016.1234478

Oh, H. J., & Lee, B. (2012). The effect of computer-mediated social support in online communities on patient empowerment and doctor–patient communication. *Health Communication*, *27*(1), 30–41. doi:10.1080/10410236.2011.567449 PMID:21797714

Piette, J. D., Resnicow, K., Choi, H., & Heisler, M. (2013). A diabetes peer support intervention that improved glycemic control: Mediators and moderators of intervention effectiveness. *Chronic Illness*, *9*(4), 258–267. doi:10.1177/1742395313476522 PMID:23585636

Reblin, M., & Uchino, B. N. (2008). Social and emotional support and its implication for health. *Current Opinion in Psychiatry*, *21*(2), 201–205. doi:10.1097/YCO.0b013e3282f3ad89 PMID:18332671

Robinson, J. D., Turner, J. W., Levine, B., & Tian, Y. (2011). Expanding the walls of the health care encounter: Support and outcomes for patients online. *Health Communication*, *26*(2), 125–134. doi:10.1080/10410236.2010.541990 PMID:21294020

Roblin, D. W. (2011). The potential of cellular technology to mediate social networks for support of chronic disease self-management. *Journal of Health Communication*, *16*(sup1), 59-76.

Rosland, A. M., Heisler, M., & Piette, J. D. (2012). The impact of family behaviors and communication patterns on chronic illness outcomes: A systematic review. *Journal of Behavioral Medicine*, *35*(2), 221–239. doi:10.1007/s10865-011-9354-4 PMID:21691845

Ross, C., Orr, E. S., Sisic, M., Arseneault, J. M., Simmering, M. G., & Orr, R. R. (2009). Personality and motivations associated with Facebook use. *Computers in Human Behavior*, *25*(2), 578–586. doi:10.1016/j.chb.2008.12.024

Sarasohn-Kahn, J. (2008). *The wisdom of patients: Healthcare meets online social media ihealth reports*. Accessed December 16, 2016 from http://www.chcf.org/topics/chronicdisease/index.cfm?itemID=133631

Shapiro, J. (2009). *Patients turn to online community for help healing*. National Public Radio.

Strine, T. W., Chapman, D. P., Balluz, L., & Mokdad, A. H. (2008). Health-related quality of life and health behaviors by social and emotional support. *Social Psychiatry and Psychiatric Epidemiology*, *43*(2), 151–159. doi:10.1007/s00127-007-0277-x PMID:17962895

Taylor, S. E., Klein, L. C., Gruenewald, T. L., Gurung, R. A. R., & Fernandes-Taylor, S. (2003). Affiliation, social support, and biobehavioral responses to stress. In J. Suls & K. A. Wallston (Eds.), *Social Psychological Foundations of Health and Illness* (pp. 314–331). doi:10.1002/9780470753552.ch12

Uchino, B. N., Cacioppo, J. T., & Kiecolt-Glaser, J. K. (1996). The relationship between social support and physiological processes: A review with emphasis on underlying mechanisms and implications for health. *Psychological Bulletin*, *119*(3), 488–531. doi:10.1037/0033-2909.119.3.488 PMID:8668748

van Dam, H. A., van der Horst, F. G., Knoops, L., Ryckman, R. M., Crebolder, H. F., & van den Borne, B. H. (2005). Social support in diabetes: A systematic review of controlled intervention studies. *Patient Education and Counseling*, *59*(1), 1–12. doi:10.1016/j.pec.2004.11.001 PMID:16198213

Wallston, B. S., Alagna, S. W., DeVellis, B. M., & DeVellis, R. F. (1983). Social support and physical health. *Health Psychology*, *2*(4), 367–391. doi:10.1037/0278-6133.2.4.367

Yardi, S., Romero, D., Schoenebeck, G., & Boyd, D. (2009). Detecting spam in a twitter network. *First Monday*, *15*(1). doi:10.5210/fm.v15i1.2793

KEY TERMS AND DEFINITIONS

Caregivers: Individuals who provide care for another person, especially those who are chronically ill.

Chronic Illness: An illness or disease that continually affects an individual; this must be dealt with all the time, rather than an acute illness that will resolve over time.

Emoji Reactions: This image-based reaction allows user on Facebook to select an icon to reflect their reaction to a message. Options include reactions such as: love, haha, wow, sad, and angry.

Emotional Support: A form of social support that centers on emotional factors such as acceptance and helping the recipient feel as though he or she is not alone.

Facebook: A social media platform that allows individuals to follow organizations' pages, join groups focused on similarities, and connect with friends, who are either known in person or solely online.

Informational Support: A form of social support that focuses on providing information relating to a specific topic.

Retweet: A message that did not originate from the person who posted it on Twitter (i.e., this is a form of sharing a message).

Social Support: An individual receiving help of some sort—such as caring, information, or tangible resources—from others, whether it is perceived or actually enacted.

Tweet: A short message (containing 140 characters or fewer) posted by a Twitter user that contains content such as text, photos, or a link to another source.

Twitter: A social media platform that allows individuals to send short messages (i.e., "tweets") that contain 140 characters or fewer.

Type 1 Diabetes (T1D): A chronic autoimmune illness that affects individuals' metabolic functioning.

Chapter 4
Social Support Through Digital Media?
Breast Cancer Groups at Facebook

Aslıhan Ardıç Çobaner
Mersin University, Turkey

Mine Gencel Bek
University of Siegen, Germany

ABSTRACT

This chapter aims to analyze the use of online support groups for breast cancer in Turkey. After describing the general characteristics of such groups, the authors closely analyze the two Facebook groups on breast cancer. The analysis focuses on how the patients read the illness and their struggle to cope with the illness; how social support mechanisms are used; and which aims and motivations are foregrounded. Both quantitative and qualitative techniques are used in the research. Informed by the international research literature, the chapter also tries to underline the similarities and differences of online social media in the Turkish context. Although the main purpose of the groups is to share information, emotional empathy and shared personal experience are also obvious.

DOI: 10.4018/978-1-5225-3716-8.ch004

Copyright © 2018, IGI Global. Copying or distributing in print or electronic forms without written permission of IGI Global is prohibited.

INTRODUCTION

It is full of friends here, "fate" friends who worry about each other, pray for each other and share recommendations. (Breast Cancer Information Group)

Cancer is one of the common diseases in Turkey following the increasing industrialization, urbanization and the changes in life-styles in the last few decades. Breast cancer is the most common cancer among women in both Turkey and the world. One in four female cancer patients in Turkey has breast cancer. 42.5 per cent of breast cancer patients are aged between 15 and 49, according to the Department of Health records (Sağlık Bakanlığı, 2014, p 40). The decreasing role of the state in public health and the rising privatization have been especially associated with the "reform" processes in the age of globalization and neo-liberalism (Keyder, 2007, p 23). The inequalities increased further with a new understanding on health, according to which health is no longer seen as part of human rights, the responsibility of the state, but, instead, is reduced to an issue of individual responsibility. Thus, protecting health, avoiding harmful habits, evaluating treatment types during illnesses, achieving correct information and appropriate treatment are all seen as the responsibility of the individual. The media is a prominent sphere in which this new understanding and the discourse of health finds space. Since the 1990s, the media has become particularly important for information on protection from illnesses (Terzioğlu, 2011, p 114). In the last decade the Internet has become a space for patients to search for and share information on health issues (54.1 per cent in 2011 and 65.9 per cent in 2016) (TUIK, 2011; 2016). In parallel with global trends, the use of the Internet and the social media networks such as Facebook, Twitter and Linkedn increased in recent years in Turkey. According to Turkish Statistics Institute (TUIK), Internet use in the whole population was 45 per cent in 2011 and 61.2 per cent in 2016. Facebook is the most used social media network in Turkey, with 32 per cent of all social media use in 2016 (Ayvaz, 2016).

This chapter aims to analyze the use of the online support groups on breast cancer through their Facebook pages by focusing on how the patients read the illness and the struggle to cope with the illness; how social support mechanisms are used. The study is not gender blind; on the contrary, it has a gender perspective in the analysis.

BACKGROUND

Online Health Communities: Breast Cancer Groups on Facebook

The use of social networks in seeking social support has been an issue much investigated in recent years (Shpigelman and Gill, 2014, p. 610). Social support groups can be useful for patients in several ways: First, they provide an opportunity for patients to share their experiences. The doctor has limited time to listen to patients and the increasing neo-liberalization and commercialization processes and the current power hierarchies also play a part. For private hospitals and clinics, patients are seen as customers. The doctors are not only responsible for saving lives but also for increasing profit. For public hospitals and clinics, the doctors do their job in its narrowest sense, but neglect the psychological aspects and sufficient communication with the patients. The accountability of the public system to citizens overall is not sufficiently developed in Turkey. The doctors do not share their patients' experience. When patients meet others with the same illness, they feel less lonely in their battle. The main function of social support groups is information exchange which can increase their knowledge and strengthen them in the treatment process. The patients are not only receivers of social support; they also help others, which affects their psychology positively (Van Uden-Kraan, 2008, p. 10). However, active participation in such groups is not always possible because of reasons such as geographical distance, fear of stigmatization or even the lack of such groups. Currently there is a general lack of social support in Turkish hospitals, both public and private.

Since the 1990s, online social support groups have got around such obstacles through chat rooms, listservs, bulletin boards, newsgroups and web forums and now probably outnumber face-to-face groups; they are accessible 24 hours a day; and are economically advantageous and anonymous (Van Uden-Kraan, 2008, p. 11). Social network sites can be used to support relationships in contexts where life conditions isolate people (Steinfield, Elison &Lampe, 2008). They enable members to participate passively through just reading and accessing information without joining any discussion. This can decrease loneliness and depression while enhancing their general condition. However, there are still obstacles such as illiteracy and access to internet connection. Another disadvantage is the quality and the validity of the information. And, since there is no official guide or professional moderator, conversations within the groups can sometimes contain negative, violent and aggressive aspects. Also, the uncertainty about the timing of the possible replies to questions can also be a worry and can even negatively influence the treatment process (Van Uden-Kraan, 2008, p.11).

Klemm et. al (2005) analyzed messages posted over a 2-month period on an online cancer caregiver listserv. According to that, supportive and hopeful statements were common among online participants. Besides this, there were also emotional/physical/psychological responses which contained anger, weakness, exhaustion, grief, and sadness. A review of the literature on on-line cancer support groups revealed that online cancer support groups helped patients cope more effectively with their disease (Klemm et.al 2003). By relying on their analysis on 2 years of content from a popular Twitter-based cancer community, Gall Myrick et. al (2016) reveal that the most common type of social support was information expression, followed by information reception and emotional support expression, with emotional support reception representing the least common type of social support.

Even though there is some research on the advantages and disadvantages of online social support, there is little literature on the positive and negative dimensions of patient participation in the online support groups. The literature focuses on social support groups started by health professionals, health associations or organizations and neglects the groups established by patients themselves (Van Uden-Kraan, 2008, pp. 11-12). Still, it is possible to list some research comparing online support groups with face-to-face groups. Research by Bender, Katz, Ferris, Oh & Jadad (2013) includes a questionnaire involving 73 attendees at a Canadian support training program examining when and why they used online support, as well as interviews with 12 people comparing online support with traditional face-to-face support. The research showed that online support was used by one third of the respondents, mostly (73.9 per cent) during the treatment and primarily for information (91.3 per cent) and symptom management (69.6 per cent) and less for emotional support (47.8 per cent). Emotional support was catered for by the face-to-face support groups. According to the research, half of the non-users declared that they did not need online support. Online communities, the authors argue, fill gaps in supportive care by addressing the unmet needs of breast cancer patients. Research by Fogel, Albert, Schnabel & Ditkoff (2002) focused on internet use and social support among women with breast cancer in New York City. Interview analysis from 188 participants showed that 42 per cent of patients used the Internet for medical information and also showed that Internet use was associated more for social support and to counter loneliness than for other purposes. Shaw et al. (2000) reveal that women patients considered the computer-mediated support group— part of a program called Comprehensive Health Enhancement Support System (CHESS)—as an "additional and unique source of support" for women with breast cancer. The computer-mediated social support groups can complement both the information from health care providers and the support of family and friends. The interviews with 12 women show that the computer-supported group had many functions, including emotional support, encouragement and information. Hearing the similar problems of others, sharing diagnoses similar to their own and seeing that they survived give patients a sense of hope.

Barbara Sharf (1997) explored a Canadian online discussion group, Breast Cancer List, by using participant-observation and discourse analysis in a comparison with face-to-face social groups. Availability, experience and expertise are seen as some of the main advantages of the list compared to face-to-face social support groups. The research identified three functions of the list: Exchange of information, social and psychological 'cyber' support, and personal empowerment, which makes them informed and leads them to take action. This research will be quoted throughout the chapter, with some specific remarks on gender. Some studies discuss the gender differences in the use of on-line social support groups: While men seek for information, women tend to share their experience and encourage others (Klemm et al 2005).

Research

Facebook as a social network allows members to not only connect with the other members but also share their memory or their current lives in a multi-modal way, including writing, photos or video (Eisenlauer, 2014, pp 309-310). This chapter explores the characteristics of the online support groups/communities of breast cancer patients and their relatives or companions through the analysis of their Facebook pages, with a special focus on how they "read" the illness with these questions:

1. What are the general characteristics of the breast cancer patient groups' Facebook pages (including their name, visual appearance and the membership structures)?
2. What are their main aims: Seeking funding, support and/or increased awareness?
3. What are the characteristics of the posts being shared?
4. How is social support being asked for and read/interpreted? What is the role of the experts in this process?
5. How are illness, health, survival and death being read and interpreted in these pages? Does reading differ according to age and socio-cultural levels? What are the most discussed topics? What is the role of gender relations?

Methodology

The messages and comments of the users give important clues to how they present/portray themselves and their identities. This research adapted content analysis as a starting technique and followed with an ethnographic analysis. For this research, in January 2017, Turkish Facebook groups were found by searching "meme kanseri" (breast cancer). The identities are protected as shown below in Figure 1.

The research identified the four largest groups that aim to provide social support and solidarity and regularly and actively send posts *(Meme Kanseri Bilgilendirme Grubu, MetAmazon-Metastazik Meme Kanseri Dayanışma Grubu, Metastazik Meme Kanseri (phase 4) and Lokal İleri Meme Kanseri (phase 3).* In parallel with the ethnographic methodology, the chosen groups' pages were observed during a one month period (1-31 January 2017) and the entire posts and comments made to the posts were copied and archived as a file by using the "*PrintScreen*" function of computer. Participants were informed and their consent gained ethically by the system administrators during the research process. All the posts (221) were analyzed according to the research questions listed above and the participants are anonymized here. The conversations have been translated.

Figure 1. Example to search on Facebook with the words of "meme kanseri"

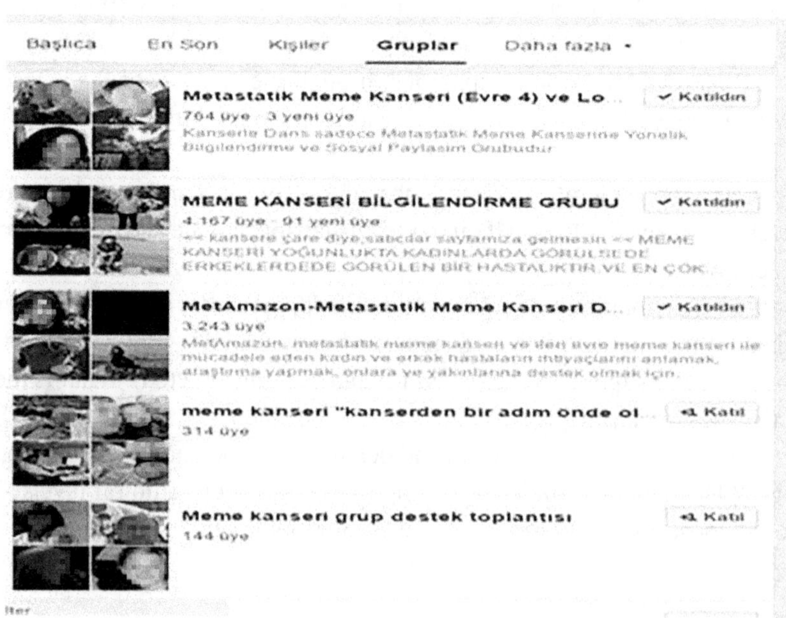
Başlıca
En Son
Kişiler
Gruplar
Daha fazla
Metastatik Meme Kanseri (Evre 4) ve Lo...
✓ Katıldın
764 üye · 3 yeni üye
MEME KANSERİ BİLGİLENDİRME GRUBU
✓ Katıldın
4.167 üye · 91 yeni üye
MetAmazon-Metastatik Meme Kanseri D...
✓ Katıldın
3.243 üye
meme kanseri "kanserden bir adım önde ol...
+1 Katıl
314 üye
Meme kanseri grup destek toplantısı
+1 Katıl
144 üye

The General Characteristics of Breast Cancer Groups on Facebook in Turkey

According to the research, 19 group pages were accessed (6 closed and 13 open groups). Groups with fewer than 10 members were not included in the research. The information showing their name, member number, aim and whether open or closed are given in Table 1.

Analysis of Group Pages

The pages, in total 19, of the largest four group established for social support were chosen and were analyzed over a one month period. (*Meme Kanseri Bilgilendirme Grubu, MetAmazon-Metastazik Meme Kanseri Dayanışma Grubu, Met Meme (Metastazik Meme Kanseri (Phase 4) ve Lokal İleri Meme Kanseri (Phase 3) ve AMAZON KADINLARI-MEME KANSERİ İLE MÜCADELE GRUBU).* Table 2 shows the characteristics of these four groups:

According to observations, only the two of these groups were identified as groups who regularly keep postings. Thus, the data of this research was produced from these two social support groups actively sharing a total of 221 posts and comments *(Meme Kanseri Bilgilendirme Grubu-Breast Cancer Information Group- and Metastazik Meme Kanseri (Phase 4) and Lokal İleri Meme Kanseri (Phase 3)- Met Meme (Phase 4) and Local Advanced Breast Cancer (Phase 3)* (Table 3). For the first group, BCIG and, for the second, MET will be used as abbreviations.

This study is based on the content analysis of two on-line social support groups. A coding schema was developed with the inspiration of the categories in the study of Van Uden-Kraan (2008). Each post/message is coded according to characteristics such as gender, age (young, middle-aged or elderly), their role (patient, patient relative/ friend, group organizer, health professional) and themes (illness or the implications of illness), based on the information being shared and their profile. The coding of 221 posts by 100 users shows that most of the participants are women (98 per cent) and young (34 or younger) (53 per cent).

There are only three participants over 65 the main participants are patients (71 per cent), 17 per cent are relatives. In some cases, group organizers are also patients (2 per cent), relatives (2 per cent) or health professionals (3 per cent). The majority of participants (75 per cent) shared only one post.

There are participants from all stages. More than half of them are in treatment (59 per cent) and those that participated the least are either undiagnosed or post diagnosis.

Table 1. The general characteristics of breast cancer groups on Facebook

No	Groups	Member Numbers (20 Jan. 2017)	Situation (Open -O- or Closed -C-)	Aim
1	*Meme Kanseri Bilgilendirme Grubu*	4165	C	Support
2	*MetAmazon-Metastazik Meme Kanseri Dayanışma Grubu*	3267	O	Support
3	*Meme kanseri*	1993 (no longer active)	O	Awareness
4	*Meme kanseri*	1901	C	Advertisement and promotion (of a 'metaphysic bio-enery expert')
5	*Metastazik Meme Kanseri (Evre 4) ve Lokal İleri Meme Kanseri (Evre 3)*	774	C	Support
6	*MEME KANSERİ*	615 (no longer active)	O	Awareness and Information
7	*MEME KANSERI (BREAST CANCER) / CARCINIMA/MAMMELLA*	552 (not regular)	O	Support
8	*AMAZON KADINLARI-MEME KANSERİ İLE MÜCADELE GRUBU*	470 (no longer active)	O	Support
9	*Inframed DITI Center /MEME KANSERİ Kaderiniz olmasın*	415	O	Advertisement and promotion (of a device and treatment)
10	*Meme kanseri "kanserden bir adım önde olun"*	314 (no longer active)	O	Support
11	*HER 2 pozitif meme kanseri*	274 (no longer active)	C	Support
12	*HYPERLINK "https://www.facebook.com/groups/475690872612694/?ref=br_rs"MEME KANSERİ FARKINDALIK* HYPERLINK "https://www.facebook.com/groups/475690872612694/?ref=br_rs"	168	C	Support
13	*Meme kanseri grup Support toplantısı*	144 (mostly by a women doctor)	O	Support
14	*MEME KANSERİ İLE MÜCADELE*	212 (not regular)	O	Awareness and Information
15	*Meme Kanseri ERKEN TEŞHİS*	211 (not regular)	O	Promotion
16	*ANNELER ÖLMESİN MEME KANSERİ VE HASTALIKLARI PLATFORMU*	221 (not regular)	O	Promotion
17	*Meme kanseri ile mücadele*	71	C	Support
18	*Meme kanseri ... Evet guzel hanimlar... bu yıl için yine zaman geldi...Gogus*	70	C	Support
19	*Meme Kanseri ve Meme Rekonstrüksiyonu*	50 (not regular)	O	Awareness and Information

Table 2. Four social support group pages

Meme Kanseri Bilgilendirme Grubu The Number of Member: 4167 Closed group.
MetAmazon-Metastazik Meme Kanseri Dayanışma Grubu The Number of Member: 3243 Open group.
Met Meme (Metastazik Meme Kanseri (Phase 4) ve Lokal İleri Meme Kanseri (Phase 3)) The Number of Member *764* Closed group.
AMAZON KADINLARI-MEME KANSERİ İLE MÜCADELE GRUBU The Number of Member 438 Open group.

Table 3. Two social support group pages

Groups	Posts		Total Members		Total Comments	Total Likes
	n	%	n	%		
Breast Cancer Information Group (BCIG) (Meme Kanseri Bilgilendirme Grubu)	105	47.5%	4167	70%	1410	1721
Met Meme (Phase 4) and Local Advanced Breast Cancer (Phase 3) (Met Meme (Metastazik Meme Kanseri (Evre 4) ve Lokal İleri Meme Kanseri (Evre 3)	116	52.5%	764	30%	511	1388
Total	221	100%	5931	100%	1921	3109

The Themes of the Posts

The themes are coded as "the illness," "the implications of illness" and "chit chat." The first theme, illness, the dominant theme—especially in the first group, covers the posts on protection from illness, early diagnosis and awareness, symptoms, diagnosis, treatment, medicine and alternative treatments, interaction with health experts and associations. Everyday talk is seen mostly in the second group: implications of the illness. The first theme is mostly in the form of questions. Participants ask about the replies of others who have experienced a similar situation or used the same medicine: It is interesting that the patients do not want to read official notes about the possible effects of the medicine but want the "ordinary" voices of the others:

Anyone feeling tired after radiotherapy? Easier than chemotherapy but still feel tired too. My throat is dry too. (BCIG)

Table 4. Participants

Participants	Groups: Breast Cancer Information Group (n=74)	Groups: Met Meme (Phase 4) and Local Advanced Breast Cancer (Phase 3) (n=26)	Total (N=100)
Gender (n, %)			
Women	73 (98.6 %)	25 (96.2 %)	98 (98 %)
Men	1 (1.4 %)	1 (3.8 %)	2 (2 %)
Age (n, %)			
Young (<34)	39 (52.7 %)	14 (53.8 %)	53 (53 %)
Middle (35-64)	27 (36.5 %)	9 (34.6 %)	36 (36 %)
Elderly (>65)	1 (1.4 %)	2 (7.7 %)	3 (3 %)
Unknown	7 (9.5 %)	1 (3.8 %)	8 (8 %)
Primary role (n, %)			
Patient	59 (79.7 %)	12 (46.2 %)	71 (71 %)
Patient relative	11 (14.9 %)	6 (23.1 %)	17 (17 %)
Moderator/Organizer (Total)	3 (4.2 %)	6 (23.1 %)	9 (9 %)
Activist+Moderator	0	1 (3.8 %)	1 (1 %)
Patient+Moderatör	1 (1.4 %)	2 (7.7 %)	2 (2 %)
Patient relative +Moderator	1 (1.4 %)	1 (3.8 %)	2 (2 %)
Health professional+Moderator	1 (1.4 %)	2 (7.7 %)	3 (3 %)
Unknown	1 (1.4 %)	2 (7.7 %)	3 (3 %)
Illness stage (n, %)			
Undiagnosed	3 (4.1 %)	1 (3.8 %)	4 (4 %)
Post diagnosed	4 (5.4 %)	0	4 (4 %)
In treatment	46 (62.2 %)	13 (50 %)	59 (59 %)
Post treatment	16 (21.6 %)	7 (27 %)	23 (23 %)
Other*	5 (6.7 %)	5 (19.2 %)	10 (10 %)

Table 5. The Themes of the posts

Themes	Groups: Breast Cancer Information Group	Groups: Met Meme (Phase 4) and Local Advanced Breast Cancer (Phase 3)	Total (N=221)
The illness	96 (91.4 %)	48 (41.4 %)	144 (65.2 %)
The implications of illness	6 (5.7 %)	29 (25 %)	35 (15.8 %)
Chit Chat	3 (2.9 %)	39 (33.6 %)	42 (19 %)
Total	**105**	**116**	**221**

Friends, it has been 10 days since I have chemotherapy and still muscle and joint pains and I am in phase 2, is it normal according to you? (BCIG)

Anyone used Arimidex 1mg and what are the possible side effects? (BCIG)

Hello I have read that walking is good for lenfodem. I try to walk regularly but should I move my arm with lenfodom or keep it up? I do not know that. I would be happy if anyone knowing this can share. (MET)

Sharing information on doctors and/ or health institutions is seen more in the comments through questions and recommendations on a "good doctor," "good hospital":

Friends, do you know a doctor who is very experienced on bone metastasis? Can you help? Thank you. (BCIG)

I am at Hacettepe hospital now. For your information, Dr. Kadri opened his private clinic. He is a very good doctor.(BCIG)

This can be seen as solidarity in an increasingly commercialized health sector in the neo-liberal age. Other issues besides good doctors include the attitude of "some doctors," differences between the doctors and their treatments, the operation of the health system and the treatments:

Their approaches are not good, rather than supporting, some of them ruin people. (MET)

I do not understand these doctors. They keep replying vaguely. It would be better if they spoke in a more clear and understandable way. Some keep testing us and change the medicines during chemotherapy while my doctor has not done tests for months, claiming that the real results will be revealed when the therapy ends. What if it does not work? I think they just have the mentality as if we were already dead 😢crazy questions in my mind. (MET)

The doctors act according to their own wishes. I asked why are you not doing any tests even though this is my second cancer? Then he asked for a BT test... One of the doctors said 'You are reading too much into this." I said yes. I experienced the second cancer even though I was being monitored by 6 doctors. Whoever gets a doctor's diploma, they just think that they are the emperors. (BCIG)

Hello friends, my mother's liver has metastasized according to dynamic MR, not the Pet one. Anyone experienced that? What kind of treatment do doctors recommend in this situation? They told us that she can have an operation but we could not be sure because of lesionsbeing small. She was about to have therapy on her breasts but doctors are divided. Some say yes to that, some say no. We are in between in every sense. (BCIG)

Do not believe in the lie of chemotherapy. People are used as an experiment... damnation on this world...damnation to such doctors. (BCIG)

Chemotherapy is nothing but torturing the body. Other than lenfoma and lecomia, surgical operation and radiotherapy is sufficient. More is commercial profit. (BCIG)

Such critical remarks are responded to in these groups. The participants underline the importance of trusting doctors and not worrying excessively.

Sharf (1997) observed a Canadian online discussion group, Breast Cancer list, and analyzed the conversations that took place. According to these, women tend to explain their own thinking, decisions and experiences and are very careful not to make direct recommendations (p. 74). Sharf shows the influence of gender on the communicative style and argues that the women's culture generated through these interactions appears to have resulted in a style and sensibility of communication characteristics of female dominated talk in other settings. Hardly any postings go without some form of acknowledgement, and most often encouragement. The often-cited practice of "flaming," i.e., making rude or abusive remarks of others, is not generally found in women-dominated discussion groups, this list being no exception. (p. 76)

Despite this, she also mentions that sometimes "hurt and anger are expressed" and gives examples. In the Turkish research discussed in this chapter, even though the style is also based on respect and understanding, there are a few aggressive posts. What is especially striking in the example here is that it comes from a moderator. She reacts to a member attempting to post an alternative herbal treatment:

Friends please forget about this or that herb thing...I deleted a comment now...This or that person suggests something on his page blah blah...Do not do it for god's sake. We are fed up saying this but you are in mostly cyber money traps. We do not read what is written here. If our friend who wrote this had read it, she would not suggest that this!!!!!!!! I know the gentleman she recommended from Istanbul. Do not do it for god's sake. Do not believe in everything in cyberspace and believe in and run into it. THESE MEN HAVE SUCH A LIFE WITH THE MONEY THEY EARNED FROM US, YOU SHOULD SEE IT... YOU CAN GET ANGRY AT ME BUT THOSE

WHO SPEND TIME IN THESE CYBER TRAP PAGES AND SPEND MONEY ON THIS OR THAT HERB I WILL CALL IGNORANT...Enough is enough. Whatever you call me, it does not matter. You will kill yourself not because of cancer but by running after these foolis things...NOTE: My dear, who is full of consciousness, these words are not aimed at you. (BCIG) [1]

It is interesting to see that cyberspace is conceived negatively here even though the current conversations and interactions take place in cyberspace. Sharf's (1997) article has several quotations from husbands or partners of cancer patients in the list, rather different from the groups in Turkey, where gender inequality is a big issue. There are no husband or partner interactions or questions within the groups. In fact, there are only two men members in the two groups. What are seen generally are questions, if not from the patients themselves, from female relatives of female patients. Most of the time these are daughters of patients. Like child care, support for patients, both physically and psychologically, is seen as the responsibility of women in Tukey. Social class is also an important parameter, and, while richer families may employ a nanny, for those households where women have to work, this responsibility is taken by the grandmothers, at least until the nursery age of 4. Thus, supporting ill health in a family can vary according to gender roles in the society.

Another thing which can show gender inequality is that sex and the changes in their own or their partners' sexual desire are the issues women openly talked about in Sharf's research (Sharf, 1997, p. 77). In the research here, however, sexuality seems taboo among participants. It is not a prominent issue being debated.

Doctors never talk about this (sexuality). If you do, they treat you, like, be grateful that you are alive, that is it (MET).

The patient who makes this statement but does not talk about this issue either. In some cases, emotion was preferred over sexual relationships

... when you are ill, just knowing that your husband is next to you. That is enough. Believe me. There isn't anything like sex in a cancer patient's life. A least this is the case for me. All I want is to put my hand on a shoulder, nothing else. (MET)

The issues on the implications of the illness are covered mostly with the changes in their bodies (hair loss, menopause) and changes in social, professional and emotional lives. Their reactions to the changes in their bodies are related to the society's reactions, to the extent that these patients are discriminated against in society.

It has been already a month since chemotherapy ended. Enough. Let my hair grow again. It is as if it would ever grow again ☹. (BCIG)

People stare at me so differently. Since I have to work, I started using a wig. When I told them of my illness, they treat me as if I was with Leprechaun'.

To which the reply comes:

Unfortunately, they are ignorant. If they knew, they would not behave like that. They can understand one day when/if their relatives experience cancer. (BCIG)

I wish they would understand us and not be scared of our masks rather than escaping from us. (BCIG)

They are so pitiful and ignorant. They do not know that the masks are to protect us from microbes. (BCIG)

Another problem that the participants complained about is that public opinion is dominated by cancer awareness and early diagnosis while ignoring the differences in cancers and treatments.

Newspapers and television channels keep praising heroes and success stories and they do not mention metastatic breast cancer, which needs ongoing treatment.... Illness can change according to people, so can treatment methods. (MET)

Besides sexuality, there are also few posts on alternative treatments. This could be related to the warnings within the groups about people exploiting patients commercially.

Some religious prayers or rituals are also occasionally seen in some posts and do not receive negative comments. For example:

A friend of mine sent me a prayer and said that she believed in it. I have not started yet. Starting tomorrow. I wanted to share it with you too. As you know we are doing whatever comes to mind: herbs, alternative medicine and so on. It is up to you. It is a matter of faith. I am going to do it. What do they say? Whoever has hope has everything... Pray for 7 days, 7 times to water and drink that water. Total, 49 prayers. To renew cells. If especially cancer patients drink, they will find their cure with the permission of God. It has been tested. Whoever can, should do it for a cure. Not necessarily just cancer patients. No harm in renewing our cells and becoming healthier. (BCIG)

The Process of Seeking Social Support

The social support mechanisms in groups can be listed as seeking information; providing information; creative content and creative expression on gratitude, friendship and thankfulness; and personal experience and empathy. The main mechanism, seeking/providing information, differs in both groups: While seeking information is considerable (67.6 per cent) in BCIG messages, the rate is lower (13,8 per cent) in more advanced MET group. Patients are the majority of information seekers on illness-related matters (diagnosis, treatment, alternative methods, health experts and institutions) (95.4 per cent). As mentioned above, questions are mostly used in information seeking:

Good morning friends. Does tamoxifen lead to an increase in vaginal discharge? (MET)

I received chemotherapy 5 days ago. I have unbelievably bad nausea. Medicines do not stop it. What can I do? I could not sleep last night. (BCIG)

Is there anyone who is diagnosed first with bone metastasis and yet had an operation? (MET)

In fact, what are sought are experiences rather than medical information:

Hello. Anyone get flu during the process of chemotherapy? What did you use as medicine, can you share? (BCIG)

Anyone had a nipple done? Satisfied? (BCIG)

Table 6. Type of social support

Type of Social Support	Groups		Total (N=221)
	Breast Cancer Information Group (n, %)	Met Meme (Phase 4) and Local Advanced Breast Cancer (Phase 3) (n, %)	
Seeking information	71 (67.6 %)	16 (13.8 %)	87 (39.4 %)
Providing information	17 (16.2 %)	53 (45.7 %)	70 (31.7 %)
Creative content/expression	2 (1.9 %)	32 (27.9 %)	34 (15.4 %)
Personal experience and empathy	15 (14.3 %)	15 (12.9 %)	30 (13.6 %)
Total	**105**	**116**	**221**

The second mechanism is providing information on illness, which is seen more in the MET group where group administrators and moderators are more active. Social support is an altruistic, multi-dimensional phenomenon with therapeutic effects, as Shaw et. al (2000) reveal in their research. According to them, as a dynamic process, social support involves a consistent progression from a position of receiving support to that of giving support. Helping other patients allowed women to "change their focus from a preoccupation with their own sickness to thinking of others" (Shaw et.al, 2000, p.?):

Since vomiting and nausea decrease sexual libido, here is some non-pharmacological advice: Avoid heavy meals, avoid synthetics and wool, wear cotton and light clothes in order to reduce high fever, avoid high temperature; decrease tea and coffee consumption; do relaxation exercises; have a warm shower before going to bed. (MET)

For the Attention of Chemotherapy Patients! Do not abandon everyday life. Do not accept yourself as someone whose life is being limited; try to continue your everyday life as much as you can. If you or your family prepare a patient's bed with the idea that "there is a patient at home" and see visitors all day in bed in your pyjamas, you could have a lot of trouble in the treatment process. (BCIG)

Hello. I am going to share useful information I have just learned. If you live in a place far from the hospital where you get treatment, the state will reimburse your and your companion's travel expenses. What is needed is to have approval from the doctor and give them the document...The main difficulty is having to repeat this every time. (BCIG)

Sharing creative content and expressions of gratitude, thankfulness and friendship through photos, visuals, memes and poems is another kind of social support. For example:

The year of 2016 has been both sad and happy for my mother and myself. We have overcome so many things together. Our active hospital adventure since April ended today There will be check-ups after this. I would like to thank you all. (BCIG)

Another social support mechanism, sharing personal experience and empathy mostly come from patients (56.7 per cent):

Hello friends, I am following all of you and your problems from a distance. You are always worried and anxious. Relax. Behave as if the problem did not exist. I applied this to my own struggle. Today was my check-up day. My results are clean.

I won this war. It is your turn now. Do not ever limit your social life. Have a little happiness. I did that and I won. I wish that the new year gives all of you health, happiness and peace. Get well soon. Love. Kisses. (BCIG)

I shared my biopsy results almost 3 weeks ago. The results are clean. Everything is OK… I would like to thank each of you for you good wishes and prayers. I wish from my God that you all will regain your health. I wish God will give all of us long and healthy lives. 😊😊. (MET)

SOLUTIONS AND RECOMMENDATIONS

The analysis will be discussed here under who shared and what; how the illness and the struggle are being signified; and the mechanisms of social support. The two groups that were analyzed have 221 posts from 100 users. Even though the numbers of the members of the groups differ, the number of total posts is similar. BCIG has 4167 members and has 47.5 per cent of the total number of posts analyzed while MET has 764 members and has 52.5 per cent of the posts analyzed. In relation to the number of members in both groups, the number of those who actively post is extremely low (1.7 per cent) while 98.3 per cent of members are just lurkers, following the posts and sometimes contributing via comments and likes. This low participation in active use can perhaps be explained by the fact that users have an illness process that is lasting and has destructive effects and are therefore not regularly active. They write when they are in need. In accordance with data that shows that online social support groups in general are mostly used by women (Van Uden-Kraan, 2008, p 33), the groups' users in this research are, as breast cancer patients, predominantly women (98 per cent). That only two men are members of the groups could be considered an extension of gender inequality. The finding that women users are mostly patients (71 per cent, while 7 per cent are patients' relatives) shows that the treatment period is the time when the patients need information the most in the whole process. Half of the users are young (53 per cent) while just 3 per cent are 65 years and above. Use of the Internet and social media by the elderly is low, although increasing in recent years in Turkey (TUIK, 2016).

Illness is painful not only for the patient who carries it in her body but also for her family, relatives and companions around her. The illness changes the perspective on life and death; the flow of everyday life; the relationships with the people and institutions. Thus, patients question their everyday life, their approach to different spiritual worlds and meaningful life and seek various types of social support. The type of online illness group analyzed in this chapter is one of these. Online social support groups provide a new social sphere for patients and their relatives through which the illness, the "correct" treatment, the side effects of medicines, alternative medicine, doctors and hospitals are discussed and many questions, replies and comments are listed.

Nineteen per cent of the posts are conversations and chats unrelated to the illness. These kinds of conversations are important to help develop trust and friendship. In Van Uden-Kraan's (2008, p 10) research, 50 per cent of the posts are like this. In Turkey, the major topics are the illness (65.2 per cent) and the results of the illness (15.8). The most common use of social support within the groups is to gain information (39.4 per cent) or to give information (31.7 per cent). Sharing personal experience is the subject of only 13.6 per cent of the posts in the groups. Research elsewhere revealed a striking difference in that sharing personal experience and empathy were high while seeking medical information was low (Van Uden-Kraan, 2008, p 34). This shows that in Turkey the priority is gaining information, which suggests that patients and their relatives are in need of medical information that is not provided sufficiently by medical institutions. According to criticism from patients' and doctors' organizations, as a result of changes in the health system, doctors can now spend less time with their patients. During a very short appointment, doctors must examine the patient, suggest and prescribe treatment and give information. This can only lead to a big communication problem between doctors and patients; there is insufficient time to ask any questions and get a satisfactory reply (Medimagazin, 2015). It is not only a matter of the time limit but also the whole mentality of health professionals, as was discussed earlier in the chapter.

It should also be mentioned that there is a problem of quality of information being shared within the groups. The information provided is based on the experience of patients or the page administrators who do not have a medical training. Only 3 per cent of members of the groups are health professionals. Having said that, the groups are important for the patients, as this post expresses very well:

It is full of friends here, "fate" friends who worry about each other, pray for each other and share recommendations. (BCIG)

For breast cancer patients, being alive means a "struggle." The treatment process is likened to a "war" or, sometimes, a "dance." The patients are seen as people who have succeeded in this process: the struggling "amazon," the "miracle" women.

I will not collapse but collapse anything that can collapse me. (BCIG)

Please do not stop praying. We do not know what is waiting for us. However, we are strong and believe that we are going to be fine. (BCIG)

I won this war, it is your turn now.... (BCIG.

We are all miracle women. Powerful, patient and, whatever happens, hopeful. (MET)

The most important thing is to be strong and to “love yourself.” This is recommended by the members very often:

Do you love yourself? Do you respect yourself and your body? Do not forget. If you do and you care for yourself, the people around you also treat you in the same way. (MET)

My doctor once told me that breast cancer loves beautiful women. We will beat that beauty!!! And it will never come back !!! (BCIG).

Death is spoken of very little within the groups. While sharing condolence messages after a person has died, there were comments showing the banality and ordinariness and even God’s judgement of death.

Continue to live. Death is for all of us. Many people die every day because of many silly reasons such as an accident or explosion. Simple reasons. Like that, suddenly. Right? Then it is not worth worrying about anything at all 😄😄*. (MET)*

Believe me ladies, when I first heard...I said OK everything is over, but I understood that I am not scared of death anymore. Everything is the judgement and the decision of God. All we can do is the duty to take sufficient care and carry on treatment. (BCIG)

Hello, my name is human...You can be called cancer...a big trouble...but you cannot harm anyone as long as my big GOD does not want it to...we get our treatment and pray. We are not scared of you. (BCIG)

FUTURE RESEARCH DIRECTIONS

The on-line support groups reveal new alliances and commonalities which would not have come together previously. There is a lack of a rights-based approach to health or a holistic conception of health, thus no politically engaged and activist participation. Still, there is a potential of transformation in and via these groups. For example, one member shares a petition which took place at change.org ‘Let’s Sign for a World without Cancer’ to stop extra payment to the private hospitals for cancer patients without private insurance. Further study could conduct face-to-face individual and focus-group interviews with the women patients to try to deepen the understanding of their experience. The findings of such a study would give a chance for the voices of the patients to be heard by medical professionals, activists and health policy makers and create a potential transformative change in the violating, oppressing or discriminating structures and practices at different micro and macro levels, such as the state, the market, the media and/or are reflected by each individual member in society.

CONCLUSION

The aim of this research is to analyze the characteristics of the posts and comments being shared on Facebook group pages established to support breast cancer patients and their relatives, friends and companions. It can be argued that the on-line social groups will increasingly gain more significance and popularity due to the problems in accessing information in the current health system in Turkey. Further research, taking into account the socio-economic, age, gender and cultural dimensions, is needed to understand the patient groups who come together in these spheres.

REFERENCES

Ayvaz, T. (2016, January 29). *İnternet ve Sosyal Medya Kullanıcı İstatistikleri 2016*. Retrieved from http://www.dijitalajanslar.com/internet-ve-sosyal-medya-kullanici-istatistikleri-2016/

Bender, J. L., Katz, J., Ferris, L. E., Oh, H., & Jadad, A. R. (2013). What is the role of online support from the perspective of facilitators of face-to-face support groups? A multi-method study of the use of breast cancer online communities. *Patient Education and Counseling*, *93*(3), 472–479. doi:10.1016/j.pec.2013.07.009 PMID:23928354

Eisenlauer, V. (2014). Facebook: A multimodal discourse analysis of (semi-)automated communicative modes. In C. Maier & S. Norris (Eds.), Interactions, Images and Texts: A Reader of Multimodality (pp. 309-317). Berlin: de Gruyter.

Fogel, J., Albert, S. M., Schnabel, F., Ditkoff, B.A., &Neugut, A. I. (2002). Use of the Internet by Women with Breast Cancer. *Journal of Medical Internet Research*, *4*(2).

Keyder, Ç. (2007). Giriş. In Ç. Keyder (Ed.), *Avrupa'da ve Türkiye'de sağlık politikaları* (pp. 7–35). İstanbul: İletişim Yayınları.

Klemm, P., Bunnell, D., Cullen, M., Soneji, R., Gibbons, P., & Holecek, A. (2003). Online cancer support groups: A review of the research literature. CIN: Computers, Informatics. *Nursing*, *21*(3), 136–142. PMID:12792194

Klemm, P., & Wheeler, E. (2005). Cancer caregivers online: Hope, emotional roller coaster, and physical/emotional/psychological responses. CIN: Computers, Informatics. *Nursing*, *23*(1), 38–45. PMID:15622203

Medimagazin. (2015, October 26). *Hastalar muayene sürelerinin kısalığından şikayetçi*. Retrieved from http://www.medimagazin.com.tr/ana-sayfa/guncel/tr-hastalar-muayene-surelerinin-kisaligindan-sikayetci-1-11-67485.html

Myrick, J. G., Holton, A. E., Himelboim, I., & Love, B. (2016). # Stupidcancer: Exploring a typology of social support and the role of emotional expression in a social media community. *Health Communication*, *31*(5), 596–605. doi:10.1080/10410236.2014.981664 PMID:26453480

Sağlık Bakanlığı (MOH). (2014). *Türkiye Kanser İstatistikleri*. Retrieved January 13, 2017, from http://kanser.gov.tr/Dosya/2017Haberler/2014-RAPOR._uzun.pdf

Sharf, B. F. (1997). Communicating breast cancer on-line: Support and empowerment on the Internet. *Women & Health*, *26*(1), 65–84. doi:10.1300/J013v26n01_05 PMID:9311100

Shaw, R. B., Mctavish, F., Hawkins, R., Gustafson, D. H., & Pingree, S. (2000). Experiences of Women with Breast Cancer: Exchanging Social Support over the CHESS Computer Network. *Journal of Health Communication*, *5*(2), 135–159. doi:10.1080/108107300406866 PMID:11010346

Shpigelman, C., & Gill, C. (2014). Facebook Use by Persons with Disabilities. *Journal of Computer-Mediated Communication*, *19*(3), 610–624. doi:10.1111/jcc4.12059

Steinfield, C., Ellison, N. B., & Lampe, C. (2008). Social capital, self-esteem, and use of online social network sites: A longitudinal analysis. *Journal of Applied Developmental Psychology*, *29*(6), 434–445. doi:10.1016/j.appdev.2008.07.002

Terzioğlu, A. (2011). Küreselleşme, Kanser ve Hastalık Anlatıları. In C. Özbay, A. Terzioğlu, & Y. Yasin (Eds.), *Neoliberalizm ve Mahremiyet Türkiye'de Beden Sağlık ve Cinsellik* (pp. 111–132). İstanbul: Metis.

TUIK. (2011). *Hanehalkı Bilişim Teknolojileri Kullanım Araştırması, 2011*. Retrieved January 3, 2017, from http://www.tuik.gov.tr/PreHaberBultenleri.do?id=8572

TUIK. (2016). *Hanehalkı Bilişim Teknolojileri Kullanım Araştırması, 2016*. Retrieved January 3, 2017, from http://www.tuik.gov.tr/PreHaberBultenleri.do?id=21779

Van Uden-Kraan, N. (2008). *Online Peer Support for Patients with Somatic Diseases* (Thesis). University of Twente. Retrieved January 12, 2017, from http://purl.utwente.nl/publications/60136

KEY TERMS AND DEFINITIONS

Alternative Treatments: These are treatments which may be used widely but are not accepted by the existing medical authorities.

Emotional Empathy: The ability to understand what another person feels during their illness.

Emotional Support: The provision of reassurance, acceptance, and encouragement in times of stress. It can have a healing effect on patients, especially on cancer patients.

Informational Support: Sharing information from one's own experience or from various resources (doctors, books, the Internet, newspaper, magazine, brochures).

Stigmatization: Patients feeling excluded as a result of the discriminatory reactions in society.

Chapter 5
Insight Into Sub-Saharan African Discussions of Anxiety and Depression Online

Seif Sekalala
Drexel University, USA

Kristin G. Maki
University at Buffalo (SUNY), USA

ABSTRACT

This chapter presents a brief review of past studies on the topics of stigma towards clinical anxiety and depression among populations of African descent in the US and Sub-Saharan Africa, as well as the efficacy of online searches for assistance and moral support. It also reports the findings of a study of nine African patients or survivors of clinical anxiety and depression who share their stories two online platforms, i.e., the website of the South African Depression and Anxiety Group (SADAG), and the www.depression-understood.org forum. Relevant themes are presented using Owen's (1984) and Mitchell's (2016) analytical frameworks.

INTRODUCTION AND BRIEF LITERATURE REVIEW

Over the past two decades, scholars have studied the existence of stigma and mistrust of professional intervention towards mental illnesses including clinical anxiety and depression among populations of African descent in the US and Caribbean, as well as Sub-Saharan Africa (SSA) e.g. Alvidrez (1999), Chamberlain et al. (2001), Diala (2001), Ojelade, McCray, Ashby, and Meyers (2011), Murry, Heflinger, Suiter

DOI: 10.4018/978-1-5225-3716-8.ch005

Copyright © 2018, IGI Global. Copying or distributing in print or electronic forms without written permission of IGI Global is prohibited.

and Brody (2010), and Nicolaidis et al. (2010). This stigma and mistrust is often complicated or exacerbated by additional factors or situations such as other chronic illnesses like HIV-AIDS (e.g., Boyes and Cluver, 2015).

However, scholars, health professionals, policy-makers, and other parties have to take note of the nuances in the studies of this stigma and mistrust. For instance, research such as Alvidrez's (1999) and Nicolaidis et al.'s (2010) has indeed revealed that white Americans (in particular, women) are more likely to seek (or *desire* to seek) professional mental health care compared to African-American and Latina women. And yet, other studies have shown that there are systemic attitudinal and structural barriers to minority groups' and SSA-descent patients' seeking and receiving professional mental health (e.g., Abera, Tesfaye, Belachew, and Hanlon 2014; Ola et al., 2014; Baron et al., 2016; Nakku et al., 2016). Also, some studies—e.g., Diala (2001)—have shown that African-American men are in fact likely to seek professional mental health help.

In light of the above challenges, vis-à-vis the provision of mental health care to SSA-descent populations, one can argue that scholars and mental health professionals should welcome supplemental or alternative ways of providing treatment and assistance to ailing or vulnerable individuals of SSA-descent. Among various demographic and ethnic populations, studies have shown that the search for assistance and moral support online from both health professionals and fellow sufferers can be efficacious. Further, the efficacy of online sources of support may be particularly beneficial among those who perceive stigma or other barriers surrounded mental health (e.g., DeAndrea, 2015).

Specific ailments for which anonymous and real identity-based online social support has been shown to be effective include cancer (Çobaner & Bek, in press; and Myrick, Holton, Himelboim & Love, 2016), major depression (De Choudhury, Gamon, Counts & Horvitz, 2013), and type 1 diabetes (Maki & O'Mally, this volume; and Huh, Neogi, Inkpen, & Pratt, 2014). The platforms on which this support is exchanged include Facebook, Twitter, and YouTube. Based on the research from the above-listed studies, it is important to note that the quality of the social support exchanged on these sites cannot be guaranteed, and it cannot substitute trained care from healthcare professionals. Scholars have also pointed out other drawbacks to online social support, compared to face-to face support (e.g., Turkle, 2011).

In this chapter, we will demonstrate the efficacy of online platforms with which clinical anxiety/depression sufferers of Sub-Saharan African (SSA)-descent can seek and provide help and support anonymously, or using their real identities. In addition to highlighting some of the general ways in which these individuals seek and share advice and support via Owen's (1984) framework, we will also make use of Mitchell's (2016) analytical framework of authentic leadership online to demonstrate how particular sufferers of clinical anxiety/depression of SSA-descent can stand out in their support of fellow sufferers.

CURRENT STUDY / MAIN FOCUS OF CHAPTER

It should be noted that as of mid-2017, online searches do not yield a sizable number of platforms—i.e., forums, websites, and social media pages—that cater specifically to African-descent patients with clinical depression and anxiety. One of the most visible exceptions in this regard is the South African Depression and Anxiety Group (SADAG), a nonprofit organization. According to SADAG's website and public Facebook page, the 20-year old non-profit organization engages in "advocacy, education and destigmatisation of mental illness" in South Africa (SADAG website), with a network of mental health professionals around the country.

It is also important to note that there are a number of systemic bottlenecks that prevent the wider use of anonymous online forums in most countries of mainland SSA by depression and anxiety patients, including the prohibitive cost of internet-connected computers and smart phones, and slow internet speeds. But of course, anxiety/depression sufferers of SSA-origin who are living in developed countries (or other countries that have widespread efficient and cost-effective online access) will not necessarily be affected by these bottlenecks. Thus, they might seek advice and support online that is geared specifically to the experiences anxiety/depression sufferers of SSA-origin. Also, educated middle- and upper-class individuals living in SSA will more than likely be able to have access to fairly efficient internet-connected computers and smart phones, and a number of current/recent reports and statistics indicate that even poor or working classes in Africa are getting better access to affordable internet-connected smart phones (Telecommunication Development Bureau/ITU, 2016).

Therefore, given the well-documented stigma that accompanies depression and anxiety among people of SSA-origin, as well as the efficacy of sharing experiences online by anxiety/depression patients (see references under "Introduction & Brief Literature Review" above), one can argue that scholars and mental health professionals should seek answers to the questions below. Moreover, by addressing these questions, scholars and practitioners will be better able to develop effective options for individuals who are faced with depression and anxiety.

RQ1: In addition to mass-awareness/education campaigns, can depression and anxiety patients of SSA-origin/heritage benefit from the wider use of anonymous online support-group forums, and if so, how?

RQ2: What are the main features of anonymous principals' stories from online support forums that can be of help to depression and anxiety patients of SSA-origin?

METHODS AND DATA COLLECTION

Analytical Frameworks

In the attempt to answer the above research questions, this study's data collection and analysis was modeled on two theoretical-methodological frameworks, namely Owen's (1984) thematic analysis method, as well as Mitchell's (2016) authentic leadership theory-based thematic analysis. Owen's (1984) method highlights three characteristics, namely recurrence, repetition, and forcefulness. He defines recurrence as the observation of at least two reports that have the same thread of meaning; repetition is the duplication of key words and phrases; and forcefulness refers to verbal or written messages representing vocal inflections or dramatic pauses that "stress or subordinate some utterances from other locutions in oral reports; it also refers to the underlining of words and phrases, the increased size of print, or use of colored marks circling or otherwise focusing on passages in the written reports" (Owen, 1984, p. 276). The themes that emerge may reflect ways in which the individuals make sense of their reality, whether they are examining their personal experiences or the norms they perceive surrounding mental health care. By examining the present study's data through this lens, a naturalistic representation of the principals' interactions with one another is afforded (Owens, 1984).

This analytical approach is complemented by the incorporation of Mitchell's (2016) framework regarding authentic leadership that draws upon Walumbwa and colleagues' (2008) work. This construct incorporates several aspects that are reflected both in the individual's psychological attributes as well as the ethical climate (Walumbwa et al., 2008). Building upon this work, Mitchell (2016) defines authentic leaders as those who nurture growth and positive development within themselves and others. They accomplish this task in several ways, specifically this growth occurs through the following four actions:

1. Developing their own and others' self-awareness;
2. Being relationally transparent;
3. Making decisions that are based upon their internalized moral perspective; and
4. Balanced processing of information, (Mitchell, 2016, p. 4).

Along with boosting personal development, Luthens and Avolio (2003) suggest that practicing authentic leadership may help others foster resilience, optimism, hope, and confidence (as cited in Mitchell, 2016). One reason is that an individual's development as an authentic leader may involve an introspective process paired with the provision of a window into this self-reflection for others. In other words, authentic leadership builds upon the iteration of common themes through which the individual stays true to his or her values and goals (Walumbwa et al., 2008). Thus, the two frameworks that were selected for the present analysis provide complementary perspectives through which the data may be understood.

DATA COLLECTION AND PROCESSING

Per Blumer's (1969) advice to researchers (as quoted in Littlejohn, 1992, p. 171), we embarked on collecting data for this study by trying to empathize with anxiety and depression sufferers of SSA-origin based on what we know about anxiety and depression sufferers from family and friends, and going through anonymous online forums for relevant advice and support resources. The particular guiding questions we had in mind during this search were: 1) what kinds of particular or specialized advice and support would an anxiety/depression patient of SSA-origin living in Africa or abroad seek, and 2) what kinds of advice and support are given by anxiety/depression patients of SSA-origin—or by other individuals—to (their fellow) anxiety/depression patients of SSA-origin?

In using these two questions as guides in this data search, we imagined that an individual of SSA-origin—either living in Africa or abroad: 1) would specifically be seeking advice and support that can cater specifically to his/her anxiety/depression, which necessarily developed against the backdrop of, or was exacerbated by his/her SSA-origin socio-cultural background, and 2) would discuss his/her struggles with anxiety and depression while necessarily interspersing those stories/discussions with said socio-cultural background-related issues. These issues will not necessarily be a feature in the stories of individuals with origins or heritages from other societies, specifically individuals from the Western world, e.g., Europe, or the USA. Arguably, whereas these countries might also have widespread stigmas and misunderstandings of anxiety and depression, one can concede that by-and-large, they have reached a critical mass vis-à-vis the widespread general acceptance/understanding that anxiety and depression are in fact diseases and have to be treated as such, so as for their victims' health to heal and/or improve.

Whereas a general online search (i.e., using Google or other search engines) for stories or testimonials of general or diverse demographics or populations of anxiety/depression patients yields a rich set of resources, our experience (at least as of this chapter's writing in June 2017), was that there is a marked dearth of advice and support from those forums, to patients in particular of SSA-origin. However, by going to the website www.depression-understood.org, we were able to find a number of conversation threads with life stories or testimonies about relevant experiences from anxiety/depression patients that reported being from a particular Sub-Saharan African country. In addition to the stories from the "depression-understood" website, we also retrieved a total of six stories or discussions from the website of the SADAG nonprofit organization.

After collecting the stories from the forum and nonprofit website, one of the authors copied and pasted them into one sheet, making no changes in grammar, syntax, and other structural features. Thereafter, he did a close reading of the stories, looking out for words and phrases that are possible markers of some of the themes he suspected to be present in the stories, e.g., persistent sadness and other negative feelings as indications of the principals' initial suspicion or discovery of their clinical depression, and belief in God or other use of religion or spirituality as a way of coping.

We also took note of the general features that all stories have in common, especially their general parts, i.e., background, known trigger or catalyst (for clinical anxiety or depressive episodes), details of the crisis, diagnosis, treatment, and coping, and conclusion, future, and advice. Finally, one of the authors used a color-coding and numbering scheme to highlight, categorize, and count the story-parts and thematic instances of Owen's (1984) and Mitchell's (2016) frameworks. All of these stories/discussions—both from the "depression-understood" forum and the "SADAG" site—can be read in their entirety in the appendix at the end of this chapter. In the sections below, we will describe and analyze these stories/discussions using: 1) a general overview/description and basic analysis of the stories/discussions, their principals, and the nature of their stories, and 2) characteristics of their stories using the frameworks introduced by Owens (1984) and Mitchell (2016).

FINDINGS, PART I: GENERAL OVERVIEW/ DESCRIPTION AND BASIC ANALYSIS OF FORUM AND SITE STORIES/DISCUSSIONS

In the data set for this study, there are a total of 15 relevant stories/discussions and responses of varying length (out of a total of 22 stories/discussions and responses) with nine principals, i.e., story-tellers of SSA-origin. From the "depression-understood" forum, the data set has a total of three Sub-Saharan African principals who are either sharing their stories to seek help, or help anxiety/depression sufferers all over the world. And from the SADAG website, there are a total of six stories or testimonials (all told in a first-person voice) from South African women and men who have all dealt with, or are still dealing with, anxiety and/or depression.

Sub-Saharan African Story-Tellers From Both Sites

The usernames (which have been replaced with similar pseudonyms to protect the individuals' identities) of the three story-tellers from the forum, in order of appearance in the data set: 1) "*Purplefairy*," 2) "*Linzi*," and 3) "*Mozmoz*." And from the SADAG website, the names of the six South-African story-tellers—also in order of their appearance in the data set—are: 1) Cor du Bruin, 2) Mary, 3) Feon, 4) Thumi Mkhize, 5) Grace Sebo, and 6) Veli Zondi.

Story-Arc(s)

As pointed out in landmark studies by Goffman (1981), Linde (1993), and Labov and Waletzky (1997) among others, life-stories and narratives can be demarcated into distinct parts, each of which has a specific and important role vis-à-vis comprehension and utility for both the principal, his/her listeners or readers, and other parties. Thus, a researcher can and arguably should attempt to similarly demarcate anxiety/depression life-stories/discussions or testimonies so as to study them with more rigor and precision.

As aforementioned, in the case of the nine SSA-origin life-stories from the forum and the SADAG website, we can demarcate a total of five parts, namely: 1) background, 2) known trigger(s) or catalyst(s) for clinical anxiety or depressive episode(s), 3) details of the crisis, 4) diagnosis, treatment, and coping, and 5) conclusion, future, and advice. One can also add a sixth part either between parts 2 and 3, or between parts 3 and 4, which we can call "reckoning and coping."

In fact, it should be pointed out in earnest that generally, the use of any classification scheme—including the one used in these stories, cannot be said to be 100% precise. Often, one can classify a story-part under two different categories, and a story might not have visible discrete parts that can be neatly classified under all the categories of a given scheme. *Linzi*'s life-story from the forum via her set of story/discussions and responses, is emblematic of this fact.

Story Backgrounds

In the context of a life-story about one's struggle with anxiety and depression, this title defines the parts of stories that discuss facts, issues, events, and other conceptual items that take place before the main watershed or landmark event(s) that trigger the discrete beginning of one or more episodes of anxiety/depression illness. All nine principals' stories from the forum and the SADAG's contain relevant exemplars in this regard. Below are three examples from *Purplefairy* (from the forum), and Cor du Bruin and Mary (from the SADAG website):

Purplefairy

Help everyone. Im 26 from xxxx and I suffer from social anxiety and it has led me to live a very depressed life. Of course none of this is visible to my family, everyone thinks I love isolating myself and I've heard some " u think you better than everyone else" comments more than I'd like to disclose. My cousin once said that i have the biggest heart.

Cor du Bruin

I first became depressed when I was 37 years old. At that stage, I was working as an Insurance Financial Advisor and was earning money on a commission basis.

Mary

In my youth, my dad always used to joke about my erratic temperament. However, overall I was a busy and confident youngster with an optimistic attitude to life.

Trigger(s) or Catalyst(s) for Clinical Anxiety/Depressive Episode(s)

This story-part emerges from the story background either suddenly, or over a period of time. For instance, a principal might lose a loved one, or a combination of factors and/or events might align to push him/her over the proverbial edge. Below are the three examples, from the same three principals' stories above:

Purplefairy

I don't necessarily like to be around a lot of people but I'm human and it bothers me that I cant make friends even though im a very caring person. I sometimes make friends in my head and imagine all the things we could do together. This drives me more and more into my depression.

Cor du Bruin

Although my business was going well, my marriage was falling apart and my ex-wife and I were in the process of getting a divorce.

Mary

Then, in my early 20's, a culmination of circumstances caused me to develop bad anxiety. I had bad reactions to medication I had to take for my allergies, was involved in a very threatening situation and was negatively affected by a close friend's terrifying experience. I seemed to handle the traumas at the time, but in the long term, they took their toll on me.

Details of the Crisis

As evidenced in the data, after the trigger(s)/catalyst(s), the principal experiences thoughts/feelings, behaviors, and events that recounted later as the constitutive scenes in his/her story of the struggle against anxiety/depression. These are set in a given time-period. Below are three examples, also taken from the same three principals' stories above:

Purplefairy

My trust in people is very fragile and even though I think I'm forgiving, people around me have told me to learn to let things go. Meeting new people is the hardest thing unless I drink something for the nerves, that's how I met my exes and all of them were convinced I had a drinking problem.

Cor du Bruin

I sunk into a deep depression. The last thing on earth I wanted to be facing was a divorce case. Thankfully, I won the divorce case and got custody of my son, then aged ten, and my daughter, aged six. However, the depression had already set in and I was starting to lose income every month as a result of my poor performance. Within the next $5^1/_2$ years, I experienced a total of 20 different traumas which really affected me. The traumas included the death of both my father and my mother, two very bad car accidents, the death of three of our household pets and the loss of all my money in the bank. I had lost almost everything except my house.

Mary

The situations for my second bout of depression were very similar to those of my first. I experienced another traumatic birth and we moved to a different city where I didn't know anyone. The future became very uncertain and this was the worst episode I had ever had. I remember going on a family holiday and feeling suicidal

I was experiencing unbelievable anxiety and terrible insomnia. It was about this time that I realised the negative effect my mood was having on my children.

Diagnosis, Treatment, and Coping

This is arguably the climax of the story (with the denouement as the "conclusion, future and advice" story-part below). The principal, having somehow realized in earnest that they might be suffering from clinical anxiety/depression, seeks and gets an official diagnosis and treatment regimen. Along with this, the principal has developed coping mechanisms, which—coupled with the treatment regimen—can help them live more comfortably. As aforementioned, story-part classification schemes are not perfect, and stories are not always neatly divisible into one's classifications. A case in point here is *Purplefairy*'s story, which happens not to have a visible discrete "diagnosis, treatment, and coping" part. But Cor du Bruin's and Mary's stories do, as shown below:

Cor du Bruin

Finally, I went to see my local doctor who gave me a combination of medications to take... It helped a lot to get in touch with the Depression and Anxiety Support Group who have a referral list of medical professionals that are in the "know" about anxiety and depression. The Support Group can be contacted on (011) 783-1474/6 from 8am to 8pm Monday to Saturday.

Mary

This motivated me to go and visit a specialist in Pretoria who gave me medication and a short therapy course. It was the best thing I ever did. The depression lifted and I felt in control of my life again.

Conclusion, Future, and Advice

In this story-part, the principal discusses his/her state of mind and living conditions in the aftermath of treatment. At this point, principals may also discuss their vision and plans for their future. Often, they also give advice to people who struggle with clinical anxiety/depression. In this regard once again, *Purplefairy*'s story does not offer a good exemplar. Below are the examples from Cor du Bruin's and Mary's stories:

Cor du Bruin

I now have a very competent psychiatrist and psychologist to help me through my bad patches. It also helped to realise that I had to start working on myself again. I started to read a lot of books on depression and enrolled at RAU to study Christian counselling.

I feel that I am now coping and enjoying life again. My business has picked up and I have good relationships with my two children. I really enjoy reaching out to other sufferers and counselling them. I think one needs discipline to overcome depression. Often people live too much in the past, and they have to learn how to replace negative thoughts with positive ones. Time, self-knowledge, exercise and spirituality are all important in beating depression. I am now involved with the group and run my own support group in Southdale.

Mary

I started working as a Senior Primary teacher at the beginning of 1997. I find my work as a teacher very fulfilling and also help run a support group for depression and anxiety sufferers in Witbank. I have learnt through my experience that one shouldn't be afraid to ask for help and support. I waited too long before I opened up to anyone about how I was feeling. At the same time, however, I am continually working on myself. You've got to be prepared to put the effort in to recover. I believe in a holistic approach to recovery – body, mind and spirit are all equally important in my eyes.

Reckoning and Coping

As we mention above, one can add this element either between parts 2 and 3, or between parts 3 and 4. It describes a point in which the principal recounts his/her memories of the events, thoughts/feelings, and behaviors that helped them realize that they might be suffering from clinical anxiety/depression. These recollections also include the coping mechanisms that the principal states having used to deal with their perceived anxiety/depression before the official diagnosis, or after the official diagnosis during time-periods or events wherein the treatment and usual coping mechanisms are not working. Below are the relevant examples of this story-part from Cor du Bruin and Mary's stories/discussions:

Cor du Bruin
(Before his diagnosis:)

I began to sleep the whole day. I used to shake so much that I couldn't hold a pen or write in front of other people.

(After his diagnosis:)

Unfortunately, I had a bad reaction to the pills. For a long time, I was very disillusioned with the medical health professionals I encountered. Over my 15 year period of depression, I have "fired" over 3 psychiatrists, 4 therapists and 9 GP's!

Mary
(Apparently, all her instances of this story-part are before her diagnosis.)

I developed panic attacks which then developed into severe agoraphobia. I was afraid to leave my house. At that stage I was dating my would-to-be husband who was very supportive of them. Luckily I found a self-help book on phobias and managed to work my way through it on my own...

Depression set in for months on end, but I hid if from my husband and my relatives. I wasn't really sure what was happening to me. Eventually, I opened up to my husband who encouraged me to go and visit a local female GP. I was given some pills for a short period. The depression abated only to resurface three years later with the birth of my second baby.

Principals' Roles

The nine principals in this data set play two main roles, namely: 1) advice and support seekers, and 2) advice and support givers. By default, all six individuals from the SADAG website are advice and support givers, as their stories are narrated after they have all managed to get treatment, as well as advice and support from other sources. As for the three individuals on the forum, *Linzi* is both a seeker and giver, whereas *Purplefairy* and *Mozmoz* are seekers.

By far, *Linzi* plays the most prolific role as an advice and support giver. She shares extensive details of her story, and she earnestly and severally confesses to having felt severely depressed and having negative thoughts about herself and her life. She also points out that she is "not perfect," and she even discloses that once attempted to commit suicide. These qualities thus mark hers as a quintessential story of an authentic leader, based on Mitchell's (2016) framework.

FINDINGS, PART II: CHARACTERISTICS OF PRINCIPALS' STORIES USING THE OWENS (1984) AND MITCHELL (2016) ANALYTIC FRAMEWORKS

Owen's (1984) Framework

Using Owen's (1984) thematic analysis scheme, we can identify at least five major discrete themes or topics among eight of the nine SSA story-tellers, excluding *Linzi*. For *Linzi*, we can also identify five themes; however, these themes are slightly different from the ones identified within the other principals. For the eight principals, the themes we can discuss here are: 1) Anxiety/Depression, 2) Known Causes/Triggers, 3) Isolation, 4) Coping Before and After Diagnosis & Treatment, and 5) Seeking Treatment and Help. For *Linzi*, the themes are: 1) Difficulty of Accessing Professional Health Care & Treatment, 2) Known Causes/Triggers, 3) Coping Before and After Diagnosis & Treatment, and 4) Advice.

Anxiety/Depression

As defined by Owen's (1984) scheme, the recurrence of the meaning associated with this theme or topic can be identified in the posts or stories/discussions of all eight principals in this context. Below are some specific exemplars from all eight posts:

Purplefairy

Help everyone. Im 26 from [Sub-Saharan City and country] and I suffer from social anxiety and it has led me to live a very depressed life...

Cor du Bruin

... my marriage was falling apart and my ex-wife and I were in the process of getting a divorce. I sunk into a deep depression...

Mary

...Then, in my early 20's, a culmination of circumstances caused me to develop bad anxiety...

Feon

If I look back, I would probably say that I've suffered from mild depression my whole life – kind of like the "Sunday afternoon blues"

Thumi Mkhize

My story starts last year in February when I began to experience bad family problems. I reacted by becoming very depressed...

Grace Sebo

...It was a very big shock to me as she was one of my closest friends and I would have trusted her with anything. I slipped into a very bad depression after I found out.

Veli Zondi

In 1995 my father died, and shortly afterwards I began to suffer from severe headaches, sleeplessness, lethargy and a depressed mood...

Mozmoz

I've been coping with depression for about 6 or 7 years now...

Known Causes/Triggers

All eight principals explicitly discuss what caused or triggered their depression, to the best of their non-professional evaluation—most principals have also talked to mental health professionals. Some of these causes can be seen from the exemplars above:

- **Isolation:** This theme refers to the desire or practice of being alone, and/or not socializing or interacting with family, friends, and strangers. Two principals—i.e., *Purplefairy* and Thumi Mkhize—explicitly discuss this action in this context, whereas one principal—i.e., *Mozmoz*—indirectly discusses it:

Purplefairy

...Of course none of this is visible to my family, everyone thinks I love isolating myself...

Thumi Mkhize

...I reacted by becoming very depressed and avoiding people...

Mozmoz

I decided to join since I'm too shy to talk to people face to face...

It should be noted that in our evaluation, Cor du Bruin's statement "I used to shake so much that I couldn't hold a pen or write in front of other people," does not qualify as isolation per se. Rather, it sounds like a form of social anxiety that he experienced in public, but that did not cause him to purposefully limit interactions with others

Coping Before and After Diagnosis and Treatment

This theme can be identified in six of the eight stories/discussions. The exemplars included below highlight this theme:

Purplefairy

...I used to break down in tears begging God to make me normal just like everyone else...its good to know that and I'm not alone. ☺ [sic]

Cor du Bruin

1)...I began to sleep the whole day...

2)...I started to read a lot of books on depression and enrolled at RAU to study Christian counselling...

Mary

...I found a self-help book on phobias and managed to work my way through it on my own...

Thumi Mkhize

...I went to stay with my mother in Pretoria for another restful week. I did a lot of soul searching when I was with my mother. I realised that I had to gain courage and learn how to face other people again...

Grace Sebo

...Through reading these brochures, I was finally able to understand what I was going through. That was the catalyst for my recovery...

Veli Zondi

...The workshop was very useful in that I learnt what I was really suffering from and how to deal with it. I also learnt how to handle the problems as they came...

Seeking Treatment and Help

One can argue meta-analytically that this theme is present in all these stories/ discussions by default. After all, these individuals are telling their stories so as to seek help, or to verbally continue and/or reify their healing processes. Be that as it may, it should be noted that the identifiable finite or discrete specific mentions of this theme are present in only seven out of the eight total number of stories/discussions in this set (excluding *Linzi*):

Cor du Bruin

...Finally, I went to see my local doctor who gave me a combination of medications to take...

Mary

1)...Eventually, I opened up to my husband who encouraged me to go and visit a local female GP. I was given some pills for a short period...

2)... This motivated me to go and visit a specialist in Pretoria who gave me medication and a short therapy course...

Feon

...In May 1995 I found a medication that worked for me...

Thumi Mkhize

... I was hospitalised for one week, during which time I attended a number of valuable therapeutic sessions and consulted with a psychiatrist...

Grace Sebo

... I got hold of the toll-free number for the Depression and Anxiety Support Group in Gauteng. I phoned up and was put through to a very understanding and supportive counsellor who explained to me that I could be suffering from depression. The Support Group sent me some very useful brochures on the causes, symptoms and treatment for depression...

Veli Zondi

...I eventually went to see a doctor in Pretoria who told me that I was suffering from stress. He prescribed some tablets which I began to take. A while later I heard about a workshop that the Depression and Anxiety Support Group were holding at Soweto College...

Mozmoz

...I've been in therapy and things got better...

Linzi's Themes, per Owen's (1984) Scheme

As aforementioned, when Owen's (1984) scheme is applied, *Linzi*'s themes are slightly different from those of the other eight Sub-Saharan-African principals. To recap, her themes are: 1) Difficulty of Accessing Professional Health Care and Treatment, 2) Known Causes/Triggers, 3) Coping Before and After Diagnosis and Treatment, and 4) Advice. Below are some of the instances in which each of these schemes can be identified in her stories/discussions.

Difficulty of Accessing Professional Health Care and Treatment

Linzi highlights this theme as she both seeks help from other posters on the forum, and as she encourages them to seek professional care and treatment for their anxiety/depression, and other mental illnesses. Below are the five instances that can be used as exemplars:

1. Here [in her particular SSA country] the antidepressants are getting scare...
2. ...there is even a limit for seeing a psychiatrist and the meds being described or a psychologist etc...
3. ...I don't see a psychologist because I have experienced the same like Sarah, they only "uhm, aahhh..okay" and nothing else and then you leave cheated out

of money and time and the humiliation that you are just a lab rat....they do not really care, they are just counting the hours and the money, here we pay a lot per hour and one appointment is obvious not enough...

4. …but I have lost trust in psychologists and counseling overall, the ones I have had appointments with so far (a lot of them), made me feel like a lab rat, it is if they can't wait for it to be over, because they make their money (They are very expensive per hour) and others are waiting in line…
5. …I stick to my meds (it is compulsory) and I do see the psychiatrist every 6 months to monitor me, but nobody else understands…

Known Causes/Triggers

Out of the five themes from her set of stories/discussions, this theme is probably the most extensively discussed. Below are five of the excerpts of the parts with some specific instances in which she discusses it (please note: as aforementioned, there were no changes made to any typographical, grammatical, or other features):

1. …I have been suffering with depression all my life because of a violent childhood. I tend to be hard on myself and judge myself by how others judge me, can't stop or help it…I know it is stupid, but it seems that I always attract people who will eventually abuse my emosionally/mentaly....I will start a relationship (with a man) with no exspectations but only because he seems bright and nice...usually then when it becomes serious (from both sides), after al while he wants to control me and if I do not play the role of a submussive damsel in destress, he will try to destroy me by insulting me as a woman and person because I became cold because of all the abuse....I live constantly with feelings of guild that there is something wrong with me as n woman...trust me, I always start out to be very warming an loving and dedicated, but men abuse my trust and I am clever enough to figure it out...then the trouble starts!
2. I seem to attract all the abusers, I was even married to a certified psycopath (my first love and I was 22) and was told that I was the reason he is a psycopath…
3. …Here in xxxx the white men likes their women skinny and blonde. I am on the other hand have only beautiful grey/green eyes (according to other people they are very striking) and very long black hair, but my weigh gain makes me feel like an outcast…
4. I myself grew up in a violent home with a father who was supposed to protect his little daughter, but instead I have gone to bed with a broken lip every night... he abused my mother physically, mentally, emotionally and sexually, everything a woman can be done to and I witnessed it all. The circumstances at home was so bad that the social workers put me and my brother in a foster home for 4

years so that my parents can sort out their divorce and for my mother to start over in a different town…

5. Unfortunately I was not prepared that he was a certified psychopath (I did not know then)…He used to throttle me until I am blue in the face, I had to hide my injuries/marks under a high necked shirt or something and my black marks on my arms as well. He even hunted me on his farm with a shotgun…

Coping Before and After Diagnosis and Treatment

In this context, the concept of "coping" is similar to those above under all principals' story-part classifications as well as the first set of eight's Owen (1984) themes. *Linzi* attempts to somehow effectively deal with her clinical anxiety/depression or to blunt its negative effects on her (e.g., sadness and worry), before or alongside psychological or psychiatric (pharmacological) treatment. Below are some examples of specific coping methods she mentions:

1. What I have found, like you, I keep myself busy with doing something I like very much, I also walk around and take pictures of my pets and nature…
2. At least I am very intelligent (I think so hahaha), because I am an avid reading especially about science and nature / biology and astronomy
3. I'm going to take out my African Grey parrot and take him outside on the grass... my parrot is calling me on my name and asks for…[food], he wants to eat fruit on the lawn now…
4. It helps to take my beloved African Grey parrot outside (I have clipped his wings) into the sun for a bit, because a lack of vitamin D can worsen your depression.....
5. Luckily I have an appreciation for nature and biology and animals and walk around with my mobile and take photos of nature and of my pets and forward it to whomever is interested…

Advice

Among the story-tellers from the forum, this theme is unique to *Linzi*, and it presents itself in a number of instances throughout her stories/discussions (all six of the story-tellers from the SADAG website explicitly give advice to fellow anxiety/depression sufferers). It should also be noted, that one can argue that there are some instances above the "Coping Before & After…" theme that can also count concurrently as instances of the "Advice" theme, e.g. instance 1) above. She advises her fellow story-tellers to seek treatment, and to somehow cope positively with their mental illnesses. Below are some specific examples:

1. ...I got so tired one day that I have tried to kill myself (Please NEVER do THAT!!! life is too beautiful and you will hurt your family)...
2. But just like in YOUR case, I must pick myself up and face the world and be brave and try and try again....WE must!
3. What helps the BEST for ME crying!!! every day....afterwards you feel your feeling is done and dusted. Like I said, don't let anyone into your "mood secret"....smile to everyone in the street to get smiles back....you might just brighten another sad person's day as well.
4. But don't feel isolated, I am a 42 year old woman who had never find the right man to get married to or having children with and because of toxic relationships...

Mitchell's (2016) Framework

Arguably, most of the nine SSA story-tellers from the forum and SADAG website demonstrate the qualities of an authentic leader, per Mitchell's (2016) framework. *Linzi* stands outs in this regard. In addition to the definition she uses as quoted further above (under "Analytical Frameworks" subsection), Mitchell derives six categories within which she lists some examples of the qualities of jaw surgery bloggers' authentic leadership. These categories are: 1) "Expressions providing evidence of increased self-awareness," 2) "Expressions providing evidence of the desire for and achievement of relational transparency," 3) "Commenters' expressions of appreciation for authors' relational transparency," 4) "Expressions of moral perspectives," 5) "Expressions providing evidence of balanced processing," and 6) "Commenters' expressions of hope, confidence, optimism, and resilience" (Mitchell 2016, pp. 7 to 10).

From reading through the data-set with all nine principals' stories/discussions, one can see that by writing (or talking) about their experiences with clinical anxiety and depression, these individuals: 1) attempt to get to know themselves better, 2) attempt to let fellow anxiety/depression sufferers see their strengths, weaknesses, and other qualities or aspects of their real lives, 3) express appreciation for other story-tellers'/discussants' honest revelations about their lives 4) express their moral convictions or beliefs, 5) seek to make informed decisions vis-à-vis coping mechanisms and treatment options after evaluating information gathered from their fellow sufferers, and 6) severally express "hope, confidence, optimism, and resilience" (Mitchell 2016, p. 10).

CONCLUSION

It is important to reiterate or emphasize a couple of caveats regarding this study's findings. As aforementioned, seeking help and advice online cannot and should not replace the receipt of professional mental health care, and one cannot guarantee the quality of advice found thereon. Moreover, as a qualitative intensive study—i.e., vs. an extensive study using methods such as statistical sampling, one has to bear in mind that the study's findings cannot be said to be typical of all anxiety/depression sufferers of SSA-descent. With that said, based on the insights above, it is arguable that scholars, mental-health professionals, and other concerned parties ought to at least consider the promotion of online discussions alongside professional treatment and other efficacious measures. And overall, the biggest advantage of this tool might be that when family, friends, and others do not know or believe that anxiety and depression are real and dangerous diseases, a Sub-Saharan African (or other) individual can count on it to know that 1) the conditions are indeed real and dangerous diseases, 2) one should not suffer alone or in silence, and 3) they should seek help and do their best to cope positively.

In sum, this chapter provides an analysis of personal stories posted by nine patients or survivors of clinical anxiety and depression, as shared on two online forums. The data were analyzed by incorporating Owen's (1984) thematic analysis framework in conjunction with Mitchell's (2016) framework on authentic leadership. Upon analyzing the messages, six thematic story-parts emerged: 1) story backgrounds; 2) triggers/catalysts for clinical anxiety/depression episodes; 3) details of the crisis; 4) diagnosis, treatment, and coping; 5) reckoning and coping, and 6) conclusion, future, and advice. And throughout the discourse shown within these forums, an authentic leader—as described by Mitchell (2016)—emerged. The specific attributes that led to this labeling include describing growth in self-awareness, transparent interactions and evidence of appreciation for this quality, the inclusion of a moral orientation, processing events in a balanced manner, and expressing positive outcomes such as hope and resilience (Mitchell, 2016). As evidenced by this analysis, online sources may provide a feasible way of giving and seeking mental health support for individuals of SSA-descent. Moving forward, clinicians and scholars will benefit from expanding upon this analysis in order to develop recommendations for best practices.

REFERENCES

Abera, M., Tesfaye, M., Belachew, T., & Hanlon, C. (2014). *Perceived challenges and opportunities arising from integration of mental health into primary care: A cross-sectional survey of primary health care workers in south-west Ethiopia*. BioMed Central Ltd.

Alvidrez, J. (1999). Ethnic Variations in Mental Health Attitudes and Service Use Among Low-Income African American, Latina, and European American Young Women. *Community Mental Health Journal*, *35*(6), 515–530. doi:10.1023/A:1018759201290 PMID:10863988

Baron, E., Hanlon, C., Mall, S., Honikman, S., Breuer, E., Kathree, T., ... Tomlinson, M. (2016). *Maternal mental health in primary care in five low- and middle-income countries: A situational analysis*. BioMed Central Ltd.

Boyes, M. E., & Cluver, L. D. (2015). Relationships between familial HIV/AIDS and symptoms of anxiety and depression: The mediating effect of bullying victimization in a prospective sample of South African children and adolescents. *Journal of Youth and Adolescence*, *44*(4), 847–859. doi:10.1007/s10964-014-0146-3 PMID:24996836

Choudhury, M. D., Gamon, M., Counts, S., & Horvitz, E. (2013). Predicting Depression via Social Media. In E. Kiciman, N. B. Ellison, B. Hogan, P. Resnick, & I. Soboroff (Eds.), *ICWSM. The AAAI Press*.

Çobaner, A. A. (2017). *Social Support Through Digital Media? Breast Cancer Groups on Facebook*. Manuscript in preparation.

DeAndrea, D. C. (2015). Testing the proclaimed affordances of online support groups in a nationally representative sample of adults seeking mental health assistance. *Journal of Health Communication*, *20*(2), 147–156. doi:10.1080/10810730.2014.914606 PMID:25116383

Depression Understood. (2017). Retrieved from http://www.depression-understood.org/

Diala, C. C. (2001). Racial/ethnic differences in attitudes toward seeking professional mental health services. *American Journal of Public Health*, *91*, 5. PMID:11344893

Goffman, E. (1981). Footing. In *Forms of talk. Philadelphia: University of Pennsylvania Press*. Abingdon, UK: Routledge.

Huh, J., Liu, L. S., Neogi, T., Inkpen, K., & Pratt, W. (2014). Health Vlogs as Social Support for Chronic Illness Management. *ACM Transactions on Computer-Human Interaction*, *21*(4). doi:10.1145/2630067

Labov, W., & Waletzky, J. (1967/1997). Narrative analysis. In J. Helm (Ed.), *Essays on the verbal and visual arts* (pp. 12–44). Seattle, WA: University of Washington Press.

Linde, C. (1993). *Life stories: The creation of coherence*. New York, NY: Oxford University Press.

Littlejohn, S. W. (1992). Theories of human communication. Belmont, CA: Wadsworth Pub. Co.

Luthans, F., & Avolio, B. (2003). Authentic leadership development. In K. S. Cameron, J. E. Dutton, & R. E. Quinn (Eds.), *Positive organizational scholarship: Foundations of a new discipline* (pp. 241–258). San Francisco, CA: Berrett-Koehler.

Mishra, S. I., Lucksted, A., Gioia, D., Barnet, B., & Baquet, C. R. (2009, January 01). Needs and preferences for receiving mental health information in an African American focus group sample. *Community Mental Health Journal*, *45*(2), 117–126. doi:10.1007/s10597-008-9157-4 PMID:18633704

Mitchell, M. (2016, December 31). Authentic leadership in illness blogs: What we can learn from jaw surgery bloggers. *Cogent Social Sciences*, *2*, 1.

Murry, V. M. B., Heflinger, C. A., Suiter, S. V., & Brody, G. H. (2011, January 01). Examining Perceptions About Mental Health Care and Help-Seeking Among Rural African American Families of Adolescents. *Journal of Youth and Adolescence*, *40*(9), 1118–1131. doi:10.1007/s10964-010-9627-1 PMID:21259067

Myrick, J. G., Holton, A. E., Himelboim, I., & Love, B. (2016, January 01). #Stupidcancer: Exploring a Typology of Social Support and the Role of Emotional Expression in a Social Media Community. *Health Communication*, *31*(5), 596–605. doi:10.1080/10410236.2014.981664 PMID:26453480

Nakku, J., Okello, E., Kizza, D., Honikman, S., Ssebunnya, J., Ndyanabangi, S., ... Kigozi, F. (2016). *Perinatal mental health care in a rural African district, Uganda: A qualitative study of barriers, facilitators and needs*. BioMed Central Ltd.

Ojelade, I. I., McCray, K., Ashby, J. S., & Meyers, J. (2011). Use of Ifá as a Means of Addressing Mental Health Concerns Among African American Clients. *Journal of Counseling and Development*, *89*(4), 406–412. doi:10.1002/j.1556-6676.2011.tb02837.x

Ola, B., Crabb, J., Adewuya, A., Olugbile, F., & Abosede, O. A. (2014). The State of Readiness of Lagos State Primary Health Care Physicians to Embrace the Care of Depression in Nigeria. *Community Mental Health Journal*, *50*(2), 239–244. doi:10.1007/s10597-013-9648-9 PMID:23912148

Owen, W. F. (1984). Interpretive themes in relational communication. *The Quarterly Journal of Speech*, *70*(3), 274–287. doi:10.1080/00335638409383697

South African Depression and Anxiety Group. (2017). Retrieved from http://www.sadag.org/

Turkle, S. (2012). *Alone together: Why we expect more from technology and less from each other*. New York: Basic Books.

Walumbwa, F. O., Avolio, B. J., Gardner, W. L., Wernsing, T. S., & Peterson, S. J. (2008). Authentic leadership: Development and validation of a theory-based measure. *Journal of Management*, *34*(1), 89–126. doi:10.1177/0149206307308913

KEY TERMS AND DEFINITIONS

Authentic Leadership: Leaders who nurture growth and positive development within themselves and others through their own and others' self-awareness, being relationally transparent, and making decisions that are based upon their internalized moral perspective as well as a balanced processing of information.

Clinical Anxiety and Depression: Mental-health conditions marked by consistent and serious debilitating worry, fear, sadness and hopelessness, among other symptoms.

Owen's Thematic Analytical Framework: An analytical framework for studying story themes, consisting of three main features, namely recurrence (observation of at least two reports that have the same thread of meaning), repetition (duplication of key words and phrases), and forcefulness (verbal or written messages representing vocal inflections or dramatic pauses that "stress or subordinate some utterances from other locutions in oral reports).

SADAG: Acronym for the South African Depression and Anxiety Group, a major non-profit pioneer in the support of South African patients and former patients of clinical anxiety and depression.

Story-Arc: The combined distinct parts of a story or narrative, each of which has a specific and important role vis-à-vis comprehension and utility for both the principal or protagonist, his/her listeners or readers, and other parties.

APPENDIX

Story/Discussion 1

(Source: www.depression-understood.org)
Purplefairy
Need a friend to talk to
Sat Jan 21, 2017 1:30 pm

Help everyone. Im 26 from xxxx and I suffer from social anxiety and it has led me to live a very depressed life. Of course none of this is visible to my family, everyone thinks I love isolating myself and I've heard some " u think you better than everyone else" comments more than I'd like to disclose. My cousin once said that i have the biggest heart. I don't necessarily like to be around a lot of people but I'm human and it bothers me that I cant make friends even though im a very caring person. I sometimes make friends in my head and imagine all the things we could do together. This drives me more and more into my depression. I would like something real, I just don't know how to go about it. My trust in people is very fragile and even though I think I'm forgiving, people around me have told me to learn to let things go. Meeting new people is the hardest thing unless I drink something for the nerves, that's how I met my exes and all of them were convinced I had a drinking problem. But I don't, I hate most alcoholic drinks but my anxiety is greater than any of my feelings. I used to break down in tears begging God to make me normal just like everyone else... its good to know that and I'm not alone ☺

Responses to Story/Discussion 1

nanacarol
Re: Need a friend to talk to
Mon Jan 23, 2017 6:08 pm

Hi; I'm so glad you have posted here! No, you are not alone. My youngest, when she was pregnant at 17 had issues with social anxiety. I personally don't know how it feels but I do know that it is real. Very real. Since she was pregnant meds were really not an option and she went through counseling. She would do fine going to her doctors because most in the waiting room understood. The problem was getting her started and in with a doctor. Here is an article that has a phone number you can call so you don't have to go out to take a step toward being happy and finding joy. http://bit.ly/2jKHSJT As for what others think and say. Words do hurt. Words can wound. It was easy when we were kids and another kid would say "your a snob" and we knew it wasn't true and we would just say "so". When you are ready to venture out to seek new friends, would it help to start with a small group at a local church? Maybe you could call around and ask different churches what types of groups they have and choose one that you thought would interest you and where you would feel comfortable. This is like I said, when YOU are ready.

You said you have prayed for God to make you normal. I'm here to tell you God made you exactly the way HE needed you to be.

Jeremiah 1: Tells us HE knew us before he ever created us and Jeremiah 29:11 tells us HE knows HE has the plans for us. That includes you.

You can find your way to joy and happiness and I will be cheering you on!

sunnysidedown89
Re: Need a friend to talk to
Wed May 31, 2017 10:46 pm

just posting to give you a big hug!

it sucks you're going through this and that your support group is making you feel even more alienated than

you already feel.

<3

Helloraspberries1
Re: Need a friend to talk to
Sat Jun 03, 2017 10:34 am

Hi there, sounds like things are tough at the moment. I don't know what's it like right now feeling the way you do but well done for responding here.

Yeah I know what you mean by making friends really hard. There's no easy way to or speed the process quickly. Has to come from us and only us can do it. I don't know if you are also losing interest in doing things but i know that can also trigger you to not make friends too.

Right now I think you need to be in your element and make the steps you need to reach your goals for life. I don't know what help or incouragment you need but I would start off by talking first to someone. I think you need to be happy in yourself before you do the things you wanna do. Remember it's little steps and not big ones.

Please keep talking to us

Story/Discussion 2: Response to Someone Else

(Source: www.depression-understood.org)
Linzi
Re: My concerns
Fri Dec 16, 2016 6:36 am

Hi there Jhaden84 and Sarah

Jhaden84, thank you, I am so glad you are taking care of Sarah, you have had both the same experience...she seems like a very nice person and are so far away from home.

Sorry Sarah to hear about you not getting emotional and physical help, but you MUST go and see some doctor...are there not any others in Canada? I am sure your parents will gladly assist you financially to make an appointment, I don't know how it is in Canada, but what I have heard it is a civilized country with very educated people who ears a lot of money. If you pay cash I am sure a physician of doctor will see you. I have never had the opportunity or money to travel over our borders, it is interesting to read about other people of other countries. I myself are from xxxx, that is going from a 1st world country to a 3 rd world country because of our worst government you can find on this world, it is not even illegal to talk about our bad president, because he is so stupid and the whole cabinet was in jail and has not even made matric / grade 12....they are aware that the whole country's residents hate them....so here the antidepressants are getting scare or are not even delivered in certain towns...it is scary because we all know how vital it is to take our antidepressants EVERY DAY....we also don't have free healthcare, you either pay very expensively for a medical aid fund every month and the medical aid fund has lots of excuses why it does not want to pay for most of the care we need...there is even a limit for seeing a psychiatrist and the meds being described or a psychologist etc.

I have made a plan, I have filled in a form where I declared I am jobless (I work for my partner at home) and then I have signed up for Government help, but it is NOT for free, you still pay but much less than private consultations....now I see a psychiatrist every six months, and get my meds by sitting at a State clinic with other poor people (I don't mind, I am middle class poor status anyway) in line... I pay about 260 [in country's monetary unit] for a 3 month course of pills and believe me, it is very cheap THIS way. I don't see a psychologist because I have experienced the same like Sarah, they only "uhm, aahhh..okay" and nothing else and then you leave cheated out of money and time and the humiliation that you are just a lab rat....they do not really care, they are just counting the hours and the money, here we pay a lot per hour and one appointment is obvious not enough...

So yes Sarah, I feel for you, but I am so afraid that you might have an ulcer of something else serious with your body...you might die if you do not get medical help soon!

Keep us posted Sarah, but study first ☺

Response to Story/Discussion 2

Sarah19

Re: My concerns

Fri Dec 16, 2016 1:18 pm

Hi Linzi,

I have actually been to xxxx! I went there in 2011 and got the most amazing chance to go there again in 2013. I just have to say, your country is beautiful along with the people, I have never met a people so special and unique, sincerely. I cherish both experiences in xxxx everyday and everywhere I am. To tell you all about my time there would be too long haha, but know that I am determined to go back again in the near future.

I was lucky enough to visit the xxxx area, xx, xx and xx. I have a few friends there that I've met over these couple of years. I have heard and been informed about how the healthcare there. I am so sorry to hear about the unhelpful experience you've had to go through. I can only imagine the struggle to get proper help, as you and I, are one in the same. Please continue to look for help, I feel that you are a wise person, and you'll be able to make the right decisions to take care of yourself. You're right I probably will see a physician soon lol. I don't know if I have an ulcer...but the symptoms of what the stress has caused alone should be enough of a reason to go haha. Thank you again for listening! I really, really appreciate it ☺

Story/Discussion 3

(Source: www.depression-understood.org)
Linzi
Toxic relationships

Wed Nov 30, 2016 3:49 am

Hi, I am new here!

I have been suffering with depression all my life because of a violent childhood. I tend to be hard on myself and judge myself by how others judge me, can't stop or help it.

I know it is stupid, but it seems that I always attract people who will eventually abuse my emotionally/mentally....I will start a relationship (with a man) with no exspectations but only because he seems bright and nice...usually then when it becomes serious (from both sides), after al while he wants to control me and if I do not play the role of a submussive damsel in destress, he will try to destroy me by insulting me as a woman and person because I became cold because of all the abuse....I live constantly with feelings of guild that there is something wrong with me as n woman...trust me, I always start out to be very warming an loving and dedicated, but men abuse my trust and I am clever enough to figure it out...then the trouble starts!

I seem to attract all the abusers, I was even married to a certified psycopath (my first love and I was 22) and was told that I was the reason he is a psycopath. It took me years after the divorce to learn to love myself.....I never do "desperate" when I start relationships, it is mutual always....but why do I keep having the "abusers" in my life?

Now I am in an engagement that is now broken but we still live together as "god knows what" because he can't give me a straight answer where I am in this with him....because again I am being emotionally abused and controlled financially (because he is the jealous type, so I resigned a good job 4 years back to help him in his business), I am not the vibrant, self-assured person he got to know, anymore.... HE on the other hand, if our arguments get out of control, he will threaten me that he will throw me out on the street because I am cold and he does not get any love (not true, but he does not know how to "make love", he only does cold sex....and I have talked to him nicely about that many times, but HE is always right and I am always wrong, because I am the "crazy one" one pills....

IS it because I manage my depression with pills, that even my boyfriends discriminate against me? Will I EVER be able to be with a man who will uplift me instead of taking advantage of my "weakness". Believe me, I am friendly and "normal" as most persons...I just struggle with anxiety, but anxiety follows me...

Responses (to Other Responses) to Story/Discussion 3

Linzi

Re: Toxic relationships
Thu Dec 15, 2016 7:13 am

Hi Lwoodall

Thank you for caring. I am from xxxx, we do have other helplines to phone if we feel lost...but I have lost trust in psychologists and counseling overall, the ones I have had appointments with so far (a lot of them), made me feel like a lab rat, it is if they can't wait for it to be over, because they make their money (They are very expensive per hour) and others are waiting in line. NOBODY has every given me the direction to follow to cope, they just sit there and "uhm, ahhhh, ok, how you feeling? bla bla bla) but afterwards I step out of their offices and feel cheated out of money and time. I could have talked to the walls....

I had to talk to psychiatrists as well, because it is only for them to know what kind of meds I need, but it is just for monitoring purposes, they are not really interested and you have to be quick as well because there is a looooong line of other patients waiting, again feeling of cheat.

I stick to my meds (it is compulsory) and I do see the psychiatrist every 6 months to monitor me, but nobody else understands, so I have resorted to this forum where I can talk freely and those who are not bored with me hahaha, have a choice if they want to talk back and it is for free.

It helps if I support the others here as well, it makes me put my own problems in perspective.

I do appreciate your advice, keep talking if you want to...

Story/Discussion 4

(Source: www.depression-understood.org)
TiberiuSahlean
Depression, anxiety and panic attacks
Tue Dec 13, 2016 4:25 am

For me it started 2 years ago. I remember clearly there was an earthquake at the end of November that year and on the 8th floor I was pretty badly shaken. Then I had no problem for the next 23 weeks. Suddenly, one night while I was watching a movie I started having heartaches, I felt my heart rushing and I felt I couldn't breathe. I panicked and went to a drug store then I ended up in the emergency room: of course the doctors could not find anything wrong with me but I didn't believe them. Over the following months I started having panic attacks evermore frequently, I was always afraid an earthquake would hit any minute, I couldn't stay at home because I always felt everything was shaking so I started avoiding going home. I would stay out in the city until it was just time to go to sleep and then I would get right into bed and put the blanket over my head and try to sleep. I lost interest in any activity and I couldn't bring myself to do anything. That was when I decided to move to a new apartment so in February we moved to a new place. After that all my problems stopped until about June or July when I contracted a pretty nasty urinary infection and my kidneys were hurting like crazy. Afterwards I started being afraid again: I was afraid the infection would start again, that the pain would resume so I started going to the doctors, started taking all kinds of drugs and all my problems were back. I felt dizzy, I lost my appetite, I could not bring myself to do anything, I had chest pains and with time all symptoms were worse. Again I started avoiding staying at home and I was feeling captive. I had panic attacks almost all day and from anything: air conditioning, fresh air, lack of fresh air, any kind of pain and so on. Of course during all this time I categorically refused to believe my mental health was not there and I checked for any and all diseases I could think of. By the end of September I remember I was feeling so bad that I can barely describe: it felt as if I was trapped inside a dark dungeon with no room to move and only a pinhole through which I could see the outside world; sometimes I could barely even acknowledge what was going on around me, my vision was barely there and I had to use all my efforts just to stay conscious. My weight dropped to around 100 pounds and I was starting to think that this is it: the end of the line for me. At the end of September I just couldn't take it anymore and I agreed to start seeing a psychiatrist. I was diagnosed with panic disorder and started taking meds. When I left the cabinet I wanted to cheer because I had finally found the source of my problems and at the same time burst into tears because my worse nightmare had come true: I was not a sane person, the others that had been viewing me as weird had been right all along! Although I was heavily drugged I still felt horrible and felt the need to talk to someone, to get everything off my chest. I week later I started going to a therapist. I can tell you that I can barely recalls stuff that has happened during the first year and a half of meds and therapy. I feel like I have been robbed by some part of my life. Although I don't recalls most of the stuff that happened during that period when I try to look back it's as if staring through a really dirty window; there is a feeling of emptiness and of suffering for me and the ones close to me.

I have been fortunate enough to not have any suicidal thoughts throughout this period but I have had to face my own mortality through thoughts that maybe this is the end of the line. Also, for me it's very hard to accept the fact that I may never be able to stop taking meds; I look at myself and I see that yes, I am better now and I have no more panic attacks, but I still have chest pains and I have many periods when depression sets in and I can't get myself to doing anything and nothing is of interest to me. One thing that has kept me going through all of this has been photography: the moments when I was composing and taking photos and I was all alone with the camera were the only moments I could get peace of mind; but I am afraid that maybe during a severe depression episode not even photography will save me... What will I have left then? Also I feel that the things that make me happy or that I am interested in doing are becoming less by day and this also worrying me.

Responses to Story/Discussion 4

Linzi

Re: Depression, anxiety and panic attacks
Tue Dec 13, 2016 4:50 am

Dear TiberiuSahlean

I have been depressed my whole life, it is a loooooong story if you have the time and lots of wine ☺.

Have you ever considered that you may suffer from POST-TRAUMATIC STRESS DISORDER? I have copied the link for you to read up abouthit....see if you recognize yourself in these symptoms.... You can feel free to talk about anything should you want to..... https://en.wikipedia.org/wiki/Posttraum... s_disorder posttraumatic stress disorder (PTSD)[note 1] is a mental disorder that can develop after a person is exposed to a traumatic event, such as sexual assault, warfare, traffic collisions, or other threats on a person's life.[1] Symptoms may include disturbing thoughts, feelings, or dreams related to the events, mental or physical distress to trauma related cues, attempts to avoid trauma related cues, alterations in how a person thinks and feels, and increased arousal. These symptoms last for more than a month after the event. Young children are less likely to show distress but instead may express their memories through play.[1] Those with PTSD are at a higher risk of suicide.[2]

Most people who have experienced a traumatic event will not develop PTSD.[2] People who experience interpersonal trauma (for example rape or child abuse) are more likely to develop PTSD, as compared to people who experience non-assault based trauma such as accidents and natural disasters.[3] About half of people develop PTSD following rape.[2] Children are less likely than adults to develop PTSD after trauma, especially if they are under ten years of age.[4] Diagnosis is based on the presence of specific symptoms following a traumatic event.[2]

Prevention may be possible when therapy is targeted at those with early symptoms but is not effective when carried out among all people following trauma.[2] The main treatments for people with PTSD are counseling and medication.[5] A number of different types of therapy may be useful.[6] This may occur one on one or in a group.[5] Antidepressants of the selective serotonin reuptake inhibitor type are the first-line medications for PTSD and result in benefit in about half of people.[7] These benefits are less than those seen with therapy.[2] It is unclear if using medications and therapy together has greater benefit.[2][8] Other medications do not have enough evidence to support their use and in the case of benzodiazepines may worsen outcomes.[9][10]

In the United States about 3.5% of adults have PTSD in a given year, and 9% of people develop it at some point in their life.[1] In much of the rest of the world, rates during a given year are between 0.5% and 1%.[1] Higher rates may occur in regions of armed conflict.[2] It is more common in women than men.[5] Symptoms of trauma-related mental disorders have been documented since at least the time of the ancient Greeks.[11] During the World Wars study increased and it was known under various terms including "shell shock" and "combat neurosis".[12] The term "posttraumatic stress disorder" came into use in the 1970s in large part due to the diagnoses of US military veterans of the Vietnam War.[13] It was officially recognized by the American Psychiatric Association in 1980 in the third edition of the Diagnostic and Statistical Manual of Mental Disorders (DSMIII).[14]

File:Posttraumatic stress disorder.webm
Video explanation
Contents [hide]

1 Classification
2 Risk factors
    2.1 Trauma
    2.2 Genetics
    2.3 Drug and substance abuse
3 Pathophysiology
    3.1 Neuroendocrinology
    3.2 Neuroanatomy
4 Diagnosis
    4.1 Screening and assessment
    4.2 Diagnostic and statistical manual
    4.3 International classification of diseases
    4.4 Differential diagnosis
5 Prevention
    5.1 Psychological debriefing
    5.2 Risktargeted

interventions

6 Management
    6.1 Psychotherapy
    6.2 Medication
    6.3 Other
7 Epidemiology
    7.1 United States
8 Veterans
    8.1 United States
    8.2 United Kingdom
    8.3 Canada
9 History
10 Terminology
11 Research
11.1 Psychotherapy adjuncts
12 Notes
13 References

External links TiberiuSahlean Re: Depression, anxiety and panic attacks Tue Dec 13, 2016 5:20 am Hello Linzi and thank you for your reply! I have read your link and I do seem to check a lot of the symptoms listed there... my therapist has also told me that PTSD is part of my problem (although not how much) and it is a matter we are working on. From what I read in your link the meds have also been spot on. I really have to start exercising but this is again something I just can't bring myself to do, I really have to break my will somehow.

Linzi
Re: Depression, anxiety and panic attacks
Wed Dec 14, 2016 2:51 am

Dear TiberiuSahlean

When you have time, read through all the comments posted on this forum, there are lots of people with a hectic past and present and are also AFRAID of the future... You are NOT alone.

What I have found, like you, I keep myself busy with doing something I like very much, I also walk around and take pictures of my pets and nature etc. to remind me of the beauty that still exist in this word. Look at YOUR avatar, you are a very very handsome man, just a bit too young for me....hahaha joking about the age part, but really you are very handsome (by us women standards)! There are people writing here with selfloath, I myself can't look at myself in the mirror or shop windows, because I used to be a VERY attractive woman who turned heads because I did kickboxing for a long time about 10 years ago and was well built, besides my good genes....I am very humble, make no mistake, I just mention here for the sake of what I am going through now: since my toxic relationship I am still in now, I have gained about 40 kg, you can make the sums, only 4 yours ago was was a pretty 64 kg...I looked at my engagement photos and other photos that were taken when me and now ex fiance started out our relationship....now my love life is affected because I can't even undress before him, I have serious self-esteem issues now and I feel like starving myself because no healthy eating and exercise I try still, seems to work, because the stress hormone Cortisol and my antidepressants are the cause of my "fattest I have ever ever been in my life"! Other people say I don't look so bad and I am still very attractive, but I DO NOT belief them because I think that they are only saying it to make me feel better.

I WILL maybe someday loos all the weight, I have lost about 3 kg the past two months, which are too slow for me but like I have mentioned the meds and stress counters that. Here in xxxx the white men likes their women skinny and blonde. I am on the other hand have only beautiful grey/green eyes (according to other people they are very striking) and very long black hair, but my weigh gain makes me feel like an outcast. At least I am very intelligent (I think so hahaha), because I am an avid reading especially about science and nature / biology and astronomy me, there is very little I DON'T know about those topics. AND I have a great sense of humor! When my very old cats (I have other interesting pets as well) barf all over the place, I sing our xxxx national anthem hahahaha....but my fiance don't think it is very funny even if I clean up quickly when my pets mess.

Try to keep your chin up, don't too many projects too soon, because if you are depressed, it will overwhelm you!

I really understand all that people are going through, that is why we all joined this forum.

Keep us posted regularly about how you feel...

Linzi
Re: Depression, anxiety and panic attacks
Wed Dec 14, 2016 3:00 am

Sorry about about all the spelling and grammar mistakes, it is not because I can't spell, but it is because I get so involved in my story that I don't realize my fingers do something else....hehehe and the reason I am xxxx maybe and does not notice..... my avatar is Linzi, it means "little cat / kitten" in xxxx which is my home language.

TiberiuSahlean
Re: Depression, anxiety and panic attacks
Wed Dec 14, 2016 5:47 am

Hello again Linzi. Please call me Tibi or Tiberiu. Thank you for the compliments, you are making me blush [blushing emoticon] and you are right you are really funny and I enjoyed reading your posts!

On a more serious note I have read some of the posts on this forum and I will continue to do so. I can relate very well with the part about antidepressants and gaining weight, I was usually around 60 kg but since I started taking meds I have been gaining weight and now I am at 80 kg; I know that does not sound bad but from my perspective it has put a lot of pressure on me, I don't feel very well with the extra weight plus it's all in the wrong parts; and because of my issues I have a hard time exercising it's unbelievable how I want to do something but it's like I have a magnet on my back that will not let me actually do it; I get really annoyed with myself sometimes over that.

It is really sad to read the struggles other members of the forum are going through so many young, beautiful people that are denied the joys and beauty of live and, as if not enough, even marginalized by our own kind as if we had a contagious disease... It's very nice to hear from all of you and I really am thankful for your responses!

Linzi
Re: Depression, anxiety and panic attacks
Wed Dec 14, 2016 8:56 am

I am smiling now because YOU are reaching out now and it is great!

When I have first join this forum end November, I thougt I was going to encounter weirdos who drinks blood, lick windows and torture small animals and so....not at all! We are all just normal beautiful minded people who struggle with bad issues...I cry every single day, but at least I can still feel...

Now I have finished my glass of wine, it is very very hot in my town, we have water shortages, my partner (I still don't know WHAT he is of me, because he can't give me a straight answer) is on holiday with his friends for a few days and I enjoy my own company.

I'm going to take out my African Grey parrot and take him outside on the grass... his wings I clip often so that he does not fly away....it is 15:49 now in xxxx, my parrot is calling me on my name and asks for "kos" (food), he wants to eat fruit on the lawn now....we must look for some shade first....I will take a plunge in our half filled swimming pool later (we have strict orders that during this draught, we are NOT allowed to waste water and can't even wash cars), because I am alone for few days I don't have to feel shy because nobody from outside can see me.

Take care young man, be proud! Will talk again!

Story/Discussion 5

(Source: www.depression-understood.org)
labellevie
Bipolar Depression
Sat Dec 10, 2016 3:49 pm

Hi everyone,

I have recently experienced a manic episode a few months ago and was hospitalized. I lost my job because of it and I have been bouncing from job to job because of my illness, not ever being satisfied with what I am doing. I have a degree in history and french and haven't been able to find suitable work other than waitressing. I decided I must go back to school to get a career. I finally decided on going back to school to be a social worker. The issue I have though is, I am a victim to my moods. I am so depressed at the moment and I recently quit my last job as a concierge. I am 27 and have really no real professional work experience. I feel like such a failure. And I have no money at the moment. I have to find a new job soon to pay rent but I just don't want to get out of the bed, ever. I feel so unmotivated, uninspired and uninterested in life. It is the complete opposite of who I am normally. I don't know how long this will last, but I have been isolating myself. I wish there was a place I could go and just be. Depression makes me so lazy, I don't want to see anyone or do anything. It's overwhelming. I don't know how to recover other than give it time. I don't feel like anything helps. I was told it takes 18 months to fully recover after a manic episode. It's like recharging a battery, all my neurotransmitters where used up in the episode. I just want to have a fulfilling career, surrounded by good friends with many interests and hobbies. Right now though, I feel such gloominess. I know staying in bed all day isn't an answer, but it's all I want to do.

Has anyone been so depressed they just gave up on having a job? I am in a circumstance I don't have a choice but to work. And that anxiety drives me crazy. I wish I could heal without having to worry about bills. I don't know, maybe I need to try harder and fake it more. I just am tired of living at this point.

Does anyone have any advice? I greatly appreciate support.

Response to Story/Discussion 5 (No Counter-Response as of 06-13-17)

Linzi

Re: Bipolar Depression
Sun Dec 11, 2016 5:26 am

Hello Labellevie

May I know (you don't have to talk about it if you don't want to...) if you have always been this way? How was your childhood and circumstances? Did anything VERY dramatic happened to you that made you this depressed?

I myself grew up in a violent home with a father who was supposed to protect his little daughter, but instead I have gone to bed with a broken lip every night...he abused my mother physically, mentally, emotionally and sexually, everything a woman can be done to and I witnessed it all. The circumstances at home was so bad that the social workers put me and my brother in a foster home for 4 years so that my parents can sort out their divorce and for my mother to start over in a different town. (I am from xx, xxxx). When I was grade 6, we got to live with my mother again and go to school in Paarl. (The foster home was in another town nearby)

But when I was in matric (grade 12), I have met a man three years older than me and from the first time I have met him I was smitten with his intelligence, because I grew up without friends always with my nose in books because I was so shy. I am mad for an intelligent guy, I ignored the fact that he was an unattractive wine farmer, but he had a charismatic personality. Needles to say, I have lost my virginity at 17 that year to him. Needles to say if you are such a young lady when it happens to you, you fall in love deeply...he was my very first love.

Unfortunately I was not prepared that he was a certified psychopath (I did not know then), I was told by his desperate and ashamed mother that I was the one causing his problem and violent outburst! I believed everything that I was accused of because I thought less of myself my whole childhood. Off course a shy barely speaking and scared naive 17 year old will NEVER start a fight, especially when I am afraid of him. Oh, I was VERY afraid of him, a psychopath MUST always be right or else there is trouble. He used to throttle me until I am blue in the face, I had to hide my injuries/ marks under a high necked shirt or something and my black marks on my arms as well. He even hunted me on his farm with a shotgun. We broke our relationship for a year while he gets therapy, but I was sooooo stupid to take him back and we got married when I was 22. We went to live and work in another town because his father sold the farm as it was time for his father to retire and my ex wanted to do diesel mechanics. We were married for a year (had a 5 year toxic relationship) and one evening he destroyed basically everything in the house and then I have realized he will NEVER change. It was a struggle to get him to divorce, but I did NOT get anything out of this divorce, I had to start over back in my old town.

Needless to say, with a childhood like I had and my experience with a psychopath (you value yourself as you are been told), my self esteem was nonexistent! It was so difficult keeping a job myself because I felt stupid and could not concentrate and I felt my bosses and coworkers was conspiring and picking on me. I felt like going back to bed every time the alarm goes off for work....I HATED everything and everybody and even eating....and I was only 24 years young....but I had never ever felt how it is to be confident and pretty and without stress. I still had no friends, I did not know HOW to talk to people....

Eventually I fell in love again a few times in my life, unfortunately always toxic relationships again because I needed to be needed....you can imagine yourself instead of being with someone who values me and takes care of me, it was the other way around and again I was not taken care of as a woman. It is a loooooong story if you have time and lots of wine I still don't have much friends at the age of 42, I am not married again and have no children. I am living with my ex fiance, because he can't decide if he wants to marry me or not. Unfortunately, I gave up a good job (the first one I have actually like) because he is so jealous and wanted me to come work for him from the rented home we are living in currently. Now because I am on antidepressants and have a history of permanent depression and anxiety, it is always MY fault when we fight of have a disagreement. I got so tired one day that I have tried to kill myself (Please NEVER do THAT!!! life is too beautiful and you will hurt your family) in front of him now he has more reason to think I am grazy and that I am the one destroying our relationship....I have had a talk with him and I have explained to him that he treats me like a dirty cloth most of the time that is why I became cold in bed because he does not listen to me and I feel dirty and foreplay for a woman begins in the head garbage in, garbage out.....the more he blames me for everything, the more I build a wall.

You see Labellevie, I am not a bad person, I have never been into drugs, I don't do sex with every man I meet, I am not white trash, I do not cheat ever on my partner and is most honest and friendly and loving. I just suffer from anxiety and my partners so far does not understand it, WILL NOT understand it and I seem to attract the dangerous, childish ones....I never feel good enough and at my age all the "good men" are married already, it seems.....

I am a psychological mess myself, I am also struggling to get work because the market is flooded with others also looking for work in my field (in xxxx there are not much opportunities for a white person)...and our Government is a corrupted mess (you can look up xxxx news on the internet).

But back to me....it is very very scary to be in a toxic relationship AND be dependent on your partner and being blamed for it....

It is very scary for me to to back to work after 4 years of staying home doing something else by helping my partner in his graphic design business....I have never had a good self-esteem and now I must try to sell myself in interviews all over again. I used to be very attractive and built like a sportswoman (I was a kickboxer 10 years back) and felt good about my appearance, but NOW at 42 I became overweight from a beautiful 64 kg to a 110 kg because of STRESS and anxiety (the stress hormone cortisol, makes you fat). When not having friends and a good job and being in a toxic relationship and not meeting other people and just clean up everyday and putting up with your partners moods bla bla bla.....I don't even want to show my face in public.

But just like in YOUR case, I must pick myself up and face the world and be brave and try and try again....WE must!

It helps to take my beloved African Grey parrot outside (I have clipped his wings) into the sun for a bit, because a lack of vitamin D can worsen your depression.....

I am not perfect, I cry everyday, I just hide it from people so that I don't get labelled...I take my pills (against my will, but it helps) every morning and sing a song while doing it....I make a joke out of everything and it becomes easier and funnier and even when I still can't look in the mirror at myself because I am so fat now, I dress neatly and put on a little makeup (just a little) and try to be friendly to everyone and make a point of smiling to strangers, because you do not know how they might suffer themselves....

I would like to know how YOU became so upset and depressed?...will you share it with me?

Story/Discussion 6

(Source: www.depression-understood.org)

sparks

Long term panic disorder, agoraphobia, depression and social phobia: really need help with a very difficult fight

Tue Dec 13, 2016 2:31 pm

Hi everyone

I'll keep it brief for now.

I'm a 26 year old female from the UK. I'm completely isolated with these conditions and it feels like all I've ever known. I've had hospitalisations as a teenager for depression. I'm a fairly intelligent person who used to be curious and care about things at one time I thought I was going to do lots of things and make the most of my life, but I have just been consumed by these illnesses in a world full of people who ave hardly any idea what they even are.

I've been almost totally housebound with panic disorder/agoraphobia from the age of 18, which I should still find terrifying and astounding, but at the moment I'm just numb to it all. I haven't had friends on any level since I was about 18. The social phobia returned full vengenance after a slighty more manageable period and I quickly developed panic disorder, when every second outside the house or around people was marked with that absolute terror and torture that is panic. I didn't even get a break: it just seemed constant, and the actual 1530 min panic attacks I get are not really that different from how I feel all the time. I often feel that I was just one of those people that were born 'weird'. I'm recently pushing for tests to rule out being on the autistic spectrum as I never really knew why I've had this intense fear of people since childhood and always felt so different all the time. I see no one day in day out. I had one person in my life at one point, my partner who really was just incredible and did everything he could but had to give up a couple of years ago and left me. Right now I'm studying with the Open Uni which, alongside the fact that I get financial support for these debilitating mental illnesses, is the one good thing in my life.

I don't want to kill myself. I want 26 to be the start of my life where I try to build some kind of livable and full-filling live for myself however I can. I want to get out there and make friends and be well enough to support myself and not be in this day-to-day hellish existence anymore.

Knowing how to do that is the issue. I get support from the mental health services, but the flat effect from the depression, and the panic and social fears make it so difficult to talk to and cooperate fully with them, despite trying desperately to. My parents have really tried recently and I feel that they're suffering from burnout and feel helpless. But until I can deal with this panic disorder monster and the terror of people that stops me from being able to make connections I don't know how anything can change. I am literally unable to say a word to another soul except from my parents and support worker. I live this hidden life and I'm sick to death of pretending that these illnesses don't really exist and having people not realise how serious it all is.

I've been forcing myself out, on my own several times a day recently. Every second I feel full of this deep dread, physically filling my insides until I actually feel like I'm drowning in it. I'm trapped in this fog, and barely have any idea of what's going on around me. I get this partial paralysis from the panic which gets worse the closer I am to other people. It feels like there's a force field coming from them which sezies up my muscles the closer they get. Sometimes part of me feels outside my body. I get all the panic attack-type delusions of losing control in different ways. I can't think properly. I can barely speak. Sometimes I feel like my brain's actually going to explode and I often feel like I'm going to die. I can't feel my legs, or they ache like I have the flu. Usually the only thing that 'soothes' me when I'm in that horrible state is imagining jumping off a bridge.

I've been trying to get to the library all week. I get about half way into town until it is physically and psychologically impossible to get any further. I am in total agony. My mind can't even imagine me going further, even if someone blindfolded me to reduce the stimulus causing the symptoms and pushed me in a wheelchair. I keep returning and usually can't get much further than the first time. I think about what other people have done at 26 and think how I've basically spent eight years either at home or venturing out to get to the local park or shop. It would almost be funny if it wasn't totally heartbreaking and alienating.

I was in touch with someone on a different forum and was speaking to him regularly but I think due to how scared and lonely I was, I was putting to much onto him. We had good conversations but he was probably too kind and accomodating. We were talking totally as friends but his wife got upset (which I feel awful about) and so we don't speak anymore. This felt like one lifeline and now it's gone. I obviously can't throw myself onto people, but I can't get well in this situation, totally on my own. I want to remember who I was and think about who I can be. I can't give up, but I desperately need help. The thing is, you need to have something to offer to make friends and so when something consumes you the way it has me you're out of luck.

Thanks for reading.

Response to Story/Discussion 6

Linzi

Re: Long term panic disorder, agoraphobia, depression and social phobia: really need help with a very difficult fight

Wed Dec 14, 2016 3:46 am

Dear Sparks

Please DO NOT feel alone. Agoraphobia is for real, I think all of us depressed people has a little trouble with that too, but not so severe as yours.

As I am typing here, I feel very nauseous of stress and depression and my pills are making me fat, I have gained 40 kg over 4 years because of stress hormone Cortisol that also contributes to weigh gain. You can picture yourself, I used to be a very pretty 64 kilograms and were very attractive to the point of turning heads because I was fit (I was a kick boxer for a very long time 10 years ago).....and now I am weighing more than the average man (104 kg) and I can't even look at myself in the mirror or shop windows...I loath myself, I have tried eating better and I go to the gym still, but I am so ashamed of myself and feels if everyone (they are all so slim) is checking me out, because I am the only one wearing men's tracksuit pants as the ladies pants don't look good on me....and I feel as I am the fattest...You know what, it is affecting my already toxic relationship with my ex fiance (he is still trying to work out if he wants me anymore or not) as well, because I feel so "rubbish" that I don't even want to undress in front of him and then he will say the nastiest things that you can say to a woman....THAT is f& up, but I am really really ashamed of myself...I feel like putting my fingers down my throat to barf out all of my meals, but I have read the stomach acid eats away your teeth....here in xxxx the men like their women skinny and blonde...I have only striking grey/green eyes left with my sense of humor....*

Sparks, I have serious issues and nowadays the same symptoms maybe of Agoraphobia, I don't feel like going out as well anymore, I am so great full that I am healthy but my weight...weight and self esteem....I really loath myself and don't know if somebody will ever love me when my partner leaves me....

STORIES/DISCUSSIONS 7 TO 9

Source: http://www.sadag.org/index.php?option=com_content&view=article&id=98:depressed-but-still-succesful-in-the-working-world-three-true-stories&catid=61&Itemid=143

Depressed, But Still Successful in the Working World: Three True Stories

Too often, depression sufferers are stigmatised as weak and unstable individuals. The truth of the matter is that many depression sufferers are well-qualified individuals with responsible jobs. We spoke to three depression sufferers who are still successful in the working world. They told us about the courage and strength it takes to overcome the trauma of a depressive disorder.

[Story 7] Cor du Bruin, 52, is an Insurance Broker Who Has Suffered From Depression for 15 Years. He is Divorced and lives with his two children.

I first became depressed when I was 37 years old. At that stage, I was working as an Insurance Financial Advisor and was earning money on a commission basis. Although my business was going well, my marriage was falling apart and my ex-wife and I were in the process of getting a divorce. I sunk into a deep depression. The last thing on earth I wanted to be facing was a divorce case.

Thankfully, I won the divorce case and got custody of my son, then aged ten, and my daughter, aged six. However, the depression had already set in and I was starting to lose income every month as a result of my poor performance. Within the next $5^1/_2$ years, I experienced a total of 20 different traumas which really affected me. The traumas included the death of both my father and my mother, two very bad car accidents, the death of three of our household pets and the loss of all my money in the bank. I had lost almost everything except my house.

I began to sleep the whole day. I used to shake so much that I couldn't hold a pen or write in front of other people. I experienced terrible anxiety and frequent suicidal thoughts. Finally, I went to see my local doctor who gave me a combination of medications to take. Unfortunately, I had a bad reaction to the pills. For a long time, I was very disillusioned with the medical health professionals I encountered. Over my 15 year period of depression, I have "fired" over 3 psychiatrists, 4 therapists and 9 GP's!

It helped a lot to get in touch with the Depression and Anxiety Support Group who have a referral list of medical professionals that are in the "know" about anxiety and depression. The Support Group can be contacted on (011) 783-1474/6 from 8am to 8pm Monday to Saturday. I now have a very competent psychiatrist and psychologist to help me through my bad patches. It also helped to realise that I had to start working on myself again. I started to read a lot of books on depression and enrolled at RAU to study Christian counselling.

I feel that I am now coping and enjoying life again. My business has picked up and I have good relationships with my two children. I really enjoy reaching out to other sufferers and counsellingthem. I think one needs discipline to overcome depression. Often people live too much in the past, and they have to learn how to replace negative thoughts with positive ones. Time, self-knowledge, exercise and spirituality are all important in beating depression. I am now involved with the group and run my own support group in Southdale.

[Story 8] Mary Is a 35-Year Old Senior Primary Teacher Who Has Suffered Sporadically From Depression for the Last 12 years. She Lives With Her Husband and Two Children.

In my youth, my dad always used to joke about my erratic temperament. However, overall I as a busy and confident youngster with an optimistic attitude to life. Then, in my early 20's, a culmination of circumstances caused me to develop bad anxiety. I had bad reactions to medication I had to take for my allergies, was involved in a very threatening situation and was negatively affected by a close friend's terrifying experience. I seemed to handle the traumas at the time, but in the long term, they took their toll on me. I developed panic attacks which then developed into severe agoraphobia. I was afraid to leave my house. At that stage I was dating my would-to-be husband who was very supportive of them. Luckily I found a self-help book on phobias and managed to work my way through it on my own. Soon, everything seemed to stabilise again and I got married.

Then, in 1990, I had to deal with another series of traumas. The traumatic birth of my first child coupled with the fact that our baby contracted a rare disease that could have been fatal, created a worrying scenario. As well as this, we moved and I found that I didn't know anyone. Depression set in for months on end, but I hid if from my husband and my relatives. I wasn't really sure what was happening to me. Eventually, I opened up to my husband who encouraged me to go and visit a local female GP. I was given some pills for a short period. The depression abated only to resurface three years later with the birth of my second baby.

The situations for my second bout of depression were very similar to those of my first. I experienced another traumatic birth and we moved to a different city where I didn't know anyone. The future became very uncertain and this was the worst episode I had ever had. I remember going on a family holiday and feeling suicidal I was experiencing unbelievable anxiety and terrible insomnia. It was about this time that I realised the negative effect my mood was having on my children. This motivated me to go and visit a specialist in Pretoria who gave me medication and a short therapy course. It was the best thing I ever did. The depression lifted and I felt in control of my life again. I started working as a Senior Primary teacher at the beginning of 1997.

I find my work as a teacher very fulfilling and also help run a support group for depression and anxiety sufferers in Witbank. I have learnt through my experience that one shouldn't be afraid to ask for help and support. I waited too long before I opened up to anyone about how I was feeling. At the same time, however, I am continually working on myself. You've got to be prepared to put the effort in to recover. I believe in a holistic approach to recovery – body, mind and spirit are all equally important in my eyes.

[Story 9] Feon, 52, Is a Practicing Chartered Accountant Who Has Suffered With Depression for the Past Eight Years. He is Divorced and lives With His One Son.

If I look back, I would probably say that I've suffered from mild depression my whole life – kind of like the "Sunday afternoon blues". However, I've always functioned pretty well and coped with everything that has come my way. In 1991, I was working as a group management accountant at a listed company, when my wife began to institute divorce proceedings against me. She started threatening that I would never see my children again, and this triggered off a major depression. My work suffered as a result, and I eventually went to se a therapist who told me that I seemed to be suffering from depression. I was very stubborn and denied it, but eventually I agreed to go and see a psychiatrist. The psychiatrist confirmed that I was clinically depressed and tried me on a variety of medications.

In May 1995 I found a medication that worked for me. Things have improved drastically since then. I have started up my own accounting practice from home which is going well. In retrospect, I feel that my experience of depression has been a very good growth experience. I've become a lot more aware of other people's feelings. I've also learnt so much more about depression and can recognise it in others. As a result of this, I've been able to help a lot of people close to me who are suffering from depression. You can never really fight for somebody else, but you can be supportive and understanding in your approach.

I really don't view depression as something to be ashamed of – to me its like somebody who has a problem with gall stones or kidney stones. I believe that depression is far more prevalent than most people realize.

STORY/DISCUSSION 10 TO 12

Source: http://www.sadag.org/index.php?option=com_content&view=article&id=163:true-stories-of-career-women-who-beat-depression&catid=61&Itemid=143

True Stories of Career Women Who Beat Depression

Too often, depression sufferers are stigmatised as weak and unstable individuals. The truth of the matter is that many depression sufferers are well-qualified individuals with responsible jobs. We spoke to three successful career women who told us about the courage and strength it takes to overcome the trauma of a depressive disorder.

[Story 10] Thumi Works as a Teacher at a Middle School. She Is Married With a Son and Daughter

My story starts last year in February when I began to experience bad family problems. I reacted by becoming very depressed and avoiding people. I also began to experience strange physical symptoms such as shortness of breath and dizziness. Before long my work began to suffer and the principal decided to give me some leave. I was hospitalised for one week, during which time I attended a number of valuable therapeutic sessions and consulted with a psychiatrist. After my hospitalisation, I went to stay with my mother in Pretoria for another restful week. I did a lot of soul searching when I was with my mother. I realised that I had to gain courage and learn how to face other people again. I left my mother's house a completely different person. I am now completely healthy and working hard as a teacher. I am also studying in my spare time and will be graduating in April. My advice to other depression sufferers is to try and stop putting the blame on themselves. Instead, they should have courage and walk tall.

[Story 11] Sebo, 25, Works at Standard Bank as a Senior Officer. She Lives With Her Mom, Dad and Two Sisters.

At the beginning of last year, a very traumatic incident occurred with a friend of mine. I discovered that my friend was using my ID and CV as her own, and was working in a very comfortable job under the pretense of being me. It was a very big shock to me as she was one of my closest friends and I would have trusted her with anything. I slipped into a very bad depression after I found out. I couldn't eat or sleep and I lost a lot of weight. The hardest thing was that there was no one I could share my agony with. After the court hearing in June last year, I felt I had to speak to someone about what I was going through. I got hold of the toll-free number for the Depression and Anxiety Support Group in Gauteng. I phoned up and was put through to a very understanding and supportive counsellor who explained to me that I could be suffering from depression. The Support Group sent me some very useful brochures on the causes, symptoms and treatment for depression. Through reading these brochures, I was finally able to understand what I was going through. That was the catalyst for my recovery. I have slowly been able to piece my life back together over the last year or so. Although I will always be hurt over the betrayal of my friend, I am starting to trust people again and feel stronger very day. The Support Group can be contacted weekdays from 8am to 7pm and Saturdays from 8am to 5pm on (011) 783-1474/6 or (011) 884-1797.

[Story 12] Zondi, 36, Is a Teacher at a Primary School. She Lives by Herself.

In 1995 my father died, and shortly afterwards I began to suffer from severe headaches, sleeplessness, lethargy and a depressed mood. I eventually went to see a doctor in Pretoria who told me that I was suffering from stress. He prescribed some tablets which I began to take. A while later I heard about a workshop that the Depression and Anxiety Support Group were holding at Soweto College. The workshop was very useful in that I learnt what I was really suffering from and how to deal with it. I also learnt how to handle the problems as they came. What my experience taught me is that people don't know enough about depression in xxxx. In total, I suffered with depression for 3 years. I think it is very important that people are made more aware about depression and the symptoms and treatment. I would also recommend depression sufferers consult professionals about their disorders.

Anyone can have depression but, these days there is no need for people to suffer unnecessary anguish. Help is readily available, either through medication, psychotherapy or support groups, depending on the severity of the individual's illness.

Clinical depression often goes untreated because people don't recognise the many symptoms. They may know some symptoms, such as sadness and withdrawal, but they are unaware of others, including anxiety, irritability and sleeplessness. As with many illnesses, if treatment is needed, the earlier it begins, the more effective it can be. Early treatment also increases the likelihood of preventing serious recurrences. Joining a patient support group can be very helpful during the recovery process. Support group members share their experience with the illness, learn coping skills and exchange information on community providers.

STORY/DISCUSSION 13

(Source: www.depression-understood.org)

DDJ

What happens after "therapy" is finished?

Sun Dec 11, 2016 12:34 pm

I joined this site months ago, have not posted since as it has been too difficult to do anything but get through the days. Am still seeing a very good therapist (every 2 weeks now). Amoung everything else I am wondering what is next. I feel like I should put on the "I'm all better now" coat and move on....put this last 2...? 3 years in a box, tape it shut and stop focusing on me stuff.

It is strange but I look around at my family, friends and work and my inside person just says "nothing matters.

Time to give up thinking they do." (No I am not hearing voices...just a dispondent inner self)

Thinking if I stop seeing her, stop the meds (Zoloft)....everything will go away.....

Responses to Story/Discussion 13

Linzi

Re: What happens after "therapy" is finished?
Mon Dec 12, 2016 3:20 am

Hi DDJ

I suggest you take your medication and stop thinking too much of it. Please do NOT tell people (especially your bosses and coworkers) that you suffer from depression because they WILL discriminate against you, even your boyfriends and girlfriends.... trust me, they will judge you and make you feel more bad of yourself. I speak of experience....not a lot of people these days know that I struggle with it and now I get to be treated normal with respect.

If you want to talk, rather talk to strangers like me and others on this site just to vent.

Luckily I have a great sense of humor, even if I cry inside....I look for the beauty in everything (not PERSONS because they disappoint me), I take my mobile phone outside and take random pictures of my garden of other gardens or flowers and my pets and share it with some family and discuss it rather than how I feel...I write privately my heart out in poems and put it away so that I don't see it again, maybe later when I come across it again and thinks differently about it.

Please never try suicide, you will hurt your family and yourself and life is too beautiful. There WILL be episodes that you'll feel very bad again and maybe even that it is the end of the word. Take yourself outside and sit in the sun a bit, because vitamin D makes you feel better. Take vitamin supplements for stress and try to exercise regularly to look better and feel better.

What helps the BEST for ME crying!!! every day....afterwards you feel your feeling is done and dusted. Like I said, don't let anyone into your "mood secret"....smile to everyone in the street to get smiles back....you might just brighten another sad person's day as well.

It will not be a quick fix, but keep your dignity and your head up!!!

DDJ
Re: What happens after "therapy" is finished?
Tue Dec 13, 2016 4:08 am

I am trying to be ok with the meds. (Unfortunately because I am a nurse, I know sometimes meds are needed...and that you should not stop "cold turkey". ..but there is another part of me that feels very isolated and alone on them). i go to great lengths to not vent at work. Some of my coworkers I thought were friends...we have worked together for over 30 years...I think would rather see me gone. Most days, if I let my control slip I would like to see me gone too.. Although It is very true that most of us want the emotional pain to end more than our lives. Just not sure how long the therapist will " put up with me".

Linzi
Re: What happens after "therapy" is finished?
Tue Dec 13, 2016 5:26 am

Hi DDJ

It is the therapist JOB to listen to all our crap, that is what he or she went to university for.

Therapists are so expensive here in xxxx (I don't know where you are from), because here we do not have "free" medical assistance. We have medical aid for which we pay a lot for every month, or you can register at a State Hospital and pay less for meds, but it will only be be a brief consultation because you will be one of MANY sitting in a line for counseling.

As long as you can afford to visit a therapist, keep doing so or else if you start feeling "ashamed" (I also tend to feel that I bore people after a while...), I check this site regularly because I had a very traumatic life (other people even worse as you will find if you go through all the conversations) and have been suffering from depression my whole life. Go through all the conversations posted by "Linzi" to get to know me better if you want to...

Just hold on there, we all have our ups and downs....they way you feel about your coworkers...

I have had experience with getting discriminated against that is why I advise not to talk about depression with "normal" people because they fill feel some kind of obligation and will start to avoid you or make you feel bad so to alienate you so that you don't become a burden to them.

But speaking about "normal", you would be surprised what even "normal" people go through, they are just coping better with it maybe or does not know that they also have depression or whatever...

But don't feel isolated, I am a 42 year old woman who had never find the right man to get married to or having children with and because of toxic relationships, I have to start over plenty of times in my life. I feel like a FAILURE!

Luckily I have an appreciation for nature and biology and animals and walk around with my mobile and take photos of nature and of my pets and forward it to whomever is interested. If you talk about "positive" things, you will draw people...the right positive kinds who will enjoy your company.

It may seem very selfish of me, but because I can't handle my OWN depression, I try to avoid other negative persons because I don't want to belong to a "club" and to be stigmatized. I would rather talk about depression and my experience on this depression forum because I will not be judged here and have a choice when I want to advise / help someone, because in a way I help myself....in real life, I want my good sense of humor to rule and make me a nice person to be with, even if I cry inside (I cry EVERY day, but at least I have some emotion, I am not dead).

You can talk as much as you like here, we all bore each other hahahahaha, I'm joking!!!

We'll speak again xox

STORY/DISCUSSION 14

(Source: www.depression-understood.org)
Mozmoz
Hi...
Mon May 13, 2013 10:51 am

Uhm... Hey there.

I decided to join since I'm too shy to talk to people face to face. I hope to make some friends here, since folks don't really care about me here.

I've been coping with depression for about 6 or 7 years now. It never really bothered me though, (sounds crazy when I say that) up until last year. I've been in therapy and things got better, up until about a week ago.

Anyway, about me. I'm 17, turning 18 this year, and I'm from xxxx. I love music, and I dj occasionally at school and parties. I also love drawing/ sketching, digital art (photoshop and 3D animation) and movies. I'm introverted and very shy, even though i try not to be. Seems like there's no getting away from that though.

So uhm yeah.. Thanks for reading.. I'm looking forward to meeting you guys.

Responses to Story/Discussion 14

hollyann
Moderator
Mon May 13, 2013 10:57 am

Hi Nice to meet you. Did something happen a week ago to trigger this into making it worse? Are you working on ways in therapy to help you socially?

hollyann
Mozmoz
Mon May 13, 2013 11:46 am

Hello hollyann. Nice to meet you too, and thanks for the quick reply.

I posted the whole story under the "my story" section. It's a bit of a long read though.

I have been on therapy last year and it did get better, until last week. Luke I said, I posted the whole story.

Section 3

Rethinking the Current Paradigm:

Analyzing Individual/Collective Agency in a Technologically Mediated Society

Chapter 6
Lonely Typers at Midnight:
Investigating the Quandaries of Millennial Illness Through Digital Ethnography of Reddit

Brandon Niezgoda
Drexel University, USA

ABSTRACT

Also known as Generation Y, Millennials—an American construct to classify those born from the early 1980 to mid-1990s—have been targeted by mainstream media as narcissistic, and internet obsessed. But as Diesing (2011) organizes, gross generalizations of the American cohort's vanity may only contain nuggets of truth. If millennials are in fact narcissistic and technologically oriented, this research attempts to understand whether this psychological assessment is innate, or deterministic. Contemporary online platforms allow users to voice their opinions and insight regarding predominant frames constructed by once exclusive media domains. Analysis of Reddit discussions through digital ethnography has worked to better understand modes of agency, or lack thereof, as this demographic navigates health problems in a technologically mediated society; providing insight for practitioners, patients, and family members in how to properly conceptualize illness to best help them, and the social order.

DOI: 10.4018/978-1-5225-3716-8.ch006

Copyright © 2018, IGI Global. Copying or distributing in print or electronic forms without written permission of IGI Global is prohibited.

INTRODUCTION

Millennials encompass, roughly, people born from the early 1980s to mid-1990s. Numerous mainstream media sources have framed the cohort negatively (Donatone, 2014; Duam, 2015; Faw, 2012; Ghose, 2013; McGrew, 2013; Smith & Aaker, 2013). In his May 2013 article, Stein classifies millennials as the "Me Me Me" generation. He uses statistics such as "40% believe they should be promoted every two years, regardless of performance," and selective findings from a 2002 study showing that only 60% of people under twenty-three want more responsibility at work, to support his claim that millennials are innately lazy and entitled.

Stein perceives millennials suffering from a constant anxiety of missing out on something better, as they interact all day almost entirely through screen. He further presents millennials as apathetic wherein "because millennials don't respect authority, they also don't resent it,"; that millennials aren't rebelling against their hardships, nor are they even sullen.

Loeb (2015) identifies millennials' relationship with consumer technology—which proliferated during their formative years— is what defines them. Their primary form of activism, rather than protests, civil disobedience or sit ins, is the Facebook campaign. Loeb further categorizes millennials as black and white minded in issues of business and society, and having already reshaped public advocacy in dramatic and influential terms, they "expect far more from the institutions that govern our society".

But it is too provincial, with insidious repercussions, to dismiss or generalize an entire age group in such a tumultuous, and complicated society. As one, if not the most consequential facet in civilization that exists beyond social construction, this research analyzes how millennials navigate their health issues in the sociological field (Bourdieau, 1980) that has been set up for them.

The specific objective of this chapter is to investigate millennials from the perspective of healthcare. Analysis of reddit discourses through six months of digital ethnography provides individual and collective insight into an "entitled" generation as online platforms offer a chance for citizens to deliberate, and contemplate frames— both mainstream, and academic.

BACKGROUND

This literature review covers six predominant points of reference for the research sample (online millennial discourses regarding healthcare): General Thoughts on Millennials, Wondering How or Why Millennials use the Internet, Millennials and Health Plans, How Millennials Experience Being a Patient, How Healthcare Providers See Millennials, and finally Millennials Use of the Web in Healthcare.

General Thoughts on Millennials

Ordun and Akun (2016) investigated links between millennial personality characteristics and associated emotional intelligence. Findings show that, depending on self-perceptions, millennials do valuate themselves relatively high on positive traits (e.g. honest, out-going, etc.) and low on negative traits (e.g. unhelpful, dishonest, etc.). According to personality characteristics and perspective, millennials were found to be highest in openness, and lowest in neuroticism. Millennials face stress from academic, social, and personal challenges. Bland, Melton, Welle & Bigham (2012) find that beyond traditional ways of coping (sleep, listening to music, relaxing), millennials surf the internet and participate in social network sites.

Millennials lack of loyalty, low expectations, and distrust that they find in the workplace, is, in turn, reproduced in a vast array of institutions. Their bewildering interactions with institutions bolster "young people's visions of themselves as completely alone, teaching them that they can depend on no one but themselves" (Silva, 2014, p. 1389). In a psychographic analysis of Generation Y college students, Woolburg & Pokrywczynski (2001) find millennials cognizant that institutions made available to past generations including social security, pensions, job security, and healthcare, may not remain for them.

How or Why Millennials Use the Internet

Despite characterizations of millennials as being internet obsessed, Leung (2013) found no real generational differences in using Facebook and blogs to satisfy social needs.

Jones and Czerniewicz (2010) chastise oversimplified characterizations of millennials as a distinct net generation (as compared to Baby Boomers). More so, he finds that the popularized discourse of a generation 'bathed in bits and bytes since birth', and separated and unique from other generations, has a wide social impact, with "echoes found in business literature and government policy" (p. 317).

Whereas similarities are found between generations, the social media use of generation Y encompasses intra-generational variance arising from environmental factors including "economic, cultural, technological and political/legal factors" and individual factors including "goals, emotions, and social norms'" (Bolton et al. 2013, p. 245).

Rather than treating the technology use of millennials as banal Jones & Healing (2010) assume interaction with technology is mediated by activity, and an initial stance. Millennials have made exceptional efforts to understand technology, wherein the picture is more complex than "the equation of exposure to new technologies and a generational change of attitudes and capacities" (344). To that point, the Uses and Gratifications Perspective has been appropriate in classifying SNS use by millennials. In forging identifies and maintaining relationships, the relatively impersonal nature of online environment is seen to facilitate young participants in negotiating the practicalities that can arise offline (Dunne, Lawlor, & Rowley, 2010).

Anderson (2010) recognizes ambitious, genuine, and sensitive practices of millennial "digital natives," including an enthusiastic embracement of social media in sharing personal information to "build friendships, form and find communities, seek help, and build their reputations (p. 2)". Beyond a rite of passage, she finds millennials will retain their willingness to share personal information (online and offline), even as they grow older and take on more responsibilities. She further recognizes that, diachronically, connected teens and young adults will both benefit and suffer due to their "hyperconnected lives" (p. 1); and that this will have a "significant impact on politics, power and control" (p. 17).

Millennials and Health Plans

Various reports categorize millennials as betrayed and alienated by Washington healthcare policy (Chastain 2013; Farris, Chong, & Danning; 2002; Furchgott-Roth & Meyer, 2015; Huang, 1997; Pallfrey, Tonniges, Greenm & Raymand, 2005; Ransford, Carrillo, & Rivera (2010)), rather than being ungrateful, or sullen about meritorious service. While millennials appreciated the premise and fundamental principle of Obamacare, they disavowed practical implementations of the law, nor did they respond well to the desperate, and patronizing marketing campaigns (Cahn & Cahn, 2006; Leonhardt & Query, 2016).

Assessing health knowledge among the millennial generation, Lloyd et al. (2013) find millennials have "advice driven knowledge,": fleeting sound bites such as don't smoke, or take your medicine. This advice driven knowledge, however, is likely to "to restrict and limit problem solving when faced with new or complex situations" (p. 41). They advocate for more research to determine not only how millennials acquire health knowledge, but if this knowledge is dynamic or static. In policy, they advocate stakeholders in health education to confront and accommodate new learning patterns of the millennial generation.

As in Diesing's 2016 report "Millenials, Who They are, What They Want, & Why You Need Them", generation Y provides particular challenges as both patients and employees.

The cultural anxieties engendered by millennials in healthcare professions have begun to tax recruiters and HR departments. Research examining expressions from stakeholders including scientists, nurses, and pharmacists has found there will be ongoing challenges in implementing a set of practices to accommodate each collective demographic, and their associated values (Keltgen, 2016). The current healthcare paradigm must be adjusted, with particular emphasis placed on substituting an aging workforce with a new generation. This needs to be done with budget austerity, and will be challenging. The key to this solution is proactivity, rather than reactivity (Gass & Bezold, 2013).

Weick (2008) regards millennials as a welcome contribution to the nurse workforce. Despite some capriciousness in their boundaryless careers, "their very resilience makes it imperative that the hospital environment be seen as welcoming and appreciative" (29). If not, they will choose to work somewhere else, and the hospital system will suffer for it. Millennials provide a technological affinity, a readiness to share/participate in creating solutions, but need to be catered to (flexibility in hours, and assignments) for these strong traits shine through.

In evaluating the primary differences of four generations silent generation, baby boomers, generation x, and generation y), Olson (2008) has investigated the pragmatic applications needed to take place so as to unleash each team members potential, and foster harmony in a synergistic way between all departments and levels in the healthcare institution. Growing up in constant contact with technology, millennials are uncomfortable in workplaces with technological debt. For workplaces and daily practices, between baby boomers and millennials, the technological divide has led to problems: in coordination, trust, communication, and overall organizational efficiency. There is a distinguished division in attitudes and work habits "between administrative staffs dominated by baby boomers, and nursing, physician, and lower administrative positions filled mostly by millennials" (237), which can have insidious implications for patients.

In reviewing literature on Millennials from the perspective of healthcare leaders, Piper (2012) recommends gatekeepers to remain cognizant of the literature portraying millennials as entitled, whether real or perceived. Adoption of social media use among public health agencies remains in the early adoption stage (Thackerary, Neigher, Smith, Van Wagener, 2012), with predominant ethical issues in using social media for healthcare issues deserving further issues (McKee, 2013). It has been noted that some Health professionals find that it would be potentially useful to integrate social media in their professional lives (George, 2011). Their indecision is marked by the Pharmaceutical marketing industries attempts to commercial social media (as they have done with television) against the FDA's (limited) imposition (Greene & Kesselheim, 2010). Social media accounts have been found to be very common among health science students (64%-96%) while increasingly rare for professional clinicians (13%-47%) (Von Muhlen & Ohno-Machado, 2012). In all, it has been situated that there are motives, barriers, and expectations for patients' and professionals' use of social media that have not been bridged (Atheunis, Neiboer, & Tates, 2013).

How Healthcare Providers See Millennials

Sarringhaus (2011) detects social media as a resource largely untapped in the healthcare field; one that presents opportunities and advantages, will innovate healthcare and create competitive advantages for adopters—if used properly.

Socio-technical integration has been recognized as one of the most important factors to transform the medical world for better and safer care. This is perhaps only rivaled by the continued integration of generation Y into the healthcare system, as the cohort has generated significant positive changes in other industries. This generation is a singularity, and ICT designers must consider generation Y's potential effects (Mills et. al., 2007).

Cowan (2010) categorizes a millennial driven transformation of primary care, where power and decision-making ability has shifted more towards the patient. Rather than the paternalistic image of the all-knowing physician, the shift provides the possible role of a partner in patient directed health decision-making as "new realities drive health professionals to interact with patients in entirely new ways" (p. 379), including internet-based information technology and social behavior shifts. Knowledge gaps between doctors and patients have dramatically shifted, with social networks to self-organize, and internet portals and Personal Health records to empower patients. Still, few doctors, and limited hospitals, have provide electronic extensions to share in the process. Many physicians oppose patients becoming self-informed, for fear that some may get it wrong.

Unresolved temporal issues of in-person care, and ambivalence towards internet accessibility are ongoing issues. Primary care services remain underproductive in all too short face-to-face encounters. In the current paradigm people who need more time with a physician are not accommodated, because patients who sometimes don't need to see the doctor to have their needs met by an overburdened system, did. Woolf et al. (2005) find that the promotion of informed choice through correcting and adapting technological solutions will supplement a human element to make the doctor/patient process work better: including increased patient autonomy, broader access to information, complex tradeoffs, and greater accommodation of personal values.

How Millennials Experience Being a Patient

As according to a survey conducted by Harris Interactive, there is a distinct disconnect of the expectations of the digitally connected Generation Y and the structural realities of healthcare's current infrastructure. A conducted survey found 54 percent find dealing with their health as frustration, 63 percent feel that they are at the mercy of their doctor's or dentists front desk staff when making an appointment, with more than fifty percent admitting they delay getting medical care because the process is a 'pain.

Concerningly the young population—as of now—is much more reluctant to seek out preventative care. The research suggests for healthcare, as an institution, to catch up technologically to other industries. As ZocDoc CEO and founder Dr. Oliver Hharraz identifies, Generation Y is feeling "powerless and frustrated by the current state of healthcare." But, despite calls to modernize the process, a national poll finds however that Americans in need of health consolation still turn to traditional lines of communication. Even if their doctors provided social media or instant messaging channels, 84% wouldn't use it.

Sullivan (2011), found millennial college students have a significant misunderstanding of asthma control, and need better medical education from their doctors or elsewhere. Most do not understand the basic processes of the ailment, exacerbated by the fact that they face a variety of barriers and limitations that prevent access to care and difficulties adapting to environmental changes, climate changes, etc. In investigating use and acceptance of social media among health educators as a means for communication, it was found that reasons for lack of use included employer monitoring/blocking of social media, belief that social media would not enhance job performance, and, that there is a difficulty of use among older health educators. (Hanson, West, Neiher Thackerary, and Barnes, 2011). Adoption of Local Health Departments Nationwide as a communication tool to educate and inform their constituents has been slow (24% with Facebook, 8% Twitter) (Harris, Mueller, Snider, 2013), and little is known about the group subscribers.

MAIN FOCUS OF THE CHAPTER

This research uses discourse analysis of Reddit discussions to analyze the experiences of millennials in contemporary healthcare, the discourses debating potential remedies, and diffusion of practices ranging from journalistic framing to government legislature (Rogers, 1962).

Issues, Controversies, Problems

A majority of academic research utilizes a top-down perspective to study millenials, particularly surveys, while mainstream media has many times cherry picked scientific data and/or historical assumptions. This methodology will be able to provide firsthand accounts of the cohort in free-flowing discussion on what it means to be a millennial suffering through illness.

Scholarship has identified online communities as a new public sphere where users may speak freely and deliberate discursive frames (Dahlberg, 2001; Papacharissi, 2002; Poor, 2005) with a particular self-referentiality in platforms like Reddit (Flock, Meinhart, Zeitfogel, & Strohmaier, 2014). Principally, the affordance of Reddit to begin discussion threads with hyperlinking to online media articles, studies provides a deliberative space to conceptualize the associated framing (i.e. millennials as lazy); whether supporting or contradicting the information.

Medical history and medical experience is sensitive. Being among other people in a non-threatening and permissive experience can empower participants, particularly cohorts with limited power and influence in the field (Ivanoff & Hultberg, 2005). Rather than one on one interviews, Reddit resembles closer a real conversation (Morgan, 1997); wherein millennials have been found to be distrustful of institutionalism.

Raw data has been categorized into themes. Themes will be categorized via social constructivism, wherein participants work to make sense of their experiences and come to new understandings of how they are to navigate, or wish to be treated, in the medical field. A comprehensive search on Reddit has been enacted.

Primary focus will be on how millennials perceive the medical industry, how they are treated within it, how they integrate contemporary technology either through the portals provided to them or through their own methods, where they see problems in the medical industry or in their own conceptualization of the medical industry, and where they feel it can be remedied.

Six months were spent participating as a "Redditor". The author himself has suffered from three medical ailments that are, stereotypically, not what you would expect from a seemingly healthy looking young man. He was diagnosed with an insulinoma, a tumor found almost exclusively in older women. In inducing lower blood sugar, an insulinoma can cause signs of lassitude that have been construed by people as stereotypical millennial laziness/narcissism (i.e. members of his collegiate cross-country team and associated coaches believed he made up his proclaimed high-school running times when he performed inadequately at the college level—blaming his failures on egotism. Following the tumor removal, he suffered from adhesions, a debilitating but "invisible" ailment found mostly in women post-pregnancy, and in 95% of abdominal surgeries. As a medical issue, researchers (Gutt, Schemmer, Mehrabi, & Büchler, 2004; Menzies & Ellis, 1990; Monk, Bergman, Montz, 1994) recommend both better public knowledge and technological processes, wherein because adhesions are caused by surgery, most doctors will refuse to perform more surgery to "fix them." With limited objectives tests to identify adhesions, patients will be left in self-doubt. Further, more communication beforehand has been recommended as sufferers of long term medical problems, both the family and patient, must be cognizant that although a primary medical incident may be over, there will be aftershocks.

Finally, the digital ethnographer as a member of generation Y (born in 1988), suffered peripheral edema caused by a rib injury, another ailment that is principally seen in older adults.

The researcher was interested in discursive patterns of medical discussion by other people who identify as millennials. A total of two hundred posts were made by the author during the time, while the majority of time was done "lurking," or reading content. As according to Pink, Horst, Postill, and Hjorth (2016) the method of digital ethnography can capture "digital rhythms," drawing attention to the mundane and hidden dimensions of how and why digital media and content matter (p.46).

RESULTS

In a method of social constructivism, five predominant themes have emerged.

Theme 1: Trying to Work Through the Pain

Reddit posts and subsequent conversations have displayed a strong resilience in millennials coping with illness, despite demoralizing circumstances. Millennials display awareness of the dire social status that they are in (socioeconomically), and wish to work through their pain.

Reddit AMA's (ask me anything) are dialogic devices where people offer insight into their lives, providing questioners the power to ask what they wish. In the sub-reddit Medical School, an AMA "I am a medical student dealing with mental illness," featured a spirited debate with fellow medical school participants eager to learn how someone has coped in such a competitive industry, and the AMA hosts as "honored" to help with their feedback.

As regarded by the AMA host, there is a strong pressure for normalization in medical education, and many do their best to not use their illness as a crutch. On the contrary, many choose not to disclose their illness because of the competitiveness. The host of the AMA did not notify the program administrators himself, but rather was called into the associate Dean's office to discuss his medical blog. No accommodations were provided, but the host was confident they would've been provided if necessary. Rather than dropping out of the competitive environment, seeking support of peers and friends (breaking the day up with exercise and coffee breaks with friends) would help. Many participants in the AMA found the blog of the author to be highly beneficial to them.

Some millennials have tried to work through the pain of illness, only to have others not allow them to show their tenacity; and thus, fall into stereotypical frames. This was construed in a thread "Redditors with Chronic illness, how do you do it? The day to day, just life? (Serious)" in the Ask Reddit sub community. A reddit member had planned to join the army after high school. But after being diagnosed with diabetes he learned that this would not happen. Others would not understand what he needed when his glucose levels would go low, and he would get occasional looks during his injections. The user was dismayed when his theater director didn't consider him for a lead role because the director felt his "diabetes could affect my attendance, even though that had never been a problem." He is afraid that one day he may "slowly wither away" in not being able to afford his medication. Yet, he refuses to complain or back down, and wanted this role.

Many have planned to work through their pain, to the point that they do not wish to bother with bureaucratic and underserving medical service. That is, as opposed to a millennial taking advantage of the system, the system takes advantage of them. For Reddit user "Skokage," even working for a healthcare company his insurance was manipulative and did not provide service worth the cost. With 1000 dollars worth of charges for tests after dropping a weight on his chest in the gym because of a $3,000-dollar deductible, the user generally refuses to go to the doctor "unless I broke something or am in fear of death." A member of the thread stated, "Those lazy millennials", amidst various posts referencing the manipulative system including "not cool with paying $500 every time I go to the doctor," and "Still in debt from the few times I did go," to showcase the absurdity of derogatory millennial frames without context. As one community member referenced, millennials face different political and social circumstances coming of age in this time rather than in the past, which make their actions contextual; "Remember when check-ups were a thing? Me neither because I'm a millennial."

Theme 2: Gaslighting Millennial Illness

The second emergent theme is the gaslighting of millennials in illness; a problem that can be associated with derogatory framing of millennials taken at face value, wherein millennials are a immoral generation corrupting a virtuous society. This was showcased in the subreddit community "Late Stage Capitalism," in a thread discussing the article "The Gaslighting of the Millenial Generation- Mental Health and Millennial Overwork". In a neo-Marxist analysis users find the derogatory frames about millennials as an ultimate scapegoating against the society that has been created, and millennials refusal to take part in the current paradigms of dehumanizing capitalism that is filled with "degrading, and sometimes downright pointless jobs." As one participant regards:

All the articles that are written about how millennials are lazy and stupid is basically the capitalists being mad that we have no money or future to buy things so they are blaming us instead of the people with the money who actually ruined the world.

The gaslighting theme of millennials is played out in sub-communities and threads on invisible illness. This was showcased in a post entitled:

Anyone diagnosed with an invisible illness at a young age; How do you handle people who insist you can't be "that sick" bc of your age? Getting pretty tired of folks older than me giving me shit over my illness bc of my age.

As "Emily1917" states, she has numerously been told, "you don't look sick." Reddit member "OpaiOctober" laments that he is constantly told:

"You're so young," you don't look sick" or "but you don't act sick.". As another user states, millenials are chastised for the invisibility of their illnesses. "I've gotten the attitude of nothing can be wrong with me because I got dressed for my appointment and am smiling. It's exhausting.

"Ivybelle" retells how a nasty receptionist would always say "you are too young to have this many problems!" after reviewing her paperwork. The receptionist would state, "You need to take better care of yourself or you will feel terrible when you get old like me!"; placing blame for "not taking care of myself."

As "Lyradunford" finds, generalized millennial age frames are at best petty in the field of healthcare, and at worse forsakening. When asked why he takes the bus and uber everywhere, his primary response has been a curt "children can get cancer; the cancer doesn't care about their age." From 17 to 25 "FalkatheMage" never received proper attention "because my parents insisted I was faking for attention."

Theme 3: Atypical Coping Methods vs. the "Typical" Millennial

Theme three addresses the atypical coping methods versus what would be expected from the typical "millennial." The primary coping method, as relative to themes one and two, is working through the illness, and transcending it (the best they can). This sometimes leaves individuals isolated, and despite the motives, may come off to others as stereotypical millennial narcissism. As a participant regards:

I constantly fight my dxs. I lost almost all of my friends because I was "too much work" and couldn't ever hang out. Now that I've dealt with everything for longer, I can push myself to do more and get out with people, as long as I rest after. I am stubborn, so I am nearly always in excruciating pain, but I refuse to let me illnesses define my actions. I'm currently in college to become a rn.

Selflessness is a key coping method that retracts framing millennials as entitled, and narcissistic. This has been exemplified in practices of the Reddit subcommunity, "r/RoastMe. The community is built upon users willing to not take themselves too seriously, and relishing in their own flaws. In particular, the sub-community works to deconstruct the invisibility of disability (that is predominant outside the digital world). In two posts "I have cerebral palsy and I'm gay I also joined Reddit just for this. ROAST. ME." And "Yes I'm in a Wheelchair give me your best," two millennials were willing to allow individuals to say whatever they want about their image and illness. Actions in the community that supported the frame of millennials as narcissistic were met with controversy and antagonism. This was epitomized recently when an individual posted what many found a too rehearsed, and too contrived post in the community; ultimately believing herself to be too perfect for anyone to find something bad about her. Users berated the woman until she cancelled her account, as they found she did not support the true message of the platform: to relish in one's flaws. As user Tyme wrote, "Lady, you came to /r/roastme and are defending yourself in reply to negative comments. Do you not understand the purpose of this sub?"

Contrary to the discourse of millenials as internet obsessed, a primary coping method has been to distance oneself from the internet (something the author himself found necessary). As in the AskReddit Thread "What is your number one top for dealing with Depression and other forms of Mental Illness?" the top answer was "Don't Check Facebook." The subsequent threaded discussion attempted to make sense the suggestion, which remains complicated. For some "Connecting with people through Facebook is one of the few things keeping me alive." Participants suggest that it is important how a platform is used. "Facebook can be a tepid social platform, or the last thread connecting you to others. Social media is crazy nuanced." For others, platforms like Facebook provide a façade of people pretending they're enjoying life, and Instagram as having the ultimate power "of making me feel like complete shit about my life."

Theme 4: Group Think

The very basis of sub-communities in Reddit is the joining together of those who, for the most part, think like you or want to discuss the same thematic issue as you. To that degree, some reddit sub-communities can work to perpetuate negative and toxic ideological views that in past societies (before the internet) would not be granted such sustenance and peer support. This has occurred in political realms, but also in medical issues.

The sub-reddit 2meirl4meirl centers on positing memes that share depressive and suicide thoughts. Even some members agree that negative opinions of being lonely and suicidal being perpetuated by others does not excuse that it is ultimately a negative path to be on. Sub-reddits like incels (involuntarily celibate men) have been seen as a cult. The insidious way the group works is to discourage truly depressed men from seeking psychological and psychiatric help they need, and instead continuously confirming their beliefs with each other. The sub-reddit Morgellons have given disparate people a forum to continuously perpetuate realities of a provenly fake mental disease. It is thanks to the community building abilities of the internet that, even though the founder of the nonprofit Morgellons Research Foundation disappeared, the disease is still continuously perpetuated.

Even more troubling is the component that the groups are able to link reddit threads to media articles that lack credibility; another symptom of a web 2.0 society that has provided a voice to media practitioners that, in the past, would be submitted to further fact checking. For support they have linked their posts to either scientific studies (that have no substance) or media figures who themselves do not have any cultural capital (a degree). One thread promoted a YouTube Video of Alex Jones of the controversial Infowars, as he perpetuated the conspiracy theory of Morgellons. Yet, as a web 2.0 entrepreneur Alex Jones makes the majority of his money through advertisements: particularly "health" related products against modern society's ills. As such, Alex Joneses' income depends on people feeling unwell, and him providing them the solution.

Theme 5: Searching for a New Supportive Paradigm

The final theme constructs millennials as searching for a new supportive paradigm in healthcare, and society as a whole. This includes utilizing web 2.0 tools in positive ways, and in particular, through helping each other.

In the thread "Any Philly ladies (or gents) have a good primary care physician" started by someone who has (too many bad experiences with Jefferson) the OP (original poster) follows up for more information about a suggestion:

"Yelp had some questionable things to say about Dr. Rowbotham; it sounds like she might be a bit curt, and that's one of the problems I've had in the past, and was hoping to avoid."

In the subreddit RedditforGrownUps, "24, male, single, no kids, need tips for finding a primary care physician" the participant is advised to take his time and use the internet resources at his disposal. He is counseled to choose a doctor and hospital that fits him, including age, gender, sick visit policy, and front desk staff.

Millennials use platforms, such as Reddit here, to make sense of the complicated paradigm where even basic procedures have been obscured with bureaucracy. This was supported in the subreddit "EverymanShouldKnow," and thread "How to set a doctor's appointment." Rather than being dismissive or self-centered, people are willing to help each other as the user should not feel bad, "Making a doctor's appointment has changed from the days of 'call any doctor, make a same day appointment. 'Thanks, insurance companies."

Many redditors are posed to support others and openly sharing knowledge to help them feel not alone; and in their actions, build communities. This was sustained in a user's post supporting her friend's video-series on rare disease promotion. In the indorsed YouTube video the woman works to situate a discourse in which millennials do not blame other generations for their ignorance. Rather she regards, for many doctors they simply situate and make sense of things based on "evidence," whereby typical symptoms would not be a rare illness (a zebra) but rather a more typical illness (a horse). She appropriates the zebra print semiology and wishes for others to do the same.

This final theme, as situated through discourse analysis, has been based upon users not lecturing people (even those who use derogatory framing or ideas), but to transcend by creating the atmosphere they haven't been granted in established institutions. As the AMA medical student regards, when he first went to a doctor "I was hoping for support and affirmation rather than a lecture." In his blog and online communities, he has found support. The creation of a potential new paradigm, however, usually regards these online communities as only a temporary solution. The host, despite knowing that he will have some bad face to face interactions, wishes to discuss these issues in person.

SOLUTIONS AND RECOMMENDATIONS

The five themes identified showcase a complicated, and confusing social landscape for millennials. Apparent is that not all millennials are the same, and that the framing device used by mainstream sources, and in academia (including this paper), is unfit for any sort of solid classification beyond age.

Some of the derogatory frames (millennials as lazy, entitled, narcissistic) have been confirmed. As with the AMA case in which Instagram model posted a too rehearsed glamorized photo clearly for publicity, there are people within the millennial generation who are indeed narcissistic, and this narcissism is showcased and supported in their social media use (Ong et al., 2011). This is exacerbated in toxic sub communities that confirm groupthink. But, even for sub-communities like Morgellons, the groups paranoia is not innate. Morgellons was not created by millennials. Further, alternative web media outlet have done their part to drive hysteria. Right-wing iconoclastic conspiracy theorists (i.e. Alex Jones of Prison Planet) who have disowned millennials themselves, similarly post and perpetuate mythologies that have been disregarded by doctors and scientists (Syed-Abdul, Fernandez-Luque, Li, Crain, and Hsu, 2013). As has been identified, in many cases Reddit community members are socially engaged, socially conscious, and quite selfless.

There are technical affordances for specific websites, that can affect user practices (i.e. in reddit the hyperlinking of—sometimes misleading informational material as a catalyst to a discussion—and the creation of different sub-communities. What would be necessary is further open communication between sub-reddits. For chapters like r/incels, more prominent than collaboration and mutual support between other sub-groups, has been feuding. Petitions to close subreddits may do more harm than good either, taking away the voice of people already so isolated. This is just one of the ongoing issues of moderation, as Massanari (2016) has investigated the complicated nature of bot integration in subreddits such as r/depression. The recent experiment r/place provided all reddit users an empty canvas where they allowed users to change blocks different colors. The purpose of the April Fools experiment was to see if individuals would work aimlessly, or if there would be collaboration. The finished product shows, for the most part, a shared sense of community. The integration of positive groups into these more negative ones could be beneficial (for instance Exercise Out of Depression members trying to contribute to r/Incels).

Reddit has provided an opportunity for individuals to share their knowledge. As with utopian views of the internet voiced by Lévy (1997) a multitude of participants post information with no other goal then to share what they know so that others may be helped (i.e. I work at a doctors office, family medicine to be specific. PM me with any questions you have, I have plenty of experience in that area"). Millennials may be so drawn to being kind online because they have not received such treatment in other places.

Results have shown that some millennials have turned online by means of the self-fulfilling prophecy. People treat millenials as internet-obsessed, and in their provincial view and associated actions, have given millenials nowhere else to turn. But millennials pose as resilient, and subdued. When the receptionist regarded the patient would be healthy if he would just take care of himself, he never would say anything back to her. "I would always want to jump the counter. It took everything I had not to say to her that I already felt worse than her since she could still work and I was disabled and trapped in my bed most days."

Reporters and writers must be ever cognizant about the effects their frames may have (McCombs, 2005). When they do publish articles, they owe it to the publics they write about to answer their questions, hear their take and listen to what they have to say. People need to be kind to "millennials" and other generations, not letting stereotypes affect their viewpoints. Such practices are discussed in Deleuze and Guattari's *A Thousand Plateaus* (1998), as the theorists ponder the pragmatics of a schizophrenic soul as able to combat some troubling aspects of contemporary modernization, and its effects. Rather than coming in with countless preconceived notions, they wish for individuals to address items with a clear mind. Many users praise the internet in its ability to provide utopian spaces, but would rather this could occur in all spaces. As the AMA medical host regards, "am an introvert by nature and writing my blog has been an outlet for my stress. That said, my experiences dealing with mental illness and talking about it with "real life" people have 100% been positive. I know this will not continue to be true, and I will have bad encounters with people, but up to now everybody has been incredibly supportive."

As time goes on, hospitals, family members, etc. must continue to recognize how their system treats patients. Millenials will work to correspond with each other, and are wary to perpetuate a system of degradation. As discursive threads promote, many would rather carry on sick then have to go to a doctor's office, or be dismissed by receptionists. Millenials are posed to support modern businesses who remain cognizant and open in how they treat patients, and are working to atone for problems with the convoluted system. Hospitals should be upfront of what type of service they provide (categorize them as modern, internet serviced, etc). This way they can get the type of service they would like.

As one Reddit user answers:

Find a doc you like who has easy access to email. We often don't have enough time during appointments to answer all questions, but emailing questions after your appointment is easy on both parties and more likely to give you the as-needed access that you want.

FUTURE RESEARCH DIRECTIONS

Future work should investigate internationally how other healthcare systems (or businesses) treat their patients, integrate technology, and how different demographics conceptualize their treatment. As a symptom of a larger cultural issue, sociological, historical, and cultural analysis should also investigate how generational cohorts are constructed, and perpetuated—as the term "millennial" has been a national edifice.

Regarded in a thread, "How to Set up a Doctor's Appointment" thread, one user laments: "Jesus. Another day on reddit, another day I'm glad I'm not American."

Literature has established that the internet practices of millennials are not only complicated, but, not exclusive to these "digital natives". In particular future research should provide more case studies detailing the communities of practice online for different platforms and associated demographics, nationalities, ailments. For instance, the researcher has spent time reading posts in Adhesions.org, a platform that is comprised of, generally, women suffering from adhesions post-pregnancy. Suggestions of the few doctor's willing to perform lysis of adhesions led to a follow up surgery. The researcher's integration into the community through digital ethnography, rather than simply "lurking," could help to further deconstruct stereotypical myths.

CONCLUSION

Discourse analysis has found five interrelated thematic discourses of millennials and health issues displayed on Reddit: 1) Trying to Work through the Pain 2) Too Young to be Sick and Millenials as to Blame for their Illness 3) Atypical Coping Methods vs. the "Typical" Millennial 4) Group-Think 5) Searching for a New Supportive Paradigm.

These five themes showcase an ambivalent relationship with technology. Far from internet obsessed, many millennials work to withdraw from technology, and sometimes, from a society that as a whole they believe to have forsaken them. Participants come to this consensus from both systematic analysis (as in Late Capitalism subreddit in which individuals find their treatment as a perpetual symptom) but for many in the small actions (someone not believing their illness). Individuals, even working within the healthcare system, find themselves lost. They turn to online communities to share what little information they have, and learn from others; as when a pharmacy school student searched for help in not knowing where to get a physical for pharmacy school. But sometimes the ability to start a group online and perpetuate negative or false ideas can be insidious (of which some members of groups like 2meirl4meirl lament).

The fifth and final theme addresses millennials understanding that a new paradigm in healthcare must be based on mutual support, beginning with each other. The mutual support can be built upon through increased activism, and future research should look into how these communities extend beyond the virtual world, and how they enact change (Ramsey, 2017) to an immoral system of communication ranging from small communicative gestures, to health plans proposed by the government despite widespread disapproval by the public (American Health Care Act of 2017). In this study, the online spaces seem to pose as symptoms, rather than illnesses.

REFERENCES

Altimier, L. (2004). Communicating with the next generation. *Newborn and Infant Nursing Reviews; NAINR*, *4*(1), 2–3. doi:10.1053/j.nainr.2003.10.001

Anderson, J., & Rainie, L. (2010). *Millennials will make online sharing in networks a lifelong habit.* Pew Research. Retrieved from Pewinternet. org website: http:// pewresearch. org/millennials

Anderson, J., & Rainie, L. (2012). *Millennials will benefit and suffer due to their hyperconnected lives*. Washington, DC: Pew Research Center.

Bland, H. W., Melton, B. F., Welle, P., & Bigham, L. (2012). Stress tolerance: New challenges for millennial college students. *College Student Journal*, *46*(2), 362.

Bolton, R. N., Parasuraman, A., Hoefnagels, A., Migchels, N., Kabadayi, S., Gruber, T., & Solnet, D. (2013). Understanding Generation Y and their use of social media: A review and research agenda. *Journal of Service Management*, *24*(3), 245–267. doi:10.1108/09564231311326987

Bourdieu, P. (1980). "Structures, Habitus, Practices," and "Belief and the Body. In *The Logic of Practice*. Stanford, CA: Stanford University Press.

Cahn, D., & Cahn, J. (2016). *When Millennials Rule: The Reshaping of America*. Simon and Schuster.

Chastian, J. (2013). *Shock! Millennials pass on Obamacare*. National Center for Policy Analysis.

Cowan, M. (2010). Millennial transformation for primary care. *Military Medicine*, *175*(6), 379–381. doi:10.7205/MILMED-D-10-00184 PMID:20572466

Dahlberg, L. (2001). The Internet and democratic discourse: Exploring the prospects of online deliberative forums extending the public sphere. *Information Communication and Society*, *4*(4), 615–633. doi:10.1080/13691180110097030

Diesing, G. (2016). Milleniala: Who they are, what they want, & why you need them. *Hospitals & Health Networks*, *90*(11), 22.

Donatone, B. (2014). A prescription for helping millennials grow up. *The Washington Post.*

Duam, M. (2015). Millennial self-esteem or narcissism? *Newsday.*

Dunne, Á., Lawlor, M. A., & Rowley, J. (2010). Young people's use of online social networking sites–a uses and gratifications perspective. *Journal of Research in Interactive Marketing*, *4*(1), 46–58. doi:10.1108/17505931011033551

Farris, R., Chong, F., & Danning, D. (2002). Generation Y: Purchasing power and implications for marketing. *Academy of Marketing Studies Journal*, *6*(1-2), 89.

Faw, L. (2012). Why Millennials are Spending More than They Earn, And Parents are Footing the Bill. *Forbes.* Retrieved from http://www.forbes.com/sites/larissafaw/2012/05/18/why-millennials-are-spending-more-than-they-earn/

Furchtgott-Roth, D., & Meyer, J. (2015). *Disinherited: How Washington is Betraying America's Young*. Encounter Books.

Gass, E., & Bezold, M. P. (2013). Generation Y, shifting funding structures, and health care reform: Reconceiving the public health paradigm through social work. *Social Work in Public Health*, *28*(7), 685–693. doi:10.1080/19371918.2011.619460 PMID:24074132

Ghose, T. (2013,). Study shows rise in teenage narcissism and sense of entitlement (posted 2013-05-06 22:14:52): A new study reinforces observations about millenials as lazy and materialistic. *The Washington Post.*

Gillespie, N. (2014). Millennials are selfish and entitled, and helicopter parents are to blame. *Time Magazine.*

Gutt, C. N., Oniu, T., Schemmer, P., Mehrabi, A., & Büchler, M. W. (2004). Fewer adhesions induced by laparoscopic surgery?. *Surgical Endoscopy and Other Interventional Techniques, 18*(6), 898-906.

Huang, F. Y. (1997). Health insurance coverage of the children of immigrants in the United States. *Maternal and Child Health Journal*, *1*(2), 69–80. doi:10.1023/A:1026266205885 PMID:10728229

Ivanoff, S. D., & Hultberg, J. (2006). Understanding the multiple realities of everyday life: Basic assumptions in focus-group methodology. *Scandinavian Journal of Occupational Therapy*, *13*(2), 125–132. doi:10.1080/11038120600691082 PMID:16856469

Jones, C., & Czerniewicz, L. (2010). Describing or debunking? The net generation and digital natives. *Journal of Computer Assisted Learning*, *26*(5), 317–320. doi:10.1111/j.1365-2729.2010.00379.x

Jones, C., & Healing, G. (2010). Net generation students: Agency and choice and the new technologies. *Journal of Computer Assisted Learning*, *26*(5), 344–356. doi:10.1111/j.1365-2729.2010.00370.x

Keltgen, J. (2016). *The impact of generational and gender effects on physician satisfaction in the US* (Doctoral dissertation). University of South Dakota.

Leung, L. (2013). Generational differences in content generation in social media: The roles of the gratifications sought and of narcissism. *Computers in Human Behavior*, *29*(3), 997–1006. doi:10.1016/j.chb.2012.12.028

Lévy, P. (1997). *Collective Intelligence* (1st ed.). Basic Books.

Lloyd, T., Shaffer, M. L., Christy, S., Widome, M. D., Repke, J., Weitekamp, M. R., & Paul, I. M. et al. (2013). Health knowledge among the millennial generation. *Journal of Public Health Research*, 2(1), 38. doi:10.4081/jphr.2013.e8 PMID:25170479

Loeb, H. (2015). *The mindset of the millennial: Disruptive & committed for the long run. Huffington Post.*

Maples, M. F., & Han, S. (2008). Cybercounseling in the United States and South Korea: Implications for counseling college students of the millennial generation and the networked generation. *Journal of Counseling and Development*, *86*(2), 178–183. doi:10.1002/j.1556-6678.2008.tb00495.x

Massanari, A. L. (2016). Contested Play. *Socialbots and Their Friends: Digital Media and the Automation of Sociality*, 110.

McGrew, M. (2013). What's a baby boomer parent to do with a millennial? *Baltimore Sun*.

Menzies, D., & Ellis, H. (1990). Intestinal obstruction from adhesions--how big is the problem? *Annals of the Royal College of Surgeons of England*, *72*(1), 60. PMID:2301905

Mills, E., Airey, C., & Yee, K. C. (2006). Generation Y in healthcare: The need for new socio-technical consideration for future technology design in healthcare. *Studies in Health Technology and Informatics*, *130*, 169–179. PMID:17917191

Monk, B. J., Berman, M. L., & Montz, F. J. (1994). Adhesions after extensive gynecologic surgery: Clinical significance, etiology, and prevention. *American Journal of Obstetrics and Gynecology*, *170*(5), 1396–1403. doi:10.1016/S0002-9378(13)90479-8 PMID:8178880

Olson, V. D. (2011). Generational diversity: Implications for healthcare leaders. *Journal of Business & Economics Research*, *6*(11). doi:10.19030/jber.v6i11.2486

Ordun, G., & Akun, A. (2016). Personality Characteristics and Emotional Intelligence Levels of Millenials: A Study in Turkish Context. *Journal of Economic and Social Studies*, *6*(1), 125. doi:10.14706/JECOSS16614

Pace, S. (2014). *Millennials, Health, and the Doctor-Patient Relationship* (Thesis). Bard College.

Palfrey, J. S., Tonniges, T. F., Green, M., & Richmond, J. (2005). Introduction: Addressing the millennial morbidity—the context of community pediatrics. *Pediatrics*, *115*(4Supplement 3), 1121–1123. doi:10.1542/peds.2004-2825B PMID:15828080

Papacharissi, Z. (2002). The virtual sphere The internet as a public sphere. *New Media & Society*, *4*(1), 9–27. doi:10.1177/14614440222226244

Parker, M. C., Ellis, H., Moran, B. J., Thompson, J. N., Wilson, M. S., Menzies, D., & Buchan, S. (2001). Postoperative adhesions: Ten-year follow-up of 12,584 patients undergoing lower abdominal surgery. *Diseases of the Colon and Rectum*, *44*(6), 822–829. doi:10.1007/BF02234701 PMID:11391142

Pink, , Horst, , Postill, , Hjorth, , & Lewis, , & Tacchi. (2016). *Digital Ethnography: Principles and Practices*. London: Sage.

Piper, L. E. (2012). Generation Y in healthcare: Leading millennials in an era of reform. *Frontiers of Health Services Management*, *29*(1), 16–28. PMID:23050334

Poor, N. (2005). Mechanisms of an online public sphere: The website Slashdot. *Journal of Computer-Mediated Communication, 10*(2).

Ransford, H. E., Carrillo, F. R., & Rivera, Y. (2010). Health care-seeking among Latino immigrants: Blocked access, use of traditional medicine, and the role of religion. *Journal of Health Care for the Poor and Underserved*, *21*(3), 862–878. doi:10.1353/hpu.0.0348 PMID:20693732

Rogers, E. M. (1962). *The Diffusion of Innovations*. Glencoe, IL: Free Press.

Sarringhaus, M. M. (2011). The great divide: Social media's role in bridging healthcare's generational shift. *Journal of Healthcare Management*, *56*(4), 235–244. PMID:21838022

Silva, J. M. (2014). Slight expectations: Making sense of the "Me me me" generation. *Sociology Compass*, *8*(12), 1388–1397. doi:10.1111/soc4.12227

Singer, P., Flöck, F., Meinhart, C., Zeitfogel, E., & Strohmaier, M. (2014, April). Evolution of reddit: from the front page of the internet to a self-referential community? In *Proceedings of the 23rd International Conference on World Wide Web* (pp. 517-522). ACM. doi:10.1145/2567948.2576943

Smith, E. E., & Aaker, J. L. (2013). Millennial searchers. *New York Times.*

Stein, J. (2013). Millennials: The me me me generation. *Time Magazine, 20*, 1-8.

Sullivan, M. F. (2011). *Asthma Management In Millenial College Students: Attitudes and Perceptions of Resources* (Doctoral dissertation). The Ohio State University, Columbus, OH.

Syed-Abdul, S., Fernandez-Luque, L., Jian, W. S., Li, Y. C., Crain, S., Hsu, M. H., & Liou, D. M. (2013). Misleading health-related information promoted through video-based social media: Anorexia on YouTube. *Journal of Medical Internet Research, 15*(2), e30. doi:10.2196/jmir.2237 PMID:23406655

Von Muhlen, M., & Ohno-Machado, L. (2012). Reviewing social media use b clinicians. *Journal of the American Medical Informatics Association, 19*(5), 777–781. doi:10.1136/amiajnl-2012-000990 PMID:22759618

Wolburg, J. M., & Pokrywczynski, J. (2001). A psychographic analysis of Generation Y college students. *Journal of Advertising Research, 41*(5), 33–52. doi:10.2501/JAR-41-5-33-52

KEY TERMS AND DEFINITIONS

Baby Boomers: A term used to denote an American Cohort born from the early 1940s to early 1960s.

Framing Theory: According to this theory of mass media, by the means of presentation media professionals predetermine interpretations of given events or given subjects to audiences, and thus, influence and bias their ways of thinking.

Gaslighting: A tactic used by a person or entity seeking to sow seeds of doubt in a targeted individual or group that makes them question their own memory or perception.

Group Think: A psychological phenomenon to classify thinking or making decisions as a group in a way that ultimately discourages creativity or individual responsibility.

Morgellons: A self-diagnosed skin condition coined by Mary Leitao in 2002 wherein patients believe sores develop that contain forms of fibers. A multi-year study by the CDC would declare "sufferers" as having no disease organisms.

Obama-Care: The informal name for the Affordable Care Act; a federal healthcare law and policy enacted by Barack Obama in 2010.

Self-Fulfilling Prophecy: A belief, or delusion, that may influence people so that there subsequent actions fulfill their confirmation.

Social Security: Developed in 1935, an existent but fading United States government program to provide support for the retired, disabled, or unemployed.

Chapter 7
Sharing Your Personal Medical Experience Online:
Is It an Irresponsible Act or Patient Empowerment?

Claudia Lisa Moeller
Istituto Alti Studi Strategici e Politici (IASSP), Italy

ABSTRACT

What happened between Mrs. Kardashian West and the FDA in 2015 is very interesting to all of us. She praised and suggested a prescribed drug against morning sickness. The FDA claimed it was a commercial and sent a warning letter to the company, which produced the drug. Kim Kardashian West changed her post and admitted it was a commercial. Was it true? Mrs. Kardashian West just expressed her personal opinion and wanted to share with her followers a piece of advice. She share her personal story, like many other Internet users, and her patient experience should have been respected. Her story shows what patient empowerment is and how the Net is a precious resource for patients to share their stories that might help other patients. For this reason, doctors should not be afraid of the Net and its potentiality.

INTRODUCTION

It is morning. You wake up; your head swirls and pounds heavily, and you can barely breathe. You are about to throw up. Luckily, your doctor prescribed you yesterday a powerful medication to prevent this bothersome nausea. You are so glad that you have finally found this drug that you want to share it with the entire world. You

DOI: 10.4018/978-1-5225-3716-8.ch007

Copyright © 2018, IGI Global. Copying or distributing in print or electronic forms without written permission of IGI Global is prohibited.

write on your webpage on a social media an enthusiastic post about the miraculous effect of this pill. No morning sickness anymore! This problem, according to your point of view, has not received the attention it deserves:

OMG. Have you heard about this? As you guys know my #morningsickness has been pretty bad. I tried changing things about my lifestyle, like my diet, but nothing helped, so I talked to my doctor. He prescribed me #Diclegis, and I felt a lot better and most importantly, it's been studied and there was no increased risk to the baby. I'm so excited and happy with my results that I'm partnering with Duchesnay USA to raise awareness about treating morning sickness. If you have morning sickness, be safe and sure to ask your doctor about the pill with the pregnant woman on it and find out more www.diclegis.com; www.DiclegisImportantSafetyInfo.com.

A couple of days later, you radically change the text and post the following:

#CorrectiveAd I guess you saw the attention my last #morningsickness post received. The FDA has told Duchesnay, Inc., that my last post about Diclegis (doxylamine succinate and pyridoxine HCl) was incomplete because it did not include any risk information or important limitations of use for Diclegis. A link to this information accompanied the post, but this didn't meet FDA requirements. So, I'm re-posting and sharing this important information about Diclegis. For US Residents Only.

Diclegis is a prescription medicine used to treat nausea and vomiting of pregnancy in women who have not improved with change in diet or other non-medicine treatments.

Limitation of Use: Diclegis has not been studied in women with hyperemesis gravidarum.

Important Safety Information

Do not take Diclegis if you are allergic to doxylamine succinate, other ethanolamine derivative antihistamines, pyridoxine hydrochloride or any of the ingredients in Diclegis. You should also not take Diclegis in combination with medicines called monoamine oxidase inhibitors (MAOIs), as these medicines can intensify and prolong the adverse CNS effects of Diclegis.

The most common side effect of Diclegis is drowsiness. Do not drive, operate heavy machinery, or other activities that need your full attention unless your healthcare provider says that you may do so. Do not drink alcohol, or take other central nervous system depressants such as cough and cold medicines, certain pain medicines, and medicines that help you sleep while you take Diclegis. Severe drowsiness can happen or become worse causing falls or accidents.

Tell your healthcare provider about all of your medical conditions, including if you are breastfeeding or plan to breastfeed. Diclegis can pass into your breast milk and may harm your baby. You should not breastfeed while using Diclegis.

Additional safety information can be found at www.DiclegisImportantSafetyinfo.com or www.Diclegis.com. Duchesnay USA encourages you to report negative side effects of prescription drugs to the FDA. Visit www.fda.gov/medwatch or call 1-800-FDA-1088.

Why did you do that? The Food and Drug Administration (FDA) sent a warning letter to the company you were praising a couple of days ago. Why is the FDA after you and your meaningless post? You are not meaningless.

BACKGROUND

How many people are going to read what you post? Just a few people? Not exactly. Indeed, your name is Kim Kardashian West. On Instagram alone, the popular picture-sharing social network, Kim Kardashian West has more than 92 million followers. Mrs. Kardashian West wrote this post a couple of years ago, on August 1, 2015,[1] while she was expecting her second child. She suffered from morning sickness, and thanks to the new drug Diclegis, she felt immediately better.

The FDA thought her original post was a concealed advertisement, and it wanted her to change it (FDA, 2015a). The FDA did not believe that what Mrs. Kardashian West posted was a sincere claim. If Mrs. Kardashian West was sponsoring a product, then she broke the rules and had to correct her first post.

FDA intervened, because Mrs. Kardashian West suggested (or sponsored) a medical pill that pregnant women can take against morning sicknesses. Only a doctor can prescribed this particular drug. In the drug facts, the side effects are: "If you take too much Diclegis® (overdose), you may have the following symptoms: restlessness, dry mouth, the pupils of your eyes become larger (dilated), sleepiness, dizziness, confusion, fast heart rate, seizures, muscle pain or weakness, and sudden and severe kidney problems" (Diclegis, 2017).

METHODOLOGY

This paper will be a philosophical one. Even if it is difficult to state what a "philosophical paper" is, the author will try to analyze an emblematic case. In particular, the author will focus her attention on what happened to Mrs. Kardashian – West. The author believes that this case is very important to the community, because it combines two fundamental questions.

The first one engages our public and private dimension on the Net. When do we become social personalities? When may our posts on Facebook or on other social medias become dangerous for the community? This is a moral question that implies that we will analyze a particular case that might be interesting for all of us. Generally, a normal Internet user is not as famous as Mrs. Kardashian – West, but every post is potentially read by millions of Internet users. For this very reason, although it might appear that Mrs. Kardashian – West is very far from us, but indeed, it is not like this.

Mrs. Kardashian –West may not be the only case in literature and in the future. For this paper, the author chose to deepen this case because it was very popular thanks to the protagonist involved and the consequences.

The second question revolves around our liberty of speech. At times of the Net, where everybody shares his or her personal experiences, can we talk openly about sensitive topics such as Medicine? Can we write only about our personal beliefs or suggestions on topics such as health? Health is individual, yet very few people have the knowledge to speak competently about health. Can we really talk online openly and without any filter about health, drugs, and cures? This is more a bioethical question that the author will try to answer in this paper.

These two questions lead us to ask ourselves if and what we mean with the concept of autonomy. When do we chose for ourselves? Can we say that we are independent, autonomous in our choices if we follow someone's suggestion? Especially in these times where Internet is full of social gurus and "influencers" are always prompt to give us pieces of advice about our lifestyle. Companies seek social media gurus' help and support in order to achieve more and more potential buyers. Social gurus' posts, as the one Mrs. Kardashian – West sometimes writes, may influence millions of people's choice. Are those, who read Mrs. Kardashian – West's posts, independent? Are their wills free? In Philosophy, Immanuel Kant is the key author when we want to discuss about heteronomy and autonomy. According to Kant, and later we will deepen this distinction, autonomous will is in a few words that will that is completely independent from anything. It is completely self-legislating. Any other principle behind our choices makes a decision heteronomous. For example, we study to get good grades. Either we study because we want to get a scholarship, or because we want our parents to let us go to that summer camp, or because we like that subject, or because we are competitive; to Kant all these reasons are heteronomous. It does not matter if someone told us to do study or not. Kant's distinction and definition is still today one of the most important and relevant in Philosophy. In this paper, we will introduce and discuss the Kantian concept of autonomy in relation to Mrs. Kardashian – West's case and our lives.

The philosophical approach will highlight those moral aspects that can have consequences on everybody's live. For this reason, the author will not discuss those Statistics and Psychological works that focus on quantitative aspects. The philosophical approach instead prefers to put the heed on a single event in order to analyze all the possible meanings, potential consequences, and suggest new strategies to face similar problems.

MAIN FOCUS OF THE CHAPTER

This case attracted author's attention because it is not clear if the FDA had the authority to step in in this case. If Mrs. Kardashian West had stated the truth in her first post, could the FDA really intervene and force her to change her post and allegedly her mind? Cannot a patient share his or her personal medical experience on the Web? This case is complicated—and therefore fascinating—because of the different aspects and topics involved, from a legal point of view to a philosophical one. We will try to analyze all these aspects to determine whether Mrs. Kardashian West did something wrong.

Regarding the legal point of view, we will try to determine whether Mrs. Kardashian West broke the rules. Many elements must be examined in order to answer this question. First, Mrs. Kardashian West wrote an advertisement, and she did not mention this fact anywhere. In addition, if her post was a commercial, it was a badly written advertisement. Indeed, a commercial concerning a drug must list all the side effects that might be caused by its consumption. First, we ask a legal question, which we will try to answer: Was Mrs. Kardashian West guilty of advertising this drug?

The second problem concerns Mrs. Kardashian West's popularity on the Web. She is not a normal Internet user.[2] She is an Internet mogul (Robehmed, 2016), and her words lead to massive consequences. Her huge number of followers is an enormous potential public: Her voice has a resonance that very few media outlets have due to her importance on the Web. Mrs. Kardashian West posted something she should not have. Why? Because of her multitude of followers. Mrs. Kardashian West traded her freedom of speech for popularity, so is she doomed to be quiet from now on? Is it fair? Mrs. Kardashian West's followers brought her to silence: If you want to be an influencer, then you must be silent. Every statement you post on your social networks will be considered a commercial. If they are commercials, then you must follow the rules related to this subject. Can influencers have a voice and state personal beliefs? Alternatively, does their and our potential public force us to stay quiet on different and sensitive topics such as health?

Those are all questions that emerged from Mrs. Kardashian West's posts. In this chapter, we will investigate these questions and try to answer them. First, we are going to analyze the legal problem. Was Mrs. Kardashian West guilty? Did the FDA have the po0Ower to intervene in this case?

Second, we will answer other questions related to the freedom of speech during this time of the Internet. If Mrs. Kardashian West expressed her personal belief, then was it a patient-empowerment claim? The last question concerning this problem is this: Was Mrs. Kardashian West eclipsing her readers' freedom of choice? These are all issues regarding Mrs. Kardashian West specifically, and all of us, because we are all Internet users.

Under a philosophical point of view, this a very interesting case. In particular, Kant's philosophy is very useful in this case. The Prussian distinction between heteronomy and autonomy may help to understand why Mrs. Kardashian West's post was not dangerous. This philosophical clarification, indeed, will help us to sort out if the "web influencers" are truly manipulating their followers. Kant's distinction between these two typologies of decision clarifies why influencers can give only advice. It is impossible to state, according to Kant, that influencers change our mind. The autonomous will is the ability to give oneself the moral law. The autonomous moral law in Kant can be summarized in the command "you must".

According to Kant, this is the only possible meaning when we speak about "autonomy". No other decisions, that we take, are autonomous. Our decisions are most of the times heteronomous, because there is always another reason under them.

The chapter will conclude with some suggestions for what patients and doctors can do with the prolific amount of health-care information available to the public in this age of the Internet.

The author's aim is to prove that Mrs. Kardashian West might have broken the rules, but she (like everybody else) is free to say whatever she wants on the Internet, especially about a topic concerning her body and her feelings. If patient empowerment exists, then patients should express and share their personal stories online, no matter how many followers they might have.

The author chose this particular case, because it is emblematic. Even if at a first glance, we may not understand how Mrs. Kardashian West has something in common with us or a normal user of the Net, in this paper the author will prove why this case is very important to all of us. Potentially, all of us can be a Kardashian with millions of followers. Where does our liberty of speech start? In this case, can a patient suggest and share her personal story on the net? This essay aims to answer, briefly, to this question.

LEGAL QUESTION: WAS SHE GUILTY?[3]

In this story, one actor is missing: the Federal Trade Commission (FTC). In truth, the FTC is the principal and responsible institution for trade and false advertising, although it did not sue or send a warning letter to Mrs. Kardashian West. The FDA, which is responsible for cases concerning food or health, accused Mrs. Kardashian West of having commercialized a medical drug in the wrong way.

Strictly, the FDA can only ask very limited questions concerning commercials: "The FDA can exercise its authority to regulate and control only those promotional activities that fall under the purview of the legal definitions of advertising and labeling" (Kale et al, 1996, p. 229).

Mrs. Kardashian West was accused of promoting a product. Because the FDA deemed her social media post a commercial, she should have listed all the drug's side effects. For this reason, the FDA asked the following in its warning letter:

Because the violations described above are serious and repeated, we request, further, that your submission include a comprehensive plan of action to disseminate truthful, non-misleading, and complete corrective messages about the issues discussed in this letter to the audience(s) that received the violative promotional materials. . . . To the extent possible, corrective messaging should be distributed using the same media, and generally for the same duration of time and with the same frequency that the violative promotional material was disseminated. (FDA, 2015a, p. 3)

How did Mrs. Kardashian West react to this letter? She abided by these admonitions and changed the text of her post. She added the hashtag "#CorrectiveAd," stated that she wrote an earlier post, and then listed all the side effects that might occur taking the medication she had endorsed.

The FDA, in fact, accused Mrs. Kardashian West of having written an advertisement, and more precisely, an endorsement. Mrs. Kardashian West was accused, and it is clearly written in the FDA warning letter sent to Diclegis, of having expressed an endorsement in the first post. In the letter, we read the following:

The social media post is false or misleading in that it presents efficacy claims for DICLEGIS, but fails to communicate any risk information associated with its use and it omits material facts. Thus, the social media post misbrands DICLEGIS within the meaning of the Federal Food, Drug, and Cosmetic Act (FD&C Act) and makes its distribution violative. 21 U.S.C. 352(a), (n); 321(n); 331(a). See 21 CFR 202.1(e)(5). These violations are concerning from a public health perspective because they suggest that DICLEGIS is safer than has been demonstrated. (FDA, 2015a, p. 1)

In the case of Mrs. Kardashian West, it may be better to ask if her post was an endorsement instead of a commercial. In American law, there are not only commercials but also endorsements. In the American legislation, the definition of commercial is left to the plain meaning rule. In other words, commercial is what normally and most commonly people will consider an advertisement. However, endorsements are easier to define than commercials.

According to the FTC (2015), an endorsement is any advertising message that consumers are likely to believe reflects the opinions, beliefs, findings, or experiences of a party other than the sponsoring advertiser, even if the views expressed by that party are identical to those of the sponsoring advertiser. The party whose opinions, beliefs, findings, or experience the message appears to reflect will be called the endorser and may be an individual, group, or institution.

Was she guilty? Had Mrs. Kardashian West the right to express her personal opinion? Those are two different questions. First, the author would like to answer the question concerning the legal aspect. Second, the author would like to analyze deeply and thoroughly the problem of whether Mrs. Kardashian West, an influencer, had the right to express her personal opinion via social media.

Since this case was settled out of court, it is clear that she recognized this was a commercial and not a personal opinion. However, we would like to ignore this fact and point out other factors that lead the author to believe that Mrs. Kardashian West spontaneously posted her personal experience.

Mrs. Kardashian West, as any Internet user might notice from other posts, adds a clear hashtag such as #adv or #advertisement, when she is promoting a product for money (Kardashian, 2016). She has no problem claiming that she earned some money for sponsoring a certain product. In this particular case, Mrs. Kardashian West did not write anywhere that it was a commercial. Only after Diclegis received an e-mail from the FDA due to her posts Mrs. Kardashian West changed her post on Instagram to state that it was an advertisement.

A particular fact drew the author's attention: It seems that no one believed this was a sincere and honest post. Everyone believed immediately that it was a commercial. No one stopped to evaluate whether it might ultimately be sincere advice given by a person with nothing to gain.

Furthermore, it was interesting to learn that the FDA scolded Mrs. Kardashian West because she shared her personal story with her followers. Indeed, if Mrs. Kardashian West had never explained her personal situation and her illness, then she would have never been in trouble. In American law, it is possible to advertise medical products without listing all the side effects. Reminder ads are particular forms of commercials that do not require quoting all the side effects.[4]

For all these reasons, the author finds it misleading to consider Mrs. Kardashian West's post as a commercial. The author thinks that accepting the FDA's accusation

(Rawlings, 2015), limits our vision on the case. Furthermore, it is more interesting (and maybe even fair) to believe Mrs. Kardashian West's words.

In addition, the author searched to see if the FTC had stepped in somehow in this case, but it appears that it did not. The author also wrote to the FTC, and this was its exhaustive reply: "There have been no public FTC legal actions against Kim Kardashian" (FTC, personal communication, February 16, 2017).

It is clear that the FTC, whose task is to control commercials, did not intervene in this case. The reason is simple: There was no evidence. The FTC general guidelines concerning celebrities and endorsements also state that you might omit to write a disclosure if a company gives you a free sample of the product for you to review (FTC, 2015). A single free sample is not a payment.

As we read in the FTC guidelines, even if Diclegis gave a free sample of the drug to Mrs. Kardashian West, then it would not have been an endorsement. Since nowhere else it is disclosed that Mrs. Kardashian West was paid for this post, FTC did not intervene consequentially. There was no reason for it to do so.

In this case, the FTC should have contacted either Diclegis or Mrs. Kardashian West. No one declared that what Mrs. Kardashian West wrote was a commercial; thus, the FDA had no right to send the warning letter to Diclegis.

In the end, was Mrs. Kardashian West guilty? Yes, if we consider her posts as two examples of commercials. In the case of her initial post, she omitted all the medication's risks, as the FDA noted in its warning letter. On the other hand, if we believe Mrs. Kardashian West's first version despite misgivings and the later corrective post, we shall say Mrs. Kardashian West was not guilty. She just expressed, too daringly, maybe, her personal beliefs. She wanted to promote a product without any reward; she thought it was the best on the market.

WHEN DOES THE FREEDOM OF SPEECH END?

What happens if your name is Alice, you have about 1,000 followers, and you write the following on your Twitter account: "Diclegis is a wonder drug @KimKardashian once endorsed that stops morning sickness and I just want everyone to know how much I love it!" (McAlexander, 2017).

Nothing, of course. Alice posted only her opinion. She mentioned a drug she tried, and it helped her. Nothing bad happened to her. The FDA did not send a letter to Diclegis because of her post. Even if this post is not that different from Mrs. Kardashian West's post. Shall we infer that when you are an influencer, you cannot have a personal opinion? What is an influencer? Today, it now seems that the Internet consists of kingdoms where new kings and queens (in most cases) lay down the rules. What is an influencer? "Individuals who have the power to affect purchase decisions of others because of their (real or perceived) authority, knowledge, position, or relationship" (*Business Dictionary*, 2017).

Mrs. Kardashian West might be an influencer in many fields, from clothes to makeup, but we are not sure how we might consider her an influencer when it comes to drugs and health problems. Mrs. Kardashian West, as the previous definition states, has no knowledge, ability, or skill in medicine. So why should we consider her in that particular moment or post an influencer?

This first objection should answer the author's question. We all might be seen in certain moments of our lives as experts. We are not experts of everything, though. In addition, Mrs. Kardashian West did not say anywhere that she was invited to take that particular drug. She said clearly to consult a doctor. Mrs. Kardashian West never tried to abuse her position; she simply told her followers about a problem she used to suffer from. As Alice above mentioned.

This detail makes Kim Kardashian West and other millions of Internet users alike. She just described how a particular drug helped her. She used to have a problem, and she found a cure. In this situation, it is difficult to state that she was an influencer. As far as we know, Mrs. Kardashian West might be an expert in many areas, just not in the medical field.

She simply shared with her millions of fans her personal story, her personal experience; ultimately, she shared a piece of advice. Mrs. Kardashian West cannot express her opinion due to the large number of followers she has; but what is the limit?[5] When are there too many followers? A billion? A million? A hundred?

If we think that the freedom of speech has boundaries—the number of followers, for example—then we must consider one pivotal aspect of the Internet, which is that it potentially makes every one of us a Kim Kardashian West. Indeed, the Internet gives the possibility to everyone to be important. Potentially, what we write and upload might be of interest to billions of people. The only hurdle on the Internet is language. The World Wide Web is the official name of the Internet; we must always remember this detail. In this way, it seems clear to me how Mrs. Kardashian West's huge number of followers cannot be a reason to put a gag on her. She is free to say whatever she wants to, like any of us. That is democracy.

If a woman experiencing morning sickness wanted to follow Mrs. Kardashian West's advice, then she would need to discuss this medication with a doctor. Mrs. Kardashian West learned about this medication thanks to her doctor. She mentioned this detail in the post, and at very end of the first text, she invited her followers to consult a doctor before making any medical decision.

For all these reasons, the author cannot really understand how someone might judge Mrs. Kardashian West's post as irresponsible. Even if her fan base on the

Internet is one of the biggest in the world, we cannot consider her as responsible for anything. Even if a woman decided to take the medication after reading Mrs. Kardashian West's post, how can we really hold her responsible for any possible harm that might follow the person's use of that drug?

We cannot. First, Mrs. Kardashian West said openly to visit a doctor. The physician, who prescribes this drug, must investigate via a medical exam if that drug is the right one for the patient.

Otherwise, if a woman chooses to take a prescribed medication without a medical prescription, she is just breaking the law. Mrs. Kardashian West never said to put your own and your baby's life at risk. She said openly to consult a doctor before taking the medication.

In both cases, it is clear that Mrs. Kardashian West is not liable for what may happen when someone reads her posts. She was simply offering advice. Alternatively, we should reconsider the concept of responsibility. It is a slippery slope condemning Mrs. Kardashian West's post. Potentially, we are all Mrs. Kardashian West. Should we then stay silent in order to avoid possible and remote consequences?[6]

On the other hand, it is clear why the FDA sent the letter. The FDA, fearing a possible increase of consumption of medication against morning sickness, tried to make Mrs. Kardashian West change her post in order to "clarify" something that did not need any further explanation. What we might infer from the FDA's behavior is that someone was concerned about the consequences of Mrs. Kardashian West's act. Because her followers are so many, it was wiser to put an alert hashtag listing all the possible side effects that a pregnant woman may face.

The author would like to point out this last detail: Would not it be more dangerous and irresponsible if Mrs. Kardashian West had spoken about a drug that is easily available without a prescription? Prescribed pharmaceuticals are available only after having consulted a physician; they are not available in supermarkets. Would not this kind of advice be more dangerous and risky? This last remark might show clearly how Mrs. Kardashian West did not want to trample on others' superior, and more qualified, authority. She simply offered advice, and she took all the necessary precautions in order not to harm anyone.

The FDA asked her to change her post because someone believed that Mrs. Kardashian West might induce all or some of her followers to buy something that might have threatened a mother's and baby's health. Should the FDA be afraid of this risk? Does this worry justify such a request? Did Mrs. Kardashian West manipulate her followers?

HETERONOMY AND AUTONOMY: PATIENTS ARE SMARTER THAN YOU THINK

This leads us to our first and most urgent philosophical question: When can we say we chose?

Can a patient really be independent? Yes, he or she can. Indeed, no matter what a celebrity or a doctor might say, the freedom and the liberty to make a decision lies only within us. After Immanuel Kant, it should be clear that heteronomy has very little to do with the commonsense[7] use of the word (Devisch & Vanheule, 2014). It does not mean, in fact, that the subject does not make his or her own decision because the person is under the influence of someone else. As Kant proved to us, heteronomy is always in the subject:

The sensible nature of rational beings in general is their existence under empirically conditioned laws and is thus, for reason, heteronomy. The supersensible nature of the same beings, on the other hand, is their existence in accordance with laws that are independent of any empirical condition and thus belong to autonomy of pure reason. (Kant, 1997, p. 38)

For Kant, heteronomy does not mean that you shift your responsibility to others. You are always responsible for your conduct. Heteronomy means only that the object and aim of the moral action is set on the deeds and more specifically on happiness:

To be happy is necessarily the demand of every rational but finite being and therefore an unavoidable determining ground of its faculty of desire. . . . he is needy and this need is directed to the matter of his faculty of desire, that is, something related to a subjective feeling of pleasure and displeasure underlying it by which is determined what he needs in order to be satisfied with his condition. But just because this material determining ground can be cognized only empirically by the subject, it is impossible to regard this problem as law, since a law, as objective, must contain the very same determining ground of the will in all cases and for all rational beings. (Kant, 1997, p.23)

For this reason, Kant insists that moral law belongs only to humankind. One can always opt to follow his or her personal happiness or pleasure, although none of this typology of behaviors are what Kant calls moral law. Notwithstanding this "pathological"[8] reason, Kant claims that those are heteronomous actions, yet it is none other than the single individual who makes his or her own decisions: "All the matter of practical rules rests always on subjective conditions, which afford it no universality for rational beings other than have a merely conditional one. . . " (Kant, 1997, p. 31).

Using Kant's words and definition, we might even see how Mrs. Kardashian West's post cannot be taken as a moral statement. Indeed, as the Prussian philosopher said, "All practical principles that presuppose an object (matter) of the faculty of desire as the determining ground of the will are, without exception, empirical and can furnish no practical laws" (Kant, 1997, p. 19).

According to Kant, it would have been impossible to consider Kardashian West's sentence as a moral command. Because her moral claim was based only on her happiness and wellness, it is impossible to review this statement as a moral law. Kant would say that her post was talking about only her personal experience; therefore, a statement like that cannot be followed by anyone outside of herself.

Furthermore, Mrs. Kardashian West never said that she wanted someone take the medication she was talking about without first consulting a doctor. She highly recommended visiting a doctor before making a decision regarding the medication.

As you can see, Mrs. Kardashian West never attempted to avoid a doctor's opinion. She simply shared her personal story and point of view as a patient. Her phenomenological[9] experience is sincere. No one can deny what she felt. Her phenomenological experience as a pregnant woman suffering from morning sickness is a truth that no doctor or institution can disagree with. Patients live experiences, and doctors cannot argue with that. That is what they feel. The Internet may be a place where patients share their stories. These personal experiences can be very useful to other patients who might be in search of a cure for their problems.

However, doctors are concerned about how individuals may use medical information available on the Internet:

As a decision support, the Internet is not only ill-constituted for the task but its flexibility makes it dangerous. Rather than enforcing a systematic approach to a decision, a search engine will likely encourage the user in pursuing shortcuts that ignore critical considerations. The patient's own preferences, wishes, and predilections will govern information search, exacerbating any pre-existing biases. (Schulz & Nakamoto, 2001, p. 67)

In this article, for example, the authors claim that a patient will never have real "background knowledge"[10] to be prepared to make his or her own decision.

This first fear is, no doubt, a real problem in this age of the Internet. On the Internet, commercials are more invasive and aggressive than on any other form of media (Lau, 2016, p. 14).[11] Because it is impossible to stop the free trade of information available on the Internet, it is better and more efficient to find a way to properly use the medical instructions found there.

Doctors should not be afraid of demanding patients. Some doctors have already noticed that patients need a professional figure to talk to and who can reassure them of the next steps.

So how do we respond to these accelerated changes in patient/consumer behavior? . . . Dispelling misinformation and quelling panic are just as important a responsibility as providing accurate information. . . . We are not simply information givers; rather, we are partners and curators who help patients build capacity for "smart consumption", to distinguish between trustworthy and unreliable sources of information. (Jirasevijinda, 2015, p. 256)[12]

Patients want to be more aware of what is going to happen to their bodies. As this research shows, the expectations are ambitious:

Patients seek online information as to complement traditional sources or to challenge their physicians. . . . Social Media marketing can prove to be a valuable tool in the hands of the people knowing how to use it. Health consumers are more mature than health providers. This situation has to change. The new environment promotes consulting enriched with informed flexibility. (Koumpouros, Toulias, & Koumpouros, 2015, p. 501)

Another study showed that patients are not fools when it comes to advertisements; they can easily identify what might be a commercial:

"Brand recognition" was reported as very important to the interviewees in navigating the health Internet. . . . A further interesting finding regarding which sites were valued and used was the low esteem in which North American sites were sometimes held as reported by our British participants. This was partly due to a perception that US sites had commercial aims and were therefore seen as "trying to sell something". (Powell, Inglis, Ronnie, & Large, 2011, p. 7)

This article goes on to say, "Health-related Internet use was seen by most of our participants as a supplement to existing health service provision rather than a replacement for it" (Powell et al., 2011, p. 8). The authors conclude that an online search for information should correspond to a doctor's consult: "The majority of online events were related to real-world consultations, whether as preparation for them or as a search for further information afterwards" (Powell et al., 2011, p. 8).

The Internet has two characteristics (Powell et al., 2011, p. 6) that doctors do not. First, it is available anytime and anywhere. Second, it is possible to get information and to seek a first form of help anonymously. These Internet qualities are different from what a doctor may offer with his or her presence and knowledge and should reassure doctors that they will not disappear because of the net. Indeed, the preparation and experience of a doctor are not endangered. Internet is only a secondary and complementary source of information.

In some studies, researches proved that patients are aware that what they might find on the Net is not always precise. What you can find online is not always accurate. For this specific reason, patients seek a first help online and a second one by their doctor. Especially, medical support is fundamental for those who suffer from particular illnesses and disease. Experts are more reliable and exhaustive. (Bevan, Sparks, Ernst, Francies & Santora, 2013, p. 23)

For all those reasons, doctors should not be afraid of what a patient can feel and they might share online about their personal medical experience. Furthermore, this is a sphere no one can deny or belittle thanks to their higher education. Besides, this is a new starting point to refuel the dialogue between doctor and patient, a new form to fight back paternalism (Lepping, Palmstierna, & Raveesh, 2016, p. 95)[13] and the constant threat to the patient's freedom of choice and status in the health-care world (Öresland, Friberg, Määttä, Öhlen, 2015).[14]

THE "PUNISHMENT": A SILENT REBELLIOUS STATEMENT

It is interesting to note what in the last post Mrs. Kardashian West wrote. Indeed, it clearly shows how she felt and according to her point of view she had done nothing wrong. Consequently, she did not need to offer an apology. This shows, and the author will prove it, how a patient felt mistreated. This FDA letter belittled her dignity, her personal story, her beliefs, and even her zeal toward a topic related to her situation.

The reader might notice that Mrs. Kardashian West is telling her personal story on her social network page. She added that she tried different strategies to avoid this illness, but nothing worked until her doctor prescribed Diclegis, and she immediately felt better. Then, she felt the urge to share her story with her followers. In addition, she said she was "partnering" with the company to "raise awareness about treating morning sickness." This last sentence is very mysterious, yet we cannot really say if Mrs. Kardashian West was not sincere with her followers.

The second corrective post is more interesting, though. Indeed, in the latter version, the reader can notice that Mrs. Kardashian West has not given any apology. Thanks to Derrida's deconstructive method (Caputo, 1997, pp. 100–105), the reader finds something very interesting in the second version of this post.

Silently and rebelliously, Mrs. Kardashian West let her followers know that she did not write a commercial. She was just sharing her personal story.

First, Mrs. Kardashian West never referred to her previous statement as a commercial. She only recalled it with a generic term such as *post*. The only time she used the term *ad* was in the hashtag. We might even highlight the first sentence of this long post: "#CorrectiveAd I guess you saw the attention my last #morningsickness post received."

In the same text, she specified that the FDA contacted the company, Duchesnay Inc., that produced the medication she took: "The FDA has told Duchesnay Inc. that my last post about DICLEGIS was incomplete . . ." Mrs. Kardashian West does not disclose that she was working for, promoting, or having other commercial relationships with Diclegis. For this very reason, the FDA should have not written to her. Furthermore, the author likes to point out again the use of the word *post* instead of *advertisement*.

As you can see, Mrs. Kardashian West never recognizes openly that she wrote an endorsement. She just called it a *post*. The author thinks that this silent yet stubborn denial to call it a different name further substantiates what the author mentioned earlier. Mrs. Kardashian West simply expressed her opinion, her relief at having found a solution to her problem. The minimal protest made of words is correct. Mrs. Kardashian West does not have to apologize: she said what she thought, she felt better thanks to a particular medication, and she prized its effects.

Derrida's method can show how, in this "corrective" message, the conflict is clear: the right of a patient to express his or her opinion because he or she is entitled to it. No one can and should take it away. Mrs. Kardashian West posted a second message that only appears at first glance to offer an apology. She is not taking back anything. Moreover, we would like to focus on the structure of this second message.

The author's last remark is how Mrs. Kardashian West met the FDA requirements. She omitted all the risk factors and the possible side effects in the first message; in the second, she listed all of them as the FDA wanted (FDA, 2015a).

More interesting, however, is this ultimate fact: Mrs. Kardashian West listed all the side effects that might occur taking this drug. FDA wanted so and medical commercial have to list all the possible side effects that a patient might feel.

However, much research proves that this a nonperforming strategy, because long texts full of information are not well remembered, especially among younger people (Davis, 2010, p. 110).[15] If this was a strategy to remedy what she posted, then it is questionable.

Last element that we did not study before is the photo uploaded in Instagram. The picture next to the post we have already mentioned in this pages. What can we say about the picture next to the text we are analyzing? The picture presents Mrs. Kardashian West holding the prescription bottle next to her face. The picture might be perceived as a commercial. A simple question arises from this particular image: What is a commercial?

This new question can lead us too far away from our main issues, but the author wants to point out a few factors. If we consider any picture (and in many case, all the positive comments about a product, whether it is a place or a food, we might read on the Internet) a commercial, then this is a trap or a loop. It is surely impossible to get out of this interpretation. What is a commercial? As we noted earlier, even American law itself is unable to offer a clear definition of a commercial. For this very reason, it is the most dangerous and biased assumption to start with this accusation. Because this post was considered a commercial, there was no way to convince someone of the opposite. Because Mrs. Kardashian West's post was labeled a commercial, she did not have any other choice but to admit that her post was an advertisement. It is impossible to define a precise aesthetic of the commercial. It is too omnifarious and broad this concept.

All these elements lead us to highlight the fact that the FDA perceived Mrs. Kardashian West's post as an advertisement. She did not offer an apology, as we proved earlier. She did not feel the urge to write down in a clear and useful way all the side effects of the medication she took.

We cannot enter someone's mind, but it is clear that this second post was very far from being a corrective advertisement.

If the Internet hides tricks and traps, then those should be the object of the FDA's investigations and worries. As other studies warned and suggest (Popovich, Smith & Hellebusch, 2013). In Mrs. Kardashian West's case, a pregnant woman shared her story; there was no need to discredit her experience. The Internet's new strategy is for patients and medical personnel to work together:

Improving health literacy in a population involves more than transmission of health information, although that remains a fundamental task. Helping people to develop confidence to act on that knowledge and the ability to work with and support others will best be achieved through more personal forms of communications, and through community-based educational outreach. (Nutbeam, 2000, p. 267)

SOLUTIONS AND RECOMMENDATIONS

Most of us do not have the reach or the influence of Mrs. Kardashian West, but this case affects all of us. We will turn to the Internet more and more extensively in the coming years.[16] Especially, younger population are already very active online and use the Net as a first source for health tips (Cotten & Gupta, 2004). Therefore, it is useless to try to silence social media users (popular or not) simply because they express their opinions. The author has proved how Mrs. Kardashian West did not write an endorsement but instead her own personal opinion. The author has proved how Mrs. Kardashian West's actions cannot be seen as irresponsible because Diclegis is a prescription medication. Without a physician's approval, it is impossible to obtain legally. Her post was simply a personal story she shared with her followers. It was her phenomenological experience as a pregnant woman.

The author thinks it is better to be with Internet side rather than against it. It is true that it is often the first resource many turn for information on how to deal with a health problem,[17] but it is also true that doctors and their medical staff[18] are regarded as the most important and influencing source in health issues. Most patients are seeking just a general overview of their illnesses or diseases on the Internet but still plan to consult their personal physicians.

FUTURE RESEARCH DIRECTIONS

The Internet is not the enemy. It is a tool. As with every tool, we should all learn how to manage it properly. This is the new task that awaits physicians, bioethicists, drug companies, hospitals, and patients. The Internet will allow a more tailored and personalized way to interact with patients. They will be able to understand what is going on with their bodies, and ultimately, to understand what it is better for them. Physicians are there to give advice and to determine the best care and treatment for their patients.

CONCLUSION

It is better to improve the dialogue between patients and physicians instead of censoring what patients feel and think. Doctors will always play a special and significant role that cannot be substituted by a machine, especially when it comes to patients, who did not study Medicine (Radalescu & Cetina, 2011). Doctors should not be afraid of being usurped by the Internet. As explained previously, patients typically search for medical information online after or before having spoken to a doctor.

Sharing your personal medical experience online is not irresponsible, because the patient is simply posting his or her story, which may be useful for other patients. Doctors should not be afraid of this possibility that patients have to tell their personal experiences, that might be useful for other patients. It is a new form of patient empowerment, because patients can collect advices from whom had their same problem.

Doctors must not be concerned about losing their jobs or their respect because their patients are more informed. Otherwise, it will end up like the doctor Fabrizio De André sang about: "In the end, I had to understand / that being a doctor is just a job / and that you cannot give away your knowledge to people / otherwise you will become ill like them / otherwise the system will make you starve." (De André, 1971).[19]

REFERENCES

Bevan, J. L., Sparks, L., Ernst, J., Francies, J., & Santora, N. (2013). Healthcare Reform Information Sources in Relation to Information Quality, Information-Seeking, and Uncertainty. In R. Ahmed & B. R. Bates (Eds.), *Health Communication and Mass Media – An Integrated Approach to Policy and Practice* (pp. 19–34). New York, NY: Routledge.

Caputo, J. D. (1997). *Deconstruction in a nutshell.* New York, NY: Fordham University Press.

Cotten, S. R., & Gupta, S. S. (2004). Characteristics of online and offline health information seekers and factors that discriminate between them. *Social Science & Medicine, 59*(9), 1795–1806. doi:10.1016/j.socscimed.2004.02.020 PMID:15312915

Davis, J. J. (2010). The effect of placement and modality on the recall of information from pharmaceutical web sites. *Journal of Medical Marketing, 10*(2), 99–114. doi:10.1057/jmm.2009.42

De André, F. (1971). Il medico. In *Non al denaro, non all'amore, né al cielo* [CD]. Milano, Italy: Produttori Associati.

Devisch, I., & Vanheule, S. (2014). Singularity and medicine: Is there a place for heteronomy in medical ethics? *Journal of Evaluation in Clinical Practice, 20*(6), 965–969. doi:10.1111/jep.12110 PMID:24387804

Diclegis. (2017). Retrieved from https://www.diclegis.com/en/diclegis/what-is-diclegis

Elkin, N. (2008). *How America searches: Health and wellness.* Retrieved from http://www.rx-edge.com/research%20pdfs/How_America_Searches_Health_and_Wellness.pdf

Federal Trade Commission. (2015). *The FTC's endorsement guides: What people are asking*. Retrieved from https://www.ftc.gov/system/files/documents/plain-language/pdf-0205-endorsement-guides-faqs_0.pdf

Food and Drug Administration. (2015a). *Warning letter*. Retrieved from https://www.fda.gov/downloads/Drugs/GuidanceComplianceRegulatoryInformation/EnforcementActivitiesbyFDA/WarningLettersandNoticeofViolationLetterstoPharmaceuticalCompanies/UCM457961.pdf

Food and Drug Administration. (2015b). *Incorrect reminder ad*. Retrieved from https://www.fda.gov/Drugs/ResourcesForYou/Consumers/PrescriptionDrugAdvertising/ucm082287.htm

Heteronomous. (2017). In *Oxford Dictionary*. Retrieved from https://en.oxforddictionaries.com/definition/heteronomous

Influencers. (2017). In *Business Dictionary*. Retrieved from http://www.businessdictionary.com/definition/influencers.html

Jirasevijinda, T. (2015). Reaching into our doctor's bag of tricks to help patients navigate health information technology. *Journal of Communication in Healthcare*, *8*(4), 255–257. doi:10.1080/17538068.2015.1126052

Kale, M., Schwendig, L. W., Culberstone, V., Cady, P. S., Sharp, W., & Adamick, B. (1996). Monitoring the regulatory process of prescribed drug advertisement. *The Journal of Pharmacy & Law*, *229*, 229–243.

Kant, I. (1997). *Critique of practical reason*. Cambridge, UK: Cambridge University Press. doi:10.1017/CBO9780511809576

Kardashian, K. [kimkardashian]. (2015, August 7). Post [Instagram page]. Retrieved from https://www.instagram.com/p/7B07j_uSww/?taken-by=kimkardashian

Kardashian, K. [kimkardashian]. (2016, August 27). Post [Instagram page]. Retrieved from https://www.instagram.com/p/BJbEC96h3a5/?taken-by=kimkardashian&hl=it

Koumpouros, Y., Toulias, T. L., & Koumpouros, N. (2015). The importance of patient engagement and the use of social media marketing in healthcare. *Technology and Health Care*, *23*(4), 495–507. doi:10.3233/THC-150918 PMID:26409912

Lau, V. (2016, November 3). Ten things for pharma marketers to know about Facebook and Instagram. *Medical Marketing and Media*. Retrieved from http://www.mmm-online.com/technology/10-things-for-pharma-marketers-to-know-about-facebook-and-instagram/article/570439/

Lepping, P., Palmstierna, T., & Raveesh, B. N. (2016). Paternalism v. autonomy—Are we barking up the wrong tree? *The British Journal of Psychiatry*, *209*(2), 95–96. doi:10.1192/bjp.bp.116.181032 PMID:27482035

Maynard, E. G. [emilygmaynard]. (2016, August 6). Post [Instagram page]. Retrieved from https://www.instagram.com/p/BIpVQd_Ag4N/?taken-by=emilygmaynard

McAlexander, A. [@alicemcalex]. (2017, February 6). Tweet [Twitter page]. Retrieved from https://twitter.com/alicemcalex/status/828600176344461312

Nutbeam, D. (2000). Health literacy as a public health goal: A challenge for contemporary health education and communication strategies into the 21st century. *Health Promotion International*, *15*(3), 259–267. doi:10.1093/heapro/15.3.259

Öresland, S., Friberg, F., Määttä, S., & Öhlen, J. (2015). Disclosing discourses: Biomedical and hospitality discourses in patient education material. *Nursing Inquiry*, *22*(3), 240–248. doi:10.1111/nin.12097 PMID:25847051

Popovic, K., Smith, C., & Hellebusch, S. J. (2013). Attitudes on the use of social media in healthcare communications. *Journal of Communication in Healthcare*, *6*(1), 22–28. doi:10.1179/1753807612Y.0000000029

Powell, J., Inglis, N., Ronnie, J., & Large, S. (2011). The characteristics and motivations of online health information seekers: Cross-selectional survey and qualitative interview study. *Journal of Medical Internet Research*, *13*(1), 1–11. doi:10.2196/jmir.1600 PMID:21345783

Radulescu, V., & Cetina, I. (2011). The impact of health care consumer education on marketing strategies of health services organization. *Procedia: Social and Behavioral Sciences*, *15*, 388–393. doi:10.1016/j.sbspro.2011.03.109

Rawlings, B. (2015). Fashion bloggers, celebrities, and other influencers' endorsements and the FTC guidelines. *Entertainment and Sports Lawyer, 32*(2). Retrieved from http://www.americanbar.org/publications/entertainment-sports-lawyer/2015/firstedition/a-practitioner_s-column.html

Robehmed, N. (2016, July 26). Kim Kardashian West, mobile mogul: The Forbes cover story. *Forbes*. Retrieved from http://www.forbes.com/sites/natalierobehmed/2016/07/11/kim-kardashian-mobile-mogul-the-forbes-cover-story/#2c7a957d77ae

Schulz, P. J., & Nakamoto, K. (2011). "Bad" Literacy, the Internet, and the Limits of Patinet Empowerment. *AI and Health Communication, Spring Symposium*, 65 – 69.

Sinnenberg, L., Buttenheim, A. M., Padrez, K., Mancheno, C., Ungar, L., & Merchant, R. M. (2017). Twitter as a tool for health research: A systematic review. *American Journal of Public Health, 107*(1), e1–e8. doi:10.2105/AJPH.2016.303512 PMID:27854532

Smith, A. (2014, February 3). 6 new facts about Facebook. *Facttank*. Retrieved from http://www.pewresearch.org/fact-tank/2014/02/03/6-new-facts-about-facebook/

Smith, D. W. (2016). Phenomenology. In E. N. Zalta (Ed.), *The Stanford Encyclopedia of Philosophy*. Retrieved from https://plato.stanford.edu/entries/phenomenology/

KEY TERMS AND DEFINITIONS

Deconstruction: Method of analyzing texts and institutions elaborated by Derrida (1930 - 2004). It is the attempt to see a picture outside of its frame. We live in a world that is in a context that already gives meaning and rules to our understanding of the thing itself.

FDA: Food and Drug Administration is a federal agency of the United States Department of Health and Human Services, one of the United States federal executive departments. The FDA is responsible for protecting and promoting public health through the control and supervision of food safety, tobacco products, dietary supplements, prescription and over-the-counter pharmaceutical drugs (medications), vaccines, biopharmaceuticals, blood transfusions, medical devices, electromagnetic radiation emitting devices (ERED), cosmetics, animal foods & feed and veterinary products.

FTC: Federal Trade Commission is an independent agency of the United States government, established in 1914 by the Federal Trade Commission Act. Its principal mission is the promotion of consumer protection and the elimination and prevention of anticompetitive business practices, such as coercive monopoly.

Kant Immanuel: German philosopher (1724 – 1804). One of the most important thinker in the Enlightenment. His texts (*Kritk der reinen Vernunft* and *Kritik der praktischen Vernunft*) are essential to modern Philosophy.

Kardashian West Kim: Socialite. She became famous thanks to gossip and a reality show about her life.

Patient Empowerment: Process to get patients more involved, more active, and aware of their health.

Phenomenology: Philosophical movement born with Husserl (1859 - 1938). Its goal is to describe and analyze the reality as we feel it.

Slippery Slope Argument: It is an argument that connects minimal (and trivial) facts to bigger and more dangerous consequences.

Social Media: Webpages where people aggregate and share their personal data. This communicating system allows people to upload (almost) infinite number of information about their lives. Those new forms want to joint personal and private aspects with a public social sphere. Facebook, Instagram, Twitter are different types of this sharing platforms.

ENDNOTES

1 Only the second, corrected, post may be available on Instagram today.

2 According to a survey by Pew Research Center, a person's average number of Facebook friends is around 200. Kim Kardashian West has more than 29 million friends on Facebook (Smith, 2014).

3 The author would like to thank Professor Jason Dinse for his precious help and patience. I would never have been able to write this brief section without him.

4 "Reminder ads give the drug's name but not the drug's use. The assumption behind reminder ads is that the audience knows what the drug is for and does not need to be told" (FDA, 2015b).

5 It is very curious that another celebrity has had the same problem. Emily Maynard Johnson (2016) wrote a post praising the effects (and the prettiness) of Diclegis. It is true that she changed her post, too, in order to add more information about the side effects of this particular drug, but it is interesting to note that Mrs. Maynard Johnson, with her 6,000 followers, did not receive a warning letter from the FDA. Not even Diclegis received a warning letter from the FDA, despite what happened with Mrs. Kardashian West.

6 See the slippery slope argument.

7 If you check the *Oxford Dictionary* (2017), the first meaning of the word is the following one: "Subject to a law or standard external to itself."

8 In Kant, "pathological" means sensitive.

9 There are several definitions about this method in philosophy. We use this very general yet clear definition: "The discipline of phenomenology may be defined initially as the study of structures of experience, or consciousness. Literally, phenomenology is the study of "phenomena": appearances of things, or things as they appear in our experience, or the ways we experience things, thus the meanings things have in our experience" (Smith, 2016).

10 "Furthermore, increasing the amount of information is incapable of enabling patients to handle this information adequately. Ever more comprehensive patient 'education' is likely to remain incomplete for fundamental reasons. . . . But only a patient's level of information can be affected, not his background knowledge" (Schulz & Nakamoto, 2001, p. 66).

11 "On a basic level, Facebook can target users by age, gender, and device, but it can target by specific interests and location as well."

12 Even if this article seems to be very positive and optimistic toward the Internet's use, its author opens and closes his reflection quoting a "bag of tricks," as if a doctor were a magician. There is no question that a physician knows more than a patient, but this word, which refers to the doctor as a magician, whose job consists of tricking people's minds and eyes, leads to think that the author does not believe that patients can actually distinguish between fake and true. As the magician tricks the spectator into believing whatever he or she wants, so the doctor lets the patient believe that he or she is choosing for himself or herself. In reality, the doctor makes the decision, and the patient is just a passive and deceived spectator.

13 There are many definitions of paternalism. The author chose the following because it is clear and concise: "Paternalism is a description of a particular type of doctor-patient or nurse-patient relationship that implies that the doctor or nurse knows what is the best for the patient and enforces that opinion on the patient. The patient in this type of relationship is not equal but in a subordinate position."

14 The author strongly recommends reading this brief on the surprising Swedish research concerning educational material given by hospitals.

15 "In sum, it is clear that the current way of presenting side effects on the bottom of web pages is ineffective (especially for younger respondents) and that even under more favorable conditions, individuals have difficulty in recalling the specific side effects associated with drug use" (Davis, 2010).

16 This chapter mainly discusses Instagram, but social networks such as Twitter and Facebook are becoming more and more popular in terms of health research (Sinnenberg et al., 2017).

17 For example, Elkin (2008) states that the first sources peopled turned to for health- and wellness-related information were the Internet (more than 60%), followed by physicians (less than 60%). Internet searches focused on the following: 50% want to find a primary care physician, 23% are looking for specialists, and nurses are third on the list. The most searched topics are symptoms (60%), treatments (58%), and diseases/conditions (56%). These data prove that Internet users often want to know how to deal with a health problem they have. They even consider if they should go to the doctor (43%), and some

(72%) are seeking more information about a particular health problem. This report may not be that recent, but it was one of the most complete and thorough for its time about how an average user seeks information on the Internet.

18 Doctors are the most important source (Elkin, 2008, p. 7): 91% believe what a specialist or a physician says, followed by pharmacists (79%) and nurses (78%).

19 There is an Italian song based on the *Anthology of Spoon River*. One of the resting corpses is a doctor. In the book, his name his Dr. Siegfried Iseman. In the Italian version translated and sung by Fabrizio de Andrè, the protagonist claims that at the beginning, he was willing to share his knowledge, but the more he worked, the more he realized that his policy was not making him a rich doctor.

Chapter 8
Social Media for Mental Health Initiatives

Gemma Richardson
Humber College, Canada

ABSTRACT

Social media has added a new dynamic for those living with mental illness. There are several benefits to using social media to obtain information and support for mental health issues, but there are also new challenges and drawbacks. This chapter explores social media for mental health initiatives, with a focus on two case studies: Facebook's suicide prevention tools and the Bell Let's Talk campaign. These case studies highlight the unique ways that social media can be harnessed to raise awareness and provide support and resources to vulnerable populations, while also providing insights into the challenges of utilizing these platforms.

INTRODUCTION

The proliferation of social media platforms has inevitably had an impact on online help seeking for mental health issues. Asynchronous message boards have been used since the early days of the Internet for mental health support and information seeking, but social media platforms have added a new dynamic. On the one hand, these platforms can be heralded as welcome ways to break down the barriers for those seeking help in several ways due to the accessibility, convenience, and geographical reach of these platforms. Some social media sites also offer user anonymity, which can potentially alleviate some of the fears around stigma. On the other hand, however, there are several problematic aspects to using social media platforms for mental health initiatives, including the potential for trolling, bullying and other negative

DOI: 10.4018/978-1-5225-3716-8.ch008

Copyright © 2018, IGI Global. Copying or distributing in print or electronic forms without written permission of IGI Global is prohibited.

interactions, and the potential for online communication to increase isolation through minimizing face-to-face social interactions. There are increasing concerns that use of social media may in fact be *contributing* to mental illness, especially among vulnerable youth.

In light of these challenges, several social media platforms have initiated mental health initiatives for users. Other organizations have decided to harness the power of social media to increase awareness and dialogue on mental illness. In this chapter, the evolution of some of these initiatives is discussed, with a particular focus on Facebook's suicide prevention efforts and the Bell Let's Talk campaign. In the summer of 2016, Facebook made its updated suicide prevention tools available globally. Users of the platform can flag posts from friends if they are worried about the potential for self-harm and several options then appear in a drop down menu (including a list of resources, sending a message of support or having the post reviewed by someone at Facebook who can then reach out with helpful information). This initiative and some of the responses to it are examined in this chapter.

The Bell Let's Talk campaign is also explored. This campaign has generated a massive amount of support in Canada each January through the use of social media platforms (and in particular hash tags) to open up the dialogue on mental health (and ultimately raise money for mental health programs with each social media share or post using the #BellLetsTalk hashtag). These two particular case studies provide insights into the involvement of social media in mental health initiatives, both the positive aspects and the criticisms arising from them. The chapter concludes with a look ahead to what is needed and how there may be a continuing evolution in how these platforms are utilized for mental health initiatives.

USE OF SOCIAL MEDIA FOR MENTAL HEALTH INITIATIVES

While social media adds new dynamics and possibilities for mental health initiatives, the use of the Internet has long had strong appeal to people with stigmatized illnesses who wish to obtain information or assistance (Klein & Wilson, 2002; Berger, Wagner & Baker, 2005). Some forms of stigma can be avoided through anonymously seeking information online about mental illness. There are social media sites that build on this appeal by allowing created identities if the user desires (including Twitter, Instagram and Reddit) while others seek to remove anonymity (including Facebook, where users are strongly encouraged to use real names and have friends and family attached to their account who can see their posts and Facebook-related affiliations).

Now not only are those living with mental illness using social media to obtain information and support, but health care providers are also turning to these platforms. Most major mental health organizations have some form of presence on social media and use these platforms for outreach. Research into how social media can be utilized by health practitioners and organizations is also gaining in popularity. The National Institutes of Health in the U.S. has awarded several million dollars in research funding to explore using social media to advance prevention and treatment of addiction (National Institutes of Health, 2014). This builds on previous research in this area, such as that from a team of Microsoft researchers who explored how social media posts could be used to detect depression in users. De Choudhury, Gamon, Counts and Horvitz (2013) found that social media posts made by Twitter users in their study contained useful information to identify the onset of major depression—opening the possibility for the development of tools for use by healthcare agencies or individuals. Their study indicated that volunteers with moderate to severe depression were more likely to post negative messages, were less socially active on Twitter and were more concerned with health and relationships.[1]

There are some clear benefits to using social media for mental health initiatives. According to the Pew Research Centre (2017), 77% of adults in the U.S. own smartphones (for adults under age 49 this percentage is much higher). This means many people have smartphones on them at all times, allowing them to access social media platforms at all times of the day. Seeking support and information through these online platforms does not limit one to conventional business hours, meaning that support and information is accessible when conventional resources are not available. The ubiquitous nature of smartphones with access to social media platforms also means that the geographic reach of mental health initiatives can be expanded to remote and underserved communities.

As noted above, much research has found that online resources are particularly attractive for individuals with stigmatized identities, as help-seeking and socialization in face-to-face situations are associated with high levels of stress for members of such groups (Parr, 2008). Many social media platforms allow for stigmatized individuals to seek help in an anonymous fashion without face-to-face interactions. The use of social media in mental health initiatives can also be viewed as empowering. Social geographer Hester Parr believes that envisioning a person living with serious mental health problems "as technically proficient, intimately networked, emotionally nuanced and socially competent challenges stigmatizing conceptualizations of the damaged, alienated and pathologized patient-subject" (2008, p. 159). Social media also allow for a unique peer-to-peer sharing that can offer those living with mental illness a sense of comradery that cannot often be found in a practitioner-patient setting. A study conducted by Hughes and Cohen (2011) indicated that those with lived experiences offer meaningful information to people with similar conditions through online forums. This sense of community can be an important aspect for those who turn to social media for information and support.

There are, of course, challenges with these open and fluid discussion-based platforms on social media. Since the early days of the internet, problems with open communities where anyone can join and comment existed. For instance Sandy Stone (1999) documents the rise and subsequent demise of CommuniTree in the early days of Internet-based discussion forums in her work *The War and Desire of Technology at the End of the Mechanical Age.* She discusses the hard lessons about what was and what was not possible in an unstructured and unprotected conferencing environment, painfully learned through direct experience with the "system bashers" (p. 117). Similar problems still exist today and have even multiplied with the advent of Web 2.0. What we would now call trolling is a major problem for those seeking support online who participate in open groups or ones linked to social media like Facebook that do not allow for more anonymous forms of online existence. There has been increasing media attention to cases surrounding cyber-bulling and suicides, as well as the fears provoked by tragic cases such as that of Nadia Kajouji, the Canadian university student who was encouraged to kill herself in 2008 by a man in an online discussion group posing as a fellow suicidal female. These are ongoing challenges for social media platforms offering mental health support: usually anyone can participate and potentially make the situation worse.

The Samaritans, a well-known British suicide prevention group, introduced an app in 2014 that alerted users whenever someone they followed on Twitter posted troubling phrases that could indicate a potential risk for suicide—only to quickly disable the app a week later when it became evident that this data could easily be used to prey on vulnerable people. The app gave no notification to those being monitored and while there was potential for people to intervene when it appeared someone was in distress based on their Twitter posts, that also meant there was potential for vulnerable people to be identified and targeted. Using social media posts to diagnose depression or identify suicidal individuals is fraught with danger. As Munmun De Choudhury, a former member of the Microsoft team studying depression, points out, "we have to think very carefully about who gets access to these tools and what the boundaries are for technology used to make judgements about individuals" (as quoted in Singer, 2014, para. 29). The Samaritans app led to public outcry over their assumption that anyone and everyone had the appropriate training and expertise to monitor social media accounts using these experimental algorithms that ultimately labelled Twitter users. There were also concerns over who had access to this information and how it could potentially be used against someone by employers or even insurance companies. This case indicated the great need for much more research on monitoring social media for intervention opportunities. The fear of being labelled by one of these algorithm-based tools is part of the larger concern around stigma and identity online when it comes to mental illness. In a Canadian study, researchers found youth interviewed about using social media to seek mental health information worried about being judged and discussed the connections between social media, bullying and stigma (Rasmussen-Pennington, Richardson, Garinger & Contursi, 2013). For these reasons, the youth in the study preferred *not* to use social media to access mental health information.

In addition to these drawbacks and concerns, there are those who question the helpfulness of social media all together and some even blame these platforms for increasing mental health issues, especially involving vulnerable young people. Technology critic Sherry Turkle (2011) laments how technological devices such as smartphones have ultimately resulted in us being "alone together" - shutting out the people right in front of us in favour of staring at a screen, where "the performance of connection seems connection enough" (p. 9). Pantic, Damjanovic, Todorovic et al. (2012) found in their study of high school students that there was a statistically significant correlation between symptoms of depression and the amount of time spent on social networking sites. Other research has indicated that some social media pose risks for potential addictive behaviour (La Barbera, La Paglia & Valsavoia, 2009; Kuss & Griffiths, 2011) or can have a negative impact on self-esteem (Mehdizadeh, 2010). While these type of studies are often picked up by media to "sound the alarm" over social media use by youth, it must be noted that there are conflicting studies and some research has actually indicated that use of Facebook can enhance self-esteem (Gonzales & Hancock, 2011) and that online communication with friends and family through social media sites is associated with a decline in depression (Bessiere, Pressman, Kiesler & Kraut, 2010). These studies do not offer conclusive evidence one way or the other, leaving the impact of social media on mental health a topic of much debate.

SUICIDE PREVENTION MEASURES ON FACEBOOK

Several social media platforms have launched their own built-in mental health initiatives to assist users. Facebook's suicide prevention initiatives are explored here, but Facebook is not the only platform to launch this type of program. The popular photo sharing platform Instagram launched a new tool in 2016 to alert them to users who may be in distress. Once a user has flagged a post for showing signs of possible self-harm or depression, Instagram then sends a message to that person with resources to offer support. They also have banned some hashtags that promote self-harm or eating disorders, and searching for other concerning hashtags will automatically bring users to a support page. The microblogging site Tumblr launched an initiative in 2015 called Post it Forward to encourage users to share their stories of bullying, mental illness and other similar issues and to post messages of kindness and encouragement in a variety of media formats. The goal of the project is to reduce stigma and encourage a positive and supportive online environment. Programs like these show that it is not just researchers and mental health organizations that are turning to these platforms, but the platforms themselves that realize they can play an important role in promoting mental health initiatives. It should be noted that while these initiatives are undertaken by private companies, they often work in partnership with government-funded organizations and charities that provide services and resources (such as Facebook's partnerships discussed below).

Facebook is one of the largest and most well-known social networks, with more than 1.23 billion daily active users worldwide as of December 2016 (Facebook Newsroom, 2017). While there are numerous studies that examine the potential imitative effect of reports of suicide in traditional media,[2] the effects of suicide notes posted to online platforms like Facebook on predisposed individuals have not been studied in any depth. As Ruder *et al.* (2011) point out, suicide notes posted to Facebook are instantly available to a large number of individuals, quite different from traditional suicide notes. This instant access by a variety of people provides opportunity for Facebook users to intervene directly or seek help from emergency services. There have been cases of individuals posting their intent to attempt suicide on Facebook as a status update, which has then prompted friends or family to take action after seeing such a post online (with some able to successfully intervene, while others were sadly too late). Examples include: a 28-year-old man in Switzerland posted his intent and the location where he planned to jump to his death but unfortunately after notifying the police his friend arrived at the location too late (Ruder et al., 2011); in Israel a police search located a 44-year-old man injured but still alive after a suicide note he posted on Facebook the day prior alerted friends (Levy-Stein, 2009); a former contestant on the television show American Idol posted what appeared to be a suicide note to Facebook, spurring his family and friends to contact the authorities, track him down and have him evaluated at a nearby hospital (Dunkerley, 2014). These examples indicate that there are cases of Facebook users actively seeking to intervene in suicide attempts of other users.

In 2011, Facebook began their partnership with the National Suicide Prevention Lifeline and the Substance Abuse and Mental Health Services Administration. This marked the first time that users who saw a suicidal comment by a friend could report this to Facebook. In March 2016, Facebook announced an update to their suicide prevention tools, including streamlined reporting, integrated suicide prevention tools to help people in real time on Facebook Live (the platform's live video streaming service), and perhaps most importantly, live chat support from crisis support professionals through Facebook's Messenger (the platform's direct messaging and live chat service). Facebook reviews content reported them and prioritizes reports of suicide. Once a post is reported as a potential suicidal statement, Facebook then sends a message to the user encouraging them to call the National Suicide

Prevention Lifeline or to join a confidential online chat session with a crisis worker. The site offers "pre-populated text messages to make it easier for people to start a conversation" (Callison-Burch, Guadagno & Davis, 2016) when trying to reach out to a friend. Users of Facebook Messenger have the option to message with a crisis support worker directly through the Messenger app. The organizations partnering with Facebook to offer this service include the National Suicide Prevention Lifeline, the National Eating Disorder Association and the Crisis Text Line. Users watching live videos on Facebook Live can reach out to someone directly who they believe is in distress or the video can be reported to Facebook. The person sharing the video that was reported will then see a set of resources on their screen: choose to reach out to a friend, contact a help line, or see tips. All of these measures may potentially reach a suicidal individual and encourage them to seek help right away.

Facebook has also now started to pilot the use of artificial intelligence to identify posts that likely include thoughts of suicide. For now this is only limited to the U.S. Once a post has been identified by the algorithm, the Community Operations team then reviews these posts and determines whether to provide resources to the person who posted the content. As mentioned earlier, algorithms that identify suicidal or depressed individuals are fraught with ethical issues. First, they are in their infancy and require a great deal more research and testing. Second, who may have access to the data gleaned by these algorithms is controversial—information that someone may have a psychiatric disorder or be suicidal can have negative consequences for employment, housing opportunities and international travel, among other aspects. Privacy protection of this data is important and having potential information about someone's mental health (whether assumed or accurate) in the hands of a for-profit company raises concern. While suicide prevention is an important goal, the ethical layers must be carefully considered with all technology-based interventions, including these updated tools available through Facebook.

BELL LET'S TALK

Perhaps one of the most common uses of social media in relation to mental health initiatives is for raising awareness. The large reach instantly available through social networking sites make them very attractive tools for stigma reduction campaigns and encouraging greater understanding of mental illness. Using social media for these campaigns bypasses an initial reliance on traditional media because news outlets usually only pick up on the content once it has already achieved a large and widespread audience. Whether through viral videos shared on YouTube or hashtags that quickly trend on Twitter (such as #StopTheStigma and #WhatYouDontSee), there are a variety of ways to use social media to increase awareness and dialogue on mental illness. The Bell Let's Talk campaign is perhaps one of the largest and most successful of the campaigns utilizing social media for this aim.

Bell Media is part of the massive Bell Canada Enterprises (BCE) media conglomerate. The company spans both media content (owning radio stations, television stations and web sites) and media distribution (providing wireless, cable, internet and home phone services). In 2010, Bell launched the Let's Talk Campaign with the purpose of opening up the national dialogue on mental health and to generate funding for mental health programs. Social media is a key component of the campaign, with the idea being that through online social networks, individuals have the power to spread a message that can potentially change minds. It also allows those living with mental illness a chance to share their own experiences. The biggest component of the campaign is a dedicated day each year in January—the Bell Let's Talk day. During this 24-hour period, Bell pledges to put 5 cents towards mental health initiatives for every call or text made on their network by Bell subscribers, as well every time a post is made on Twitter and Instagram using the #BellLetsTalk hashtag, anytime a Snapchat user sends a snap using the Bell Let's Talk geofilter, and anytime a Facebook user watches one of the Bell Let's Talk videos.

There has been a steady increase in the number of interactions on Bell Let's Talk day each year since the campaign began. Starting with 66,079,236 interactions in 2011, the campaign grew to 131,705,010 interactions in 2017 (Bell Canada, 2017). The campaign features a variety of celebrity ambassadors and has received support through the social media accounts of notable people, including the Prime Minister of Canada, pop star Justin Bieber, comedian Ellen DeGeneres and actor William Shatner, as well as dozens of other celebrities, professional athletes and Canadian politicians. As of 2017, the campaign has generated 729,065,654 interactions, raising over $86 million for mental health initiatives (Bell Canada, 2017).

There is no doubt that the Bell Let's Talk Day is an incredibly successful social media campaign and the need to talk openly about mental health problems is a message that has been spread wide and far. Not only does the campaign aim to open up dialogue and reduce stigma, but the tangible effect of raising money for actual programs makes this a very popular initiative for millions of people to get involved in. With the ease of simply retweeting or using a hashtag, social media users can participate and contribute. Going beyond awareness and emphasizing the importance of community support programs for those living with mental illness allows the campaign to escape much of the criticism of other initiatives dubbed "slackivism", whereby social media users do very little to actually contribute to concrete solutions. Social media allows for new forms of dialogue on mental health and the Bell Let's Talk Day perfectly harnesses the power of this medium.

However, this does not mean it is completely free of criticism. Each year, there are those who use the day to disparage the company behind this campaign and highlight some of the problematic aspects of this campaign. When a massive telecommunications company is behind a campaign that encourages people to use their telecommunication devices to participate, it justifiably raises some suspicions. It must be noted that the campaign and its corresponding hashtags and social media mentions are not generic—it is not "Let's Talk" but instead "*Bell* Let's Talk". The company's name is uttered in every single tweet and share. This is no doubt a massive marketing campaign, not just a campaign for mental health. Perhaps this is one of the more intriguing aspects of this campaign, as it not only raises awareness and money, but it also gets the company's name out there and attaches goodwill to their name. As the employee who oversees the Bell Let's Talk campaign told *The Globe and Mail*, the campaign has "also helped people see Bell in different, more positive light and made them think about giving Bell a second chance" (as quoted in Ladurantaye & Krashinsky Robertson, 2013, para. 5). Whether it be frustrations as a Bell customer or animosity towards the company in the increasingly concentrated Canadian mediascape, these concerns seem to be put aside by many people each year who participate in the campaign. The very tangible element of raising money for mental health programs and research no doubt helps move this beyond a marketing and awareness campaign so that more people want to participate. The hashtag does inevitably get used each year by some who are displeased with the company[3], but the vast majority are genuine interactions and participation with the campaign. As with the Facebook suicide prevention initiative, the Bell Let's Talk campaign involves a private company partnering (or in this case, providing funding) to publicly-funded organizations and programs for those living with mental illness.

LIMITATIONS AND FUTURE RESEARCH

This chapter is by no means a complete look at the current landscape for social media and mental health initiatives. Facebook's suicide prevention tools and the Bell Let's Talk campaign were used as case studies here to highlight some of the issues at stake, but there are certainly many others that warrant research and discussion. Larger studies that look at impacts of these media tools and campaigns are required—the financial outcomes are known for the Bell Let's Talk campaign but potential impacts on stigma reduction are much more difficult to measure and assess. Potential future research projects could involve surveying individuals who have sought mental health treatment and support to find out how they were directed to that service and what role, if any, social media played. While incredibly difficult to navigate both logistically and ethically, it would provide highly interesting and necessary data if individuals who have attempted suicide could also be surveyed to find out what role, if any, social media has played in their lives and whether it resulted in early intervention for suicide attempts. As mentioned earlier, the studies that have been done about the impact of social media on mental health are limited, conflicting and do not offer conclusive evidence that there is necessarily any harm being done or that these tools are beneficial, leaving this a topic of much debate.

CONCLUSION

The use of social media by those living with mental illness continues to expand, as it offers a new way to connect to seek community, support and information. Naslund, Aschbrenner, Marsch and Bartels (2016) argue that online peer-to-peer connections through social media give individuals living with mental illness a chance to challenge stigma through personal empowerment and providing hope. Individuals can learn from their peers online, provide mutual support and help promote treatment across a wide demographic (Naslund, Aschbrenner, Marsh & Bartels, 2016). Social media also appeals to health practitioners, mental health organizations and researchers. These new forms of communication can help to monitor, identify and treat mental illness, potentially changing how psychiatry is practiced in the future (Peek, 2015). While these encouraging aspects must continue to be harnessed to benefit as many as possible, it is critical that the ethical implications that come along with this use of Web 2.0 are addressed. Privacy and the safety and well-being of everyone involved must be at the forefront of any discussions about how to use social media to benefit mental health initiatives.

REFERENCES

Au, J. S., Yip, P. S., Chan, C. L., & Law, Y. W. (2004). Newspaper reporting of suicide cases in Hong Kong. *Crisis, 25*(4), 161–168. doi:10.1027/0227-5910.25.4.161 PMID:15580851

Barraclough, B., Shepherd, D., & Jennings, C. (1977). Do newspaper reports of coroners' inquests incite people to commit suicide? *The British Journal of Psychiatry, 131*(5), 528–532. doi:10.1192/bjp.131.5.528 PMID:588871

Bell Canada. (2017). *Let's Talk results and impact*. Retrieved from: http://letstalk.bell.ca/en/results-impact/

Berger, M., Wagner, T. H., & Baker, L. C. (2005). Internet use and stigmatized illness. *Social Science & Medicine*, *61*(1), 1821–1827. doi:10.1016/j.socscimed.2005.03.025 PMID:16029778

Berman, A. L. (1988). Fictional depiction of suicide in television films and imitation effects. *The American Journal of Psychiatry*, *145*(8), 982–986. doi:10.1176/ajp.145.8.982 PMID:3394883

Bessiere, K., Pressman, S., Kiesler, S., & Kraut, R. (2010). Effects of internet use on health and depression: A longitudinal study. *Journal of Medical Internet Research*, *12*(1), e6. doi:10.2196/jmir.1149 PMID:20228047

Bollen, K. A., & Phillips, D. P. (1982). Imitative suicides: A national study of the effects of television news stories. *American Sociological Review*, *47*(6), 802–809. doi:10.2307/2095217

Callison-Burch, V., Guadagno, J., & Davis, A. (2016, March 1). Building a safer community with new suicide prevention tools. *Facebook Newsroom*. Retrieved from: http://newsroom.fb.com/news/2017/03/building-a-safer-community-with-new-suicide-prevention-tools/

De Choudhury, M., Gamon, M., Counts, S., & Horvitz, E. (2013). Predicting depression via social media. *Microsoft Research & the Association for the Advancement of Artificial Intelligence*. Retrieved from: https://www.microsoft.com/en-us/research/wp- content/uploads/2016/02/icwsm_13.pdf

Dunkerley, B. (2014, August 15). Josh Gracin posts suicide note on Facebook. *Rolling Stone*. Retrieved from: http://www.rollingstone.com/music/news/josh-gracin-posts-suicide-note-on-facebook-20140815

Etzersdorfer, E., & Sonneck, G. (1998). Preventing suicide by influencing mass-media reporting: The Viennese experience 1980-1996. *Archives of Suicide Research*, *4*(1), 67–74. doi:10.1080/13811119808258290

Facebook Newsroom. (2017). *Company info*. Retrieved from: http://newsroom.fb.com/company-info/

Fekete, S., & Schmidtke, A. (1995). The impact of mass media and reports on suicide and attitudes toward self-destruction. In B. L. Mishara (Ed.), *The Impact of Suicide* (pp. 142–155). New York: Springer Publishing Company.

Gonzales, A. L., & Hancock, J. T. (2011). Mirror, mirror on my Facebook wall: Effects of exposure to Facebook on self-esteem. *Cyberpsychology, Behavior, and Social Networking*, *14*(1-2), 79–83. doi:10.1089/cyber.2009.0411 PMID:21329447

Gould, M., Jamieson, P., & Romer, D. (2003). Media contagion and the young. *The American Behavioral Scientist*, *46*(9), 1269–1284. doi:10.1177/0002764202250670

Gunnell. (1994). Reporting suicide: The effect of media coverage on patterns of self harm. *British Medical Journal*, *308*, 1446-47.

Hassan, R. (1995). Effects of newspaper stories on the incidence of suicide in Australia: A research note. *The Australian and New Zealand Journal of Psychiatry*, *29*(3), 480–483. doi:10.3109/00048679509064957 PMID:8573052

Hawton, K., & Williams, K. (2002). Influences of the media on suicide. *British Medical Journal*, *352*(7377), 1374–1375. doi:10.1136/bmj.325.7377.1374 PMID:12480830

Ho, K. K. (2016, January 31). *Let's talk about how my job at Bell gave me mental health issues and no benefits*. Retrieved from: http://www.canadalandshow.com/lets-talk-about-how-my-job-bell-gave-me-mental-health-issues-and-no-benefits/

Hughes, S., & Cohen, D. (2011). Can online consumers contribute to drug knowledge? A mixed-methods comparison of consumer-generated and professionally controlled psychotropic medication information on the Internet. *Journal of Medical Internet Research*, *13*(3), e53. doi:10.2196/jmir.1716 PMID:21807607

Kessler, R. C., & Stipp, H. (1984). The impact of fictional television suicide stories on American fatalities. *American Journal of Sociology*, *90*, 151–167. doi:10.1086/228051

Klein, J. D., & Wilson, K. M. (2002). Delivery quality care: Adolescents' discussion of health risks with their providers. *The Journal of Adolescent Health*, *30*(3), 190–195. doi:10.1016/S1054-139X(01)00342-1 PMID:11869926

Kuss, D. J., & Griffiths, M. D. (2011). Online social networking and addiction - A review of the psychological literature. *International Journal of Environmental Research and Public Health*, *8*(9), 3528–3552. doi:10.3390/ijerph8093528 PMID:22016701

La Barbera, D., La Paglia, F., & Valsavoia, R. (2009). Social network and addiction. *Studies in Health Technology and Informatics*, *144*, 33–36. PMID:19592725

Ladurantaye, S., & Robertson Krashinsky, S. (2013, February 13). "Let's Talk" campaign a boost for mental health and Bell. *The Globe and Mail*. Retrieved from: http://www.theglobeandmail.com/report-on-business/industry-news/marketing/lets-talk- campaign-a-boost-for-mental-health-and-bell/article8644553/

Levy-Stein, R. (2009). Facebook suicide threat sparks massive manhunt in Eilat. *Haaretz*. Retrieved from: http://www.haaretz.com/news/facebook-suicide-threat-sparks-massive-manhunt-in-eilat-1.3436

Mehdizadeh, S. (2010). Self-presentation 2.0L Narcissism and self-esteem on Facebook. *Cyberpsychology, Behavior, and Social Networking*, *13*(4), 357–364. doi:10.1089/cyber.2009.0257 PMID:20712493

Naslund, J. A., Aschbrenner, K. A., Marsch, L. A., & Bartels, S. J. (2016). The future of mental health care: Peer-to-peer support and social media. *Epidemiology and Psychiatric Sciences*, *25*(2), 113–122. doi:10.1017/S2045796015001067 PMID:26744309

National Institutes of Health. (2014, October 17). *Using social media to better understand, prevent and treat substance abuse.* Retrieved from: https://www.nih.gov/news- events/news-releases/using-social-media-better-understand-prevent-treat-substance-use

Pantic, I., Damjanovic, A., & Todorovic, J. (2012). Association between online social networking and depression in high school students: Behavioral physiology viewpoint. *Psychiatria Danubina*, *24*, 90–93. PMID:22447092

Parr, H. (2008). *Mental health and social space: Towards inclusionary geographies*. Malden, MA: Blackwell Publishing. doi:10.1002/9780470712924

Peek, H. (2015). Harnessing social media and mobile apps for mental health. *The Psychiatric Times*, *32*(3), 33.

Pew Research Centre. (2017). *Mobile fact sheet*. Retrieved from: http://www.pewinternet.org/fact-sheet/mobile/

Phillips, D. P. (1974). The influence of suggestion on suicide: Substantive and theoretical implications of the Werther effect. *American Sociological Review*, *39*(3), 340–354. doi:10.2307/2094294 PMID:11630757

Phillips, D. P. (1979). Suicide, motor vehicle fatalities and the mass media: Evidence toward a theory of suggestion. *American Journal of Sociology*, *84*(5), 1150–1174. doi:10.1086/226904 PMID:507276

Pirkis, J., & Blood, R. W. (2001). Suicide and the media: Reportage in nonfictional media. *Crisis*, *22*(4), 146–154. doi:10.1027//0227-5910.22.4.146 PMID:11848658

Pirkis, J., Francis, C., Blood, R. W., Burgess, P., Morley, B., & Stewart, A. et al.. (2002). Reporting of suicide in the Australian media. *The Australian and New Zealand Journal of Psychiatry*, *36*(2), 190–197. doi:10.1046/j.1440-1614.2002.01000.x PMID:11982539

Rasmussen-Pennington, D. M., Richardson, G., Garinger, C., & Contursi, M. L. (2013). "I could be on Facebook by now": Insights from Canadian youth on online mental health information resources. *Canadian Journal of Information and Library Science*, *37*(3), 183–200. doi:10.1353/ils.2013.0015

Ruder, T. D., Hatch, G. M., Amponzi, G., Thali, M. J., & Fischer, N. (2011). Suicide announcement on Facebook. *Crisis: The Journal of Crisis Intervention and Suicide*, *32*(5), 280–282. doi:10.1027/0227-5910/a000086 PMID:21940257

Singer, N. (2014, December 26). Risks in using social media to spot signs of distress. *The New York Times.* Retrieved from: https://www.nytimes.com/2014/12/27/technology/risks-in-using-social-posts-to-spot-signs-of-distress.html?_r=0

Stack, S. (1996). The effect of media on suicide: Evidence from Japan, 1955-1985. *Suicide & Life-Threatening Behavior*, *26*(2), 132–142. PMID:8840417

Stack, S. (2002). Media coverage as a risk factor in suicide. *Injury Prevention*, *8*(90004Suppl IV), 30–32. doi:10.1136/ip.8.suppl_4.iv30 PMID:12460954

Stack, S. (2005). Suicide in the media: A quantitative review of studies based on non-fictional stories. *Suicide & Life-Threatening Behavior*, *35*(2), 121–133. doi:10.1521/suli.35.2.121.62877 PMID:15843330

Stone, R. A. (1996). *The war of desire and technology at the close of the mechanical age*. Cambridge, MA: MIT Press.

Turkle, S. (2011). *Alone, together: Why we expect more from technology and less from each other*. New York: Basic Books.

Weldon, T. (2017, January 25). Grand Falls radio host says Bell Media fired her for mental health issues. *CBC News*. Retrieved from: http://www.cbc.ca/news/canada/new-brunswick/bell-media-host-mental-health-1.3950097

KEY TERMS AND DEFINITIONS

Algorithm: A set of rules or procedures a computer program carries out to complete a task. Each algorithm is a sequence of instructions.

Hashtag: A user-generated method of categorizing content on social media. By placing the # symbol before a keyword or phrase, users categorize their content into easily searchable content areas.

Mental Illness: A range of health conditions that involve thinking, mood and behaviour. Examples include depression, anxiety disorders, addictions, eating disorders and schizophrenia.

Peer-to-Peer: Can refer to decentralized computer networks sharing information between them, or (as in the case of this chapter) people who provide information or support to others with whom they share a common identity. Peer-to-peer information or support is direct between the participants and does not involve outsider experts or authority figures.

Social Media: Web site that allow users to generate content and share with others. Online forms of communication that allow for large-scale sharing, networking and discussion.

Stigma: Negative feelings, beliefs or associations to something. Can be unfair and inaccurate beliefs, but often widely held. Literally means a mark of shame.

Suicide Prevention: Efforts to intervene in the actions of a suicidal person to cease harm or potential death, or to stop suicidal thoughts from being acted upon.

ENDNOTES

1 When this type of initiative was put into actual practice, there were, however, negative consequences and public outcry (see the discussion of the Samaritans app later in the chapter).

2 See, for example, Phillips 1974, 1979; Barraclough, Shepherd & Jennings, 1977; Berman, 1988; Bollen & Phillips, 1982; Kessler & Stipp, 1984; Gunnell, 1994; Fekete & Schmidtke 1995; Hassan, 1995; Stack 1996, 2002, 2005; Etzersdorfer & Sonneck 1998; Pirkis & Blood 2001; Hawton & Williams, 2002; Pirkis et al., 2002, Gould, Jamieson & Romer 2003; Au, Yip, Chan & Law 2004; and many others.

3 For example, on the day of the January 2017 Bell Let's Talk day, CBC published a damning article about a Bell employee who claimed to have been fired for her mental illness (Weldon, 2017, January 25). Sharing this article using the #BellLetsTalk hashtag showcases some of criticisms launched at the campaign and the company behind it. The year prior, another scathing article was published by a former Bell Media employee who claimed her job with the company was incredibly stressful yet her contract did not grant her access to the employee benefits package to seek mental health support (Ho, 2016). This was also shared using the #BellLetsTalk hashtag.

Related References

To continue our tradition of advancing information science and technology research, we have compiled a list of recommended IGI Global readings. These references will provide additional information and guidance to further enrich your knowledge and assist you with your own research and future publications.

Aas, I. H. (2013). Improving patient safety with telemedicine: Exploring organizational factors. In A. Moumtzoglou & A. Kastania (Eds.), *E-health technologies and improving patient safety: Exploring organizational factors* (pp. 56–70). Hershey, PA: IGI Global. doi:10.4018/978-1-4666-2657-7.ch004

Aboelfotoh, M. H., Martin, P., & Hassanein, H. (2013). Ubiquitous multimedia data access in electronic health care systems. In D. Tjondronegoro (Ed.), *Tools for mobile multimedia programming and development* (pp. 191–227). Hershey, PA: IGI Global. doi:10.4018/978-1-4666-4054-2.ch011

Abreu, J. F., Almeida, P., & Silva, T. (2013). iNeighbour TV: A social TV application to promote wellness of senior citizens. In R. Martinho, R. Rijo, M. Cruz-Cunha, & J. Varajão (Eds.), Information systems and technologies for enhancing health and social care (pp. 1-19). Hershey, PA: IGI Global. doi:10.4018/978-1-4666-3667-5.ch001

Aceti, V., & Luppicini, R. (2013). Exploring the effect of mhealth technologies on communication and information sharing in a pediatric critical care unit: A case study. In J. Tan (Ed.), *Healthcare information technology innovation and sustainability: Frontiers and adoption* (pp. 88–108). Hershey, PA: IGI Global. doi:10.4018/978-1-4666-2797-0.ch006

Adami, I., Antona, M., & Stephanidis, C. (2014). Ambient assisted living for people with motor impairments. In G. Kouroupetroglou (Ed.), *Disability informatics and web accessibility for motor limitations* (pp. 76–104). Hershey, PA: IGI Global. doi:10.4018/978-1-4666-4442-7.ch003

Adeyemo, O. (2013). The nationwide health information network: A biometric approach to prevent medical identity theft. In I. Management Association (Ed.), User-driven healthcare: Concepts, methodologies, tools, and applications (pp. 1636-1649). Hershey, PA: IGI Global. doi:10.4018/978-1-4666-2770-3.ch081

Åkerberg, A., Lindén, M., & Folke, M. (2013). Pedometer cell phone applications and future trends in measuring physical activity. In R. Martinho, R. Rijo, M. Cruz-Cunha, & J. Varajão (Eds.), *Information systems and technologies for enhancing health and social care* (pp. 324–339). Hershey, PA: IGI Global. doi:10.4018/978-1-4666-3667-5.ch021

Al Hamouche, V. (2014). Making quality control decisions in radiology department: A decision support system for radiographers' performance appraisal using PACS. In C. El Morr (Ed.), *Research perspectives on the role of informatics in health policy and management* (pp. 48–61). Hershey, PA: IGI Global. doi:10.4018/978-1-4666-4321-5.ch004

Al-Khudairy, S. (2014). Caring for our aging population: Using CPOE and telehomecare systems as a response to health policy concerns. In C. El Morr (Ed.), *Research perspectives on the role of informatics in health policy and management* (pp. 153–166). Hershey, PA: IGI Global. doi:10.4018/978-1-4666-4321-5.ch010

Albuquerque, C. (2013). The study of social needs as a strategic tool for the innovation of the social care sector: The contribution of new technologies. In M. Cruz-Cunha, I. Miranda, & P. Gonçalves (Eds.), *Handbook of research on ICTs for human-centered healthcare and social care services* (pp. 347–365). Hershey, PA: IGI Global. doi:10.4018/978-1-4666-3986-7.ch018

Alexandrou, D. A., & Pardalis, K. V. (2013). SEMantic PATHways: Modeling, executing, and monitoring intra-organizational healthcare business processes towards personalized treatment. In A. Moumtzoglou & A. Kastania (Eds.), *E-health technologies and improving patient safety: Exploring organizational factors* (pp. 98–123). Hershey, PA: IGI Global. doi:10.4018/978-1-4666-2657-7.ch007

Algarín, A. D., Demurjian, S. A., Ziminski, T. B., Sánchez, Y. K., & Kuykendall, R. (2014). Securing XML with role-based access control: Case study in health care. In A. Ruiz-Martinez, R. Marin-Lopez, & F. Pereniguez-Garcia (Eds.), *Architectures and protocols for secure information technology infrastructures* (pp. 334–365). Hershey, PA: IGI Global. doi:10.4018/978-1-4666-4514-1.ch013

Alhaqbani, B., & Fidge, C. (2013). A medical data trustworthiness assessment model. In I. Management Association (Ed.), User-driven healthcare: Concepts, methodologies, tools, and applications (pp. 1425-1445). Hershey, PA: IGI Global. doi:10.4018/978-1-4666-2770-3.ch071

Almeida, L., Menezes, P., & Dias, J. (2013). Augmented reality framework for the socialization between elderly people. In M. Cruz-Cunha, I. Miranda, & P. Gonçalves (Eds.), *Handbook of research on ICTs for human-centered healthcare and social care services* (pp. 430–448). Hershey, PA: IGI Global. doi:10.4018/978-1-4666-3986-7.ch023

Amer, M. B., Amawi, M., & El-Khatib, H. (2013). A novel neural fuzzy approach for diagnosis of potassium disturbances. In J. Tan (Ed.), *Healthcare information technology innovation and sustainability: Frontiers and adoption* (pp. 208–218). Hershey, PA: IGI Global. doi:10.4018/978-1-4666-2797-0.ch013

Andersen, S. T., & Jansen, A. (2013). Innovation in ICT-based health care provision. In J. Tan (Ed.), *Healthcare information technology innovation and sustainability: Frontiers and adoption* (pp. 58–72). Hershey, PA: IGI Global. doi:10.4018/978-1-4666-2797-0.ch004

Angjellari-Dajci, F., Lawless, W. F., Stachura, M. E., Wood, E. A., & DiBattisto, C. (2013). Economic evaluations for service delivery in autism spectrum disorders: benefit-cost analysis for emerging telehealth systems. In M. Cruz-Cunha, I. Miranda, & P. Gonçalves (Eds.), *Handbook of research on ICTs and management systems for improving efficiency in healthcare and social care* (pp. 16–42). Hershey, PA: IGI Global. doi:10.4018/978-1-4666-3990-4.ch002

Archibald, D., MacDonald, C. J., Hogue, R., & Mercer, J. (2013). Accessing knowledge from the bedside: Introducing the tablet computer to clinical teaching. In C. Rückemann (Ed.), *Integrated information and computing systems for natural, spatial, and social sciences* (pp. 96–109). Hershey, PA: IGI Global. doi:10.4018/978-1-4666-2190-9.ch005

Archondakis, S. (2013). Static telecytological applications for proficiency testing. In V. Gulla, A. Mori, F. Gabbrielli, & P. Lanzafame (Eds.), *Telehealth networks for hospital services: New methodologies* (pp. 228–239). Hershey, PA: IGI Global. doi:10.4018/978-1-4666-2979-0.ch015

Arling, P. A., Doebbeling, B. N., & Fox, R. L. (2013). Improving the implementation of evidence-based practice and information systems in healthcare: A social network approach. In J. Tan (Ed.), *Healthcare information technology innovation and sustainability: Frontiers and adoption* (pp. 247–270). Hershey, PA: IGI Global. doi:10.4018/978-1-4666-2797-0.ch016

Arriaga, P., Esteves, F., & Fernandes, S. (2013). Playing for better or for worse?: Health and social outcomes with electronic gaming. In M. Cruz-Cunha, I. Miranda, & P. Gonçalves (Eds.), *Handbook of research on ICTs for human-centered healthcare and social care services* (pp. 48–69). Hershey, PA: IGI Global. doi:10.4018/978-1-4666-3986-7.ch003

Arslan, P. (2014). Collaborative participation in personalized health through mobile diaries. In K. Rızvanoğlu & G. Çetin (Eds.), *Research and design innovations for mobile user experience* (pp. 150–181). Hershey, PA: IGI Global. doi:10.4018/978-1-4666-4446-5.ch009

Assis-Hassid, S., Reychav, I., Pliskin, J. S., & Heart, T. H. (2013). The effects of electronic medical record (EMR) use in primary care on the physician-patient relationship. In M. Cruz-Cunha, I. Miranda, & P. Gonçalves (Eds.), *Handbook of research on ICTs for human-centered healthcare and social care services* (pp. 130–150). Hershey, PA: IGI Global. doi:10.4018/978-1-4666-3986-7.ch007

Azar, A. T. (2013). Overview of biomedical engineering. In I. Management Association (Ed.), Bioinformatics: Concepts, methodologies, tools, and applications (pp. 1-28). Hershey, PA: IGI Global. doi:10.4018/978-1-4666-3604-0.ch001

Azar, A. T., & Eljamel, M. S. (2014). Medical robotics. In I. Management Association (Ed.), Robotics: Concepts, methodologies, tools, and applications (pp. 1116-1147). Hershey, PA: IGI Global. doi:10.4018/978-1-4666-4607-0.ch054

Baladrón, C., Aguiar, J. M., Calavia, L., Carro, B., & Sánchez-Esguevillas, A. (2014). Learning on the move in the web 2.0: New initiatives in m-learning. In *K-12 education: Concepts, methodologies, tools, and applications* (pp. 1693–1714). Hershey, PA: IGI Global. doi:10.4018/978-1-4666-4502-8.ch097

Bauer, K. A. (2013). Caught in the web: The internet and the demise of medical privacy. In I. Management Association (Ed.), User-driven healthcare: Concepts, methodologies, tools, and applications (pp. 1252-1272). Hershey, PA: IGI Global. doi:10.4018/978-1-4666-2770-3.ch063

Belsis, P., Skourlas, C., & Gritzalis, S. (2013). Secure electronic healthcare records management in wireless environments. In M. Khosrow-Pour (Ed.), *Interdisciplinary advances in information technology research* (pp. 202–219). Hershey, PA: IGI Global. doi:10.4018/978-1-4666-3625-5.ch015

Benito, R. V., Vega-Colado, C., Coco, M. B., Cuadrado, R., Torres-Zafra, J. C., Sánchez-Pena, J. M., & López-Miguel, A. et al. (2013). New electro-optic and display technology for visually disabled people. In M. Cruz-Cunha, I. Miranda, & P. Gonçalves (Eds.), *Handbook of research on ICTs for human-centered healthcare and social care services* (pp. 687–718). Hershey, PA: IGI Global. doi:10.4018/978-1-4666-3986-7.ch036

Bergenti, F., Poggi, A., & Tomaiuolo, M. (2013). Using multi-agent systems to support e-health services. In M. Cruz-Cunha, I. Miranda, & P. Gonçalves (Eds.), *Handbook of research on ICTs for human-centered healthcare and social care services* (pp. 549–567). Hershey, PA: IGI Global. doi:10.4018/978-1-4666-3986-7.ch029

Berler, A., & Apostolakis, I. (2014). Normalizing cross-border healthcare in Europe via new e-prescription paradigms. In C. El Morr (Ed.), *Research perspectives on the role of informatics in health policy and management* (pp. 168–208). Hershey, PA: IGI Global. doi:10.4018/978-1-4666-4321-5.ch011

Bernardi, R. (2013). Information technology and resistance to public sector reforms: A case study in Kenya. In I. Management Association (Ed.), User-driven healthcare: Concepts, methodologies, tools, and applications (pp. 14-33). Hershey, PA: IGI Global. doi:10.4018/978-1-4666-2770-3.ch002

Bernhard, S., Al Zoukra, K., & Schtte, C. (2013). From non-invasive hemodynamic measurements towards patient-specific cardiovascular diagnosis. In *Data mining: Concepts, methodologies, tools, and applications* (pp. 2069–2093). Hershey, PA: IGI Global. doi:10.4018/978-1-4666-2455-9.ch106

Best, C., O'Neill, B., & Gillespie, A. (2013). Assistive technology for cognition: Enabling activities of daily living. In M. Cruz-Cunha, I. Miranda, & P. Gonçalves (Eds.), *Handbook of research on ICTs for human-centered healthcare and social care services* (pp. 112–129). Hershey, PA: IGI Global. doi:10.4018/978-1-4666-3986-7.ch006

Bhattacharya, P., Asanga, A. P., & Biswas, R. (2013). Stomodeum to proctodeum: Email narratives on clinical problem solving in gastroenterology. In I. Management Association (Ed.), User-driven healthcare: Concepts, methodologies, tools, and applications (pp. 1073-1091). Hershey, PA: IGI Global. doi:10.4018/978-1-4666-2770-3.ch054

Boboc, C., & Ţiţan, E. (2014). Migration of medical doctors, health, medical education, and employment in eastern and central Europe. In A. Driouchi (Ed.), *Labor and health economics in the Mediterranean region: Migration and mobility of medical doctors* (pp. 158–191). Hershey, PA: IGI Global. doi:10.4018/978-1-4666-4723-7.ch007

Botella, C., Baños, R. M., Etchemendy, E., Castilla, D., García-Palacios, A., & Alcañiz, M. (2013). An e-health system for promoting wellbeing in the elderly: The butler system. In I. Management Association (Ed.), User-driven healthcare: Concepts, methodologies, tools, and applications (pp. 838-852). Hershey, PA: IGI Global. doi:10.4018/978-1-4666-2770-3.ch042

Bradai, N., Chaari, L., & Kamoun, L. (2013). A comprehensive overview of wireless body area networks (WBAN). In J. Rodrigues (Ed.), *Digital advances in medicine, e-health, and communication technologies* (pp. 1–32). Hershey, PA: IGI Global. doi:10.4018/978-1-4666-2794-9.ch001

Brown, K. E., Bayley, J., & Newby, K. (2013). Serious game for relationships and sex education: Application of an intervention mapping approach to development. In S. Arnab, I. Dunwell, & K. Debattista (Eds.), *Serious games for healthcare: Applications and implications* (pp. 135–166). Hershey, PA: IGI Global. doi:10.4018/978-1-4666-1903-6.ch007

Brown, M. (2013). Will comparative effectiveness research lead to healthcare rationing? In I. Management Association (Ed.), User-driven healthcare: Concepts, methodologies, tools, and applications (pp. 1487-1507). Hershey, PA: IGI Global. doi:10.4018/978-1-4666-2770-3.ch074

Burlamaqui, A. M., Azevedo, S. O., Silva, I. R., Silva, S. R., Souto da Silva, G. H., & Benjamim, X. C. … Felix de Castro, A. (2013). Low cost t-health and t-social with ginga: Experience with mime TV, ImFine, and iFunnyCube interactive TV programs. In M. Cruz-Cunha, I. Miranda, & P. Gonçalves (Eds.), Handbook of research on ICTs for human-centered healthcare and social care services (pp. 303-318). Hershey, PA: IGI Global. doi:10.4018/978-1-4666-3986-7.ch015

Burns, J., Blanchard, M., & Metcalf, A. (2013). Bridging the digital divide in Australia: The potential implications for the mental health of young people experiencing marginalisation. In *Digital literacy: Concepts, methodologies, tools, and applications* (pp. 772–793). Hershey, PA: IGI Global. doi:10.4018/978-1-4666-1852-7.ch040

Buyurgan, N., Rardin, R. L., Jayaraman, R., Varghese, V. M., & Burbano, A. (2013). A novel GS1 data standard adoption roadmap for healthcare providers. In J. Tan (Ed.), *Healthcare information technology innovation and sustainability: Frontiers and adoption* (pp. 41–57). Hershey, PA: IGI Global. doi:10.4018/978-1-4666-2797-0.ch003

Cabrita, M. D., & Cabrita, M. (2014). Applying social marketing to healthcare: Challenges and opportunities. In A. Kapoor & C. Kulshrestha (Eds.), *Dynamics of competitive advantage and consumer perception in social marketing* (pp. 78–97). Hershey, PA: IGI Global. doi:10.4018/978-1-4666-4430-4.ch004

Carroll, J. M., & Rosson, M. B. (2013). Community networks: Infrastructure and models for therapeutic support. In M. Cruz-Cunha, I. Miranda, & P. Gonçalves (Eds.), *Handbook of research on ICTs for human-centered healthcare and social care services* (pp. 187–207). Hershey, PA: IGI Global. doi:10.4018/978-1-4666-3986-7.ch010

Castiglioni, I., Gilardi, M. C., & Gallivanone, F. (2013). E-health decision support systems for the diagnosis of dementia diseases. In A. Moumtzoglou & A. Kastania (Eds.), *E-health technologies and improving patient safety: Exploring organizational factors* (pp. 84–97). Hershey, PA: IGI Global. doi:10.4018/978-1-4666-2657-7.ch006

Catley, C., Smith, K., McGregor, C., James, A., & Eklund, J. M. (2013). A framework for multidimensional real-time data analysis: A case study for the detection of apnoea of prematurity. In A. Gangopadhyay (Ed.), *Methods, models, and computation for medical informatics* (pp. 16–35). Hershey, PA: IGI Global. doi:10.4018/978-1-4666-2653-9.ch002

Chaari, L., & Kamoun, L. (2013). QoS concepts and architecture over wireless body area networks for healthcare applications. In J. Rodrigues (Ed.), *Digital advances in medicine, e-health, and communication technologies* (pp. 114–130). Hershey, PA: IGI Global. doi:10.4018/978-1-4666-2794-9.ch007

Chamberlin, B., Maloney, A., Gallagher, R. R., & Garza, M. L. (2013). Active video games: Potential for increased activity, suggestions for use, and guidelines for implementation. In S. Arnab, I. Dunwell, & K. Debattista (Eds.), *Serious games for healthcare: Applications and implications* (pp. 191–212). Hershey, PA: IGI Global. doi:10.4018/978-1-4666-1903-6.ch009

Charisi, A., Korvesis, P., & Megalooikonomou, V. (2013). Similarity searching of medical image data in distributed systems: Facilitating telemedicine applications. In A. Gangopadhyay (Ed.), *Methods, models, and computation for medical informatics* (pp. 58–77). Hershey, PA: IGI Global. doi:10.4018/978-1-4666-2653-9.ch004

Chattopadhyay, A., Malhotra, K., & Chatterjee, S. (2013). Ethical guidelines for the quality assessment of healthcare. In I. Management Association (Ed.), User-driven healthcare: Concepts, methodologies, tools, and applications (pp. 1332-1347). Hershey, PA: IGI Global. doi:10.4018/978-1-4666-2770-3.ch066

Chen, J. Y., Xu, H., Shi, P., Culbertson, A., & Meslin, E. M. (2013). Ethics and privacy considerations for systems biology applications in predictive and personalized medicine. In I. Management Association (Ed.), Bioinformatics: Concepts, methodologies, tools, and applications (pp. 1378-1404). Hershey, PA: IGI Global. doi:10.4018/978-1-4666-3604-0.ch071

Chen, Y. (2013). Construction of digital statistical atlases of the liver and their applications to computer-aided diagnosis. In J. Wu (Ed.), *Technological advancements in biomedicine for healthcare applications* (pp. 68–79). Hershey, PA: IGI Global. doi:10.4018/978-1-4666-2196-1.ch008

Cheng, B., Stanley, R. J., De, S., Antani, S., & Thoma, G. R. (2013). Automatic detection of arrow annotation overlays in biomedical images. In J. Tan (Ed.), *Healthcare information technology innovation and sustainability: Frontiers and adoption* (pp. 219–236). Hershey, PA: IGI Global. doi:10.4018/978-1-4666-2797-0.ch014

Cherian, E. J., & Ryan, T. W. (2014). Incongruent needs: Why differences in the iron-triangle of priorities make health information technology adoption and use difficult. In C. El Morr (Ed.), *Research perspectives on the role of informatics in health policy and management* (pp. 209–221). Hershey, PA: IGI Global. doi:10.4018/978-1-4666-4321-5.ch012

Chowdhry, N., Ashraf, A., Chowdhry, B., Baloch, A., Ansari, A., & De Meer, H. (2013). Grid for post operative care through wireless sensor networks. In I. Management Association (Ed.), User-driven healthcare: Concepts, methodologies, tools, and applications (pp. 514-531). Hershey, PA: IGI Global. doi:10.4018/978-1-4666-2770-3.ch026

Chun, S. A., Kwon, J. H., & Lee, H. (2013). Social credential-based role recommendation and patient privacy control in medical emergency. In A. Gangopadhyay (Ed.), *Methods, models, and computation for medical informatics* (pp. 215–237). Hershey, PA: IGI Global. doi:10.4018/978-1-4666-2653-9.ch013

Cohen, J. F., Bancilhon, J., & Sergay, S. (2013). An empirical study of patient willingness to use self-service technologies in the healthcare context. In M. Cruz-Cunha, I. Miranda, & P. Gonçalves (Eds.), *Handbook of research on ICTs and management systems for improving efficiency in healthcare and social care* (pp. 378–395). Hershey, PA: IGI Global. doi:10.4018/978-1-4666-3990-4.ch019

Constantinides, P. (2013). The development of the English national health information infrastructure. In I. Management Association (Ed.), User-driven healthcare: Concepts, methodologies, tools, and applications (pp. 968-991). Hershey, PA: IGI Global. doi:10.4018/978-1-4666-2770-3.ch049

Constantinides, P. (2013). The development of a regional health information infrastructure in Greece. In I. Management Association (Ed.), User-driven healthcare: Concepts, methodologies, tools, and applications (pp. 992-1017). Hershey, PA: IGI Global. doi:10.4018/978-1-4666-2770-3.ch050

Corrigan, D., Hederman, L., Khan, H., Taweel, A., Kostopoulou, O., & Delaney, B. (2013). An ontology-driven approach to clinical evidence modelling implementing clinical prediction rules. In A. Moumtzoglou & A. Kastania (Eds.), *E-health technologies and improving patient safety: Exploring organizational factors* (pp. 257–284). Hershey, PA: IGI Global. doi:10.4018/978-1-4666-2657-7.ch016

Corritore, C. L., Kracher, B., Wiedenbeck, S., & Marble, R. (2013). Foundations of trust for e-health. In I. Management Association (Ed.), User-driven healthcare: Concepts, methodologies, tools, and applications (pp. 1167-1193). Hershey, PA: IGI Global. doi:10.4018/978-1-4666-2770-3.ch059

Costa, Â., Andrade, F., & Novais, P. (2013). Privacy and data protection towards elderly healthcare. In M. Cruz-Cunha, I. Miranda, & P. Gonçalves (Eds.), *Handbook of research on ICTs for human-centered healthcare and social care services* (pp. 330–346). Hershey, PA: IGI Global. doi:10.4018/978-1-4666-3986-7.ch017

Coughlan, J., & Brinkman, W. (2013). Design considerations for delivering e-learning to surgical trainees. In J. Rodrigues (Ed.), *Digital advances in medicine, e-health, and communication technologies* (pp. 341–350). Hershey, PA: IGI Global. doi:10.4018/978-1-4666-2794-9.ch020

D'Abundo, M. L. (2013). Electronic health record implementation in the United States healthcare industry: Making the process of change manageable. In V. Wang (Ed.), *Handbook of research on technologies for improving the 21st century workforce: Tools for lifelong learning* (pp. 272–286). Hershey, PA: IGI Global. doi:10.4018/978-1-4666-2181-7.ch018

D'Abundo, M. L. (2013). Electronic health record implementation in the United States healthcare industry: Making the process of change manageable. In I. Management Association (Ed.), User-driven healthcare: Concepts, methodologies, tools, and applications (pp. 382-395). Hershey, PA: IGI Global. doi:10.4018/978-1-4666-2770-3.ch019

D'Andrea, A., Ferri, F., & Grifoni, P. (2013). RFID technologies in the health sector. In A. Moumtzoglou & A. Kastania (Eds.), *E-health technologies and improving patient safety: Exploring organizational factors* (pp. 140–147). Hershey, PA: IGI Global. doi:10.4018/978-1-4666-2657-7.ch009

D'Astolfo, C. (2014). Investing in a "rehabilitation model" to improve the decision-making process in long-term care. In C. El Morr (Ed.), *Research perspectives on the role of informatics in health policy and management* (pp. 37–47). Hershey, PA: IGI Global. doi:10.4018/978-1-4666-4321-5.ch003

Daniel, V. M. (2013). Genomics and genetic engineering: Playing God? In I. Management Association (Ed.), Bioinformatics: Concepts, methodologies, tools, and applications (pp. 249-267). Hershey, PA: IGI Global. doi:10.4018/978-1-4666-3604-0.ch013

Dasgupta, S. S. (2013). Cyber capability framework: A tool to evaluate ICT for development projects. In M. Cruz-Cunha, I. Miranda, & P. Gonçalves (Eds.), *Handbook of research on ICTs for human-centered healthcare and social care services* (pp. 399–406). Hershey, PA: IGI Global. doi:10.4018/978-1-4666-3986-7.ch021

Davis, S. A. (2013). Global telemedicine and ehealth: Advances for future healthcare – Using a systems approach to integrate healthcare functions. In V. Gulla, A. Mori, F. Gabbrielli, & P. Lanzafame (Eds.), *Telehealth networks for hospital services: New methodologies* (pp. 15–32). Hershey, PA: IGI Global. doi:10.4018/978-1-4666-2979-0.ch002

Deng, M., Petkovic, M., Nalin, M., & Baroni, I. (2013). Home healthcare in cloud computing. In M. Cruz-Cunha, I. Miranda, & P. Gonçalves (Eds.), *Handbook of research on ICTs and management systems for improving efficiency in healthcare and social care* (pp. 614–634). Hershey, PA: IGI Global. doi:10.4018/978-1-4666-3990-4.ch032

DeVany, M., Knobloch-Ludwig, K., Penticoff, M., Assimacopoulos, A., & Speedie, S. (2013). Telehealth implementation: The voice of experience. In S. Sarnikar, D. Bennett, & M. Gaynor (Eds.), *Cases on healthcare information technology for patient care management* (pp. 126–139). Hershey, PA: IGI Global. doi:10.4018/978-1-4666-2671-3.ch008

Ding, W., Qiu, P., Liu, Y., & Feng, W. (2013). Current omics technologies in biomarker discovery. In I. Management Association (Ed.), Bioinformatics: Concepts, methodologies, tools, and applications (pp. 465-497). Hershey, PA: IGI Global. doi:10.4018/978-1-4666-3604-0.ch027

Dingli, A., Abela, C., & D'Ambrogio, I. (2013). PINATA: Taking e-health a step forward. In A. Moumtzoglou & A. Kastania (Eds.), *E-health technologies and improving patient safety: Exploring organizational factors* (pp. 173–195). Hershey, PA: IGI Global. doi:10.4018/978-1-4666-2657-7.ch012

Dogra, D. P., Nandam, K., Majumdar, A. K., Sural, S., Mukhopadhyay, J., Majumdar, B., & Mukherjee, S. et al. (2013). A tool for automatic hammersmith infant neurological examination. In J. Rodrigues (Ed.), *Digital advances in medicine, e-health, and communication technologies* (pp. 301–311). Hershey, PA: IGI Global. doi:10.4018/978-1-4666-2794-9.ch017

Doyle, J., Bertolotto, M., & Wilson, D. (2013). Towards multimodal mobile GIS for the elderly. In *Digital literacy: Concepts, methodologies, tools, and applications* (pp. 590–609). Hershey, PA: IGI Global. doi:10.4018/978-1-4666-1852-7.ch031

Dragoni, A. F. (2013). Health services through digital terrestrial television. In V. Gulla, A. Mori, F. Gabbrielli, & P. Lanzafame (Eds.), *Telehealth networks for hospital services: New methodologies* (pp. 207–227). Hershey, PA: IGI Global. doi:10.4018/978-1-4666-2979-0.ch014

Dragoni, A. F. (2013). Virtual carer: A first prototype. In V. Gulla, A. Mori, F. Gabbrielli, & P. Lanzafame (Eds.), *Telehealth networks for hospital services: New methodologies* (pp. 290–299). Hershey, PA: IGI Global. doi:10.4018/978-1-4666-2979-0.ch019

Driouchi, A. (2014). Introduction to labor and health economics: Mobility of medical doctors in the Mediterranean region. In A. Driouchi (Ed.), *Labor and health economics in the Mediterranean region: Migration and mobility of medical doctors* (pp. 1–22). Hershey, PA: IGI Global. doi:10.4018/978-1-4666-4723-7.ch001

Driouchi, A. (2014). Medical knowledge, north-south cooperation, and mobility of medical doctors. In A. Driouchi (Ed.), *Labor and health economics in the Mediterranean region: Migration and mobility of medical doctors* (pp. 376–395). Hershey, PA: IGI Global. doi:10.4018/978-1-4666-4723-7.ch015

Driouchi, A. (2014). Skilled human resources in the health sectors and impacts of new health technologies on health workforce in developing economies. In A. Driouchi (Ed.), *Labor and health economics in the Mediterranean region: Migration and mobility of medical doctors* (pp. 23–50). Hershey, PA: IGI Global. doi:10.4018/978-1-4666-4723-7.ch002

Duan, X., Wang, X., & Huang, Q. (2013). Medical manipulators for surgical applications. In J. Wu (Ed.), *Technological advancements in biomedicine for healthcare applications* (pp. 111–122). Hershey, PA: IGI Global. doi:10.4018/978-1-4666-2196-1.ch012

Dugdale, A. (2013). Australian patient organizations: Using digital technologies to engage health citizen communities in health policy. In I. Management Association (Ed.), User-driven healthcare: Concepts, methodologies, tools, and applications (pp. 853-869). Hershey, PA: IGI Global. doi:10.4018/978-1-4666-2770-3.ch043

Dunwell, I., & Jarvis, S. (2013). A serious game for on-the-ward infection control awareness training: Ward off infection. In S. Arnab, I. Dunwell, & K. Debattista (Eds.), *Serious games for healthcare: Applications and implications* (pp. 233–246). Hershey, PA: IGI Global. doi:10.4018/978-1-4666-1903-6.ch011

Durant, K. T., McCray, A. T., & Safran, C. (2013). Identifying temporal changes and topics that promote growth within online communities: A prospective study of six online cancer forums. In A. Gangopadhyay (Ed.), *Methods, models, and computation for medical informatics* (pp. 78–97). Hershey, PA: IGI Global. doi:10.4018/978-1-4666-2653-9.ch005

El-Farargy, N. (2013). Refresher training in clinical psychology supervision: A blended learning approach. In A. Benson, J. Moore, & S. Williams van Rooij (Eds.), *Cases on educational technology planning, design, and implementation: A project management perspective* (pp. 295–317). Hershey, PA: IGI Global. doi:10.4018/978-1-4666-4237-9.ch016

Enquist, H. (2013). From idea to use: lessons learned from a participatory ICT healthcare case study. In I. Management Association (Ed.), User-driven healthcare: Concepts, methodologies, tools, and applications (pp. 1037-1053). Hershey, PA: IGI Global. doi:10.4018/978-1-4666-2770-3.ch052

Ervin, K. (2014). Legal and ethical considerations in the implementation of electronic health records. In J. Krueger (Ed.), *Cases on electronic records and resource management implementation in diverse environments* (pp. 193–210). Hershey, PA: IGI Global. doi:10.4018/978-1-4666-4466-3.ch012

Escayola, J., Trigo, J., Martínez, I., Martínez-Espronceda, M., Aragüés, A., Sancho, D., . . . García, J. (2013). Overview of the ISO/IEEE11073 family of standards and their applications to health monitoring. In I. Management Association (Ed.), User-driven healthcare: Concepts, methodologies, tools, and applications (pp. 357-381). Hershey, PA: IGI Global. doi:10.4018/978-1-4666-2770-3.ch018

Facelli, J. C., Hurdle, J. F., & Mitchell, J. A. (2013). Medical informatics and bioinformatics. In I. Management Association (Ed.), Bioinformatics: Concepts, methodologies, tools, and applications (pp. 195-221). Hershey, PA: IGI Global. doi:10.4018/978-1-4666-3604-0.ch010

Fakhar, A. (2014). Beyond brain drain: A case study of the benefits of cooperation on medical immigration. In A. Driouchi (Ed.), *Labor and health economics in the Mediterranean region: Migration and mobility of medical doctors* (pp. 294–313). Hershey, PA: IGI Global. doi:10.4018/978-1-4666-4723-7.ch012

Falan, S. L., Han, B., Zoeller, L. H., Tarn, J. M., & Roach, D. M. (2013). Sustaining healthcare through waste elimination: A taxonomic analysis with case illustrations. In J. Tan (Ed.), *Healthcare information technology innovation and sustainability: Frontiers and adoption* (pp. 18–39). Hershey, PA: IGI Global. doi:10.4018/978-1-4666-2797-0.ch002

Farinha, C., & Mira da Silva, M. (2013). Identifying requirements for healthcare information systems with focus groups. In M. Cruz-Cunha, I. Miranda, & P. Gonçalves (Eds.), *Handbook of research on ICTs for human-centered healthcare and social care services* (pp. 491–510). Hershey, PA: IGI Global. doi:10.4018/978-1-4666-3986-7.ch026

Fernando, J. (2013). The protocols of privileged information handling in an e-health context: Australia. In I. Management Association (Ed.), User-driven healthcare: Concepts, methodologies, tools, and applications (pp. 737-759). Hershey, PA: IGI Global. doi:10.4018/978-1-4666-2770-3.ch036

Ferreira, L., Teixeira, A., & Cunha, J. P. (2013). Medical information extraction in European Portuguese. In M. Cruz-Cunha, I. Miranda, & P. Gonçalves (Eds.), *Handbook of research on ICTs for human-centered healthcare and social care services* (pp. 607–626). Hershey, PA: IGI Global. doi:10.4018/978-1-4666-3986-7.ch032

Fitzpatrick, J. (2013). An exploration of the experiences of migrant women: Implications for policy development of effective user driven health care delivery systems. In I. Management Association (Ed.), User-driven healthcare: Concepts, methodologies, tools, and applications (pp. 954-967). Hershey, PA: IGI Global. doi:10.4018/978-1-4666-2770-3.ch048

Fitzpatrick, J., & Ako, W. (2013). Developing community ontologies in user driven healthcare. In I. Management Association (Ed.), User-driven healthcare: Concepts, methodologies, tools, and applications (pp. 655-672). Hershey, PA: IGI Global. doi:10.4018/978-1-4666-2770-3.ch032

Flores, A. E., Win, K. T., & Susilo, W. (2013). Secure exchange of electronic health records. In I. Management Association (Ed.), IT policy and ethics: Concepts, methodologies, tools, and applications (pp. 1059-1079). Hershey, PA: IGI Global. doi:10.4018/978-1-4666-2919-6.ch048

Flores, A. E., Win, K. T., & Susilo, W. (2013). Secure exchange of electronic health records. In I. Management Association (Ed.), User-driven healthcare: Concepts, methodologies, tools, and applications (pp. 1403-1424). Hershey, PA: IGI Global. doi:10.4018/978-1-4666-2770-3.ch070

Forrestal, E. J., Cellucci, L. W., Zeng, X., Kennedy, M. H., & Smith, D. (2013). Health information technology collaboration in community health centers: The community partners HealthNet, Inc. In S. Sarnikar, D. Bennett, & M. Gaynor (Eds.), *Cases on healthcare information technology for patient care management* (pp. 171–196). Hershey, PA: IGI Global. doi:10.4018/978-1-4666-2671-3.ch011

Frederico, C. (2013). Nutrition games. In S. Arnab, I. Dunwell, & K. Debattista (Eds.), *Serious games for healthcare: Applications and implications* (pp. 167–190). Hershey, PA: IGI Global. doi:10.4018/978-1-4666-1903-6.ch008

Freitas, L., Pereira, R. T., Pereira, H. G., Martini, R., Mozzaquatro, B. A., Kasper, J., & Librelotto, G. (2013). Ontological representation and an architecture for homecare pervasive systems. In R. Martinho, R. Rijo, M. Cruz-Cunha, & J. Varajão (Eds.), *Information systems and technologies for enhancing health and social care* (pp. 215–234). Hershey, PA: IGI Global. doi:10.4018/978-1-4666-3667-5.ch015

Frigo, C. A., & Pavan, E. E. (2014). Prosthetic and orthotic devices. In *Assistive technologies: Concepts, methodologies, tools, and applications* (pp. 549–613). Hershey, PA: IGI Global. doi:10.4018/978-1-4666-4422-9.ch028

Fukami, T., & Wu, J. (2013). Image fusion method and the efficacy of multimodal cardiac images. In J. Wu (Ed.), *Technological advancements in biomedicine for healthcare applications* (pp. 47–54). Hershey, PA: IGI Global. doi:10.4018/978-1-4666-2196-1.ch006

Furdu, I., & Patrut, B. (2013). ICT applications and solutions in healthcare: Present and perspectives. In M. Cruz-Cunha, I. Miranda, & P. Gonçalves (Eds.), *Handbook of research on ICTs and management systems for improving efficiency in healthcare and social care* (pp. 559–576). Hershey, PA: IGI Global. doi:10.4018/978-1-4666-3990-4.ch029

Gabbrielli, F. (2013). Telemedicine R&D influencing incoming strategies and organization models. In V. Gulla, A. Mori, F. Gabbrielli, & P. Lanzafame (Eds.), *Telehealth networks for hospital services: New methodologies* (pp. 250–264). Hershey, PA: IGI Global. doi:10.4018/978-1-4666-2979-0.ch017

Gaivéo, J. M. (2013). Security of ICTs supporting healthcare activities. In M. Cruz-Cunha, I. Miranda, & P. Gonçalves (Eds.), *Handbook of research on ICTs for human-centered healthcare and social care services* (pp. 208–228). Hershey, PA: IGI Global. doi:10.4018/978-1-4666-3986-7.ch011

Gallo, C. (2013). A multichannel framework for multimedia content deployment in e-health environments. In M. Cruz-Cunha, I. Miranda, & P. Gonçalves (Eds.), *Handbook of research on ICTs and management systems for improving efficiency in healthcare and social care* (pp. 872–891). Hershey, PA: IGI Global. doi:10.4018/978-1-4666-3990-4.ch045

Gao, Y., Yang, W., Yang, J., Satoshi, T., & Wu, J. (2013). Neural mechanisms of audiovisual integration in integrated processing for verbal perception and spatial factors. In J. Wu (Ed.), *Biomedical engineering and cognitive neuroscience for healthcare: Interdisciplinary applications* (pp. 327–336). Hershey, PA: IGI Global. doi:10.4018/978-1-4666-2113-8.ch034

Garzo, A., Carmien, S. P., & Madina, X. (2013). Mapping input technology to ability. In I. Management Association (Ed.), User-driven healthcare: Concepts, methodologies, tools, and applications (pp. 480-501). Hershey, PA: IGI Global. doi:10.4018/978-1-4666-2770-3.ch024

Gatzidis, C. (2013). First-person shooter game engines and healthcare: An examination of the current state of the art and future potential. In S. Arnab, I. Dunwell, & K. Debattista (Eds.), *Serious Games for Healthcare: Applications and Implications* (pp. 76–89). Hershey, PA: IGI Global. doi:10.4018/978-1-4666-1903-6.ch004

Gaughan, M. (2013). The hybridized nature of America's health care system: Medicare as a case of both market and public failure. In M. Merviö (Ed.), *Healthcare management and economics: Perspectives on public and private administration* (pp. 154–164). Hershey, PA: IGI Global. doi:10.4018/978-1-4666-3982-9.ch012

Gavgani, V. Z. (2013). Information therapy (ix) service and patients' preference. In A. Gangopadhyay (Ed.), *Methods, models, and computation for medical informatics* (pp. 117–125). Hershey, PA: IGI Global. doi:10.4018/978-1-4666-2653-9.ch007

Gavgani, V. Z. (2013). Ubiquitous information therapy service through social networking libraries: An operational web 2.0 service model. In I. Management Association (Ed.), User-driven healthcare: Concepts, methodologies, tools, and applications (pp. 673-688). Hershey, PA: IGI Global. doi:10.4018/978-1-4666-2770-3.ch033

Germaine-McDaniel, N. S. (2013). The emerging hispanic use of online health information in the United States: Cultural convergence or dissociation? In I. Management Association (Ed.), User-driven healthcare: Concepts, methodologies, tools, and applications (pp. 1607-1621). Hershey, PA: IGI Global. doi:10.4018/978-1-4666-2770-3.ch079

Gholson, J., & Tennyson, H. (2013). One system of care, one electronic chart. In S. Sarnikar, D. Bennett, & M. Gaynor (Eds.), *Cases on healthcare information technology for patient care management* (pp. 55–69). Hershey, PA: IGI Global. doi:10.4018/978-1-4666-2671-3.ch003

Ghosh, B. (2013). Healthcare systems using clinical data: Addressing data interoperability challenges. In S. Sarnikar, D. Bennett, & M. Gaynor (Eds.), *Cases on healthcare information technology for patient care management* (pp. 208–223). Hershey, PA: IGI Global. doi:10.4018/978-1-4666-2671-3.ch013

Gibson, L., Sloan, D., & Moncur, W. (2013). E-health and digital inclusion. In I. Management Association (Ed.), User-driven healthcare: Concepts, methodologies, tools, and applications (pp. 197-210). Hershey, PA: IGI Global. doi:10.4018/978-1-4666-2770-3.ch011

Gillies, A. C., & Howard, J. (2013). Information as change agent or barrier in health care reform? In J. Tan (Ed.), *Healthcare information technology innovation and sustainability: Frontiers and adoption* (pp. 1–17). Hershey, PA: IGI Global. doi:10.4018/978-1-4666-2797-0.ch001

Glusker, A., & Hoelscher, E. (2014). Transitioning from print to online-only resources: The experience of a medium-sized healthcare organization library. In J. Krueger (Ed.), *Cases on electronic records and resource management implementation in diverse environments* (pp. 226–242). Hershey, PA: IGI Global. doi:10.4018/978-1-4666-4466-3.ch014

Gofuku, A., Fukumori, S., & Sato, K. (2013). A mirror visual feedback therapy system applying virtual reality technology. In J. Wu (Ed.), *Biomedical engineering and cognitive neuroscience for healthcare: Interdisciplinary applications* (pp. 73–80). Hershey, PA: IGI Global. doi:10.4018/978-1-4666-2113-8.ch008

Gomes, C., Sperandio, F., Peles, A., Borges, J., Brito, A. C., & Almada-Lobo, B. (2013). An operating theater planning decision support system. In R. Martinho, R. Rijo, M. Cruz-Cunha, & J. Varajão (Eds.), *Information systems and technologies for enhancing health and social care* (pp. 69–86). Hershey, PA: IGI Global. doi:10.4018/978-1-4666-3667-5.ch005

Grissom, T. E., DuKatz, A., Kordylewski, H. A., & Dutton, R. P. (2013). Bring out your data: The evolution of the national anesthesia clinical outcomes registry (NACOR). In A. Gangopadhyay (Ed.), *Methods, models, and computation for medical informatics* (pp. 126–145). Hershey, PA: IGI Global. doi:10.4018/978-1-4666-2653-9.ch008

Gudes, O., Kendall, E., Yigitcanlar, T., Han, J. H., & Pathak, V. (2013). Developing a competitive city through healthy decision-making. In I. Management Association (Ed.), User-driven healthcare: Concepts, methodologies, tools, and applications (pp. 808-822). Hershey, PA: IGI Global. doi:10.4018/978-1-4666-2770-3.ch040

Gugerty, B., & Maranda, M. J. (2013). The promises and challenges of health information technology. In I. Management Association (Ed.), User-driven healthcare: Concepts, methodologies, tools, and applications (pp. 57-76). Hershey, PA: IGI Global. doi:10.4018/978-1-4666-2770-3.ch004

Guimarães, C., Antunes, D. R., García, L. S., & Fernandes, S. (2013). Information challenges of the deaf in their health and social care needs. In M. Cruz-Cunha, I. Miranda, & P. Gonçalves (Eds.), *Handbook of research on ICTs for human-centered healthcare and social care services* (pp. 93–111). Hershey, PA: IGI Global. doi:10.4018/978-1-4666-3986-7.ch005

Guinalíu, M., Marta, J., & Subero, J. M. (2013). Social networks as a tool to improve the life quality of chronic patients and their relatives. In M. Cruz-Cunha, I. Miranda, & P. Gonçalves (Eds.), *Handbook of research on ICTs for human-centered healthcare and social care services* (pp. 172–186). Hershey, PA: IGI Global. doi:10.4018/978-1-4666-3986-7.ch009

Gullà, V. (2013). Leading the technological innovation in healthcare systems: The telematic medicine approach. In V. Gulla, A. Mori, F. Gabbrielli, & P. Lanzafame (Eds.), *Telehealth networks for hospital services: New methodologies* (pp. 134–153). Hershey, PA: IGI Global. doi:10.4018/978-1-4666-2979-0.ch009

Gullà, V., & Cancellotti, C. (2013). Telemedicine in emergency: A first aid hospital network experience. In V. Gulla, A. Mori, F. Gabbrielli, & P. Lanzafame (Eds.), *Telehealth networks for hospital services: New methodologies* (pp. 240–248). Hershey, PA: IGI Global. doi:10.4018/978-1-4666-2979-0.ch016

Guo, M., Yu, Y., Yang, J., & Wu, J. (2013). The crossmodal between the visual and tactile for motion perception. In J. Wu (Ed.), *Biomedical engineering and cognitive neuroscience for healthcare: Interdisciplinary applications* (pp. 99–108). Hershey, PA: IGI Global. doi:10.4018/978-1-4666-2113-8.ch011

Habib, M. K. (2014). Web-based multi-user distributed and collaborative environment supporting emergency and relief activities. In I. Management Association (Ed.), Crisis management: Concepts, methodologies, tools and applications (pp. 425-445). Hershey, PA: IGI Global. doi:10.4018/978-1-4666-4707-7.ch019

Hafeez-Baig, A., & Gururajan, R. (2013). Phenomena of adoption of wireless handheld devices: A case of healthcare setting. In H. Muga & K. Thomas (Eds.), *Cases on the diffusion and adoption of sustainable development practices* (pp. 20–43). Hershey, PA: IGI Global. doi:10.4018/978-1-4666-2842-7.ch002

Haida, M. (2013). Implications of NIRS brain signals. In J. Wu (Ed.), *Biomedical engineering and cognitive neuroscience for healthcare: Interdisciplinary applications* (pp. 120–128). Hershey, PA: IGI Global. doi:10.4018/978-1-4666-2113-8.ch013

Han, D., & Braun, K. L. (2013). Promoting active ageing through technology training in Korea. In *Digital literacy: Concepts, methodologies, tools, and applications* (pp. 572–589). Hershey, PA: IGI Global. doi:10.4018/978-1-4666-1852-7.ch030

Haniff, D. (2013). Usability engineering and e-health. In I. Management Association (Ed.), User-driven healthcare: Concepts, methodologies, tools, and applications (pp. 1446-1468). Hershey, PA: IGI Global. doi:10.4018/978-1-4666-2770-3.ch072

Hareva, D. H., Okada, H., & Oka, H. (2013). Ecological momentary assessment using a mobile phone. In J. Wu (Ed.), *Technological advancements in biomedicine for healthcare applications* (pp. 398–407). Hershey, PA: IGI Global. doi:10.4018/978-1-4666-2196-1.ch039

Harnett, B. (2013). Patient centered medicine and technology adaptation. In I. Management Association (Ed.), User-driven healthcare: Concepts, methodologies, tools, and applications (pp. 77-98). Hershey, PA: IGI Global. doi:10.4018/978-1-4666-2770-3.ch005

Hatton, J. D., Schmidt, T. M., & Jelen, J. (2013). Adoption of electronic health care records: Physician heuristics and hesitancy. In R. Martinho, R. Rijo, M. Cruz-Cunha, & J. Varajão (Eds.), *Information systems and technologies for enhancing health and social care* (pp. 148–165). Hershey, PA: IGI Global. doi:10.4018/978-1-4666-3667-5.ch010

Heinrichs, L., Fellander-Tsai, L., & Davies, D. (2013). Clinical virtual worlds: The wider implications for professional development in healthcare. In K. Bredl & W. Bösche (Eds.), *Serious games and virtual worlds in education, professional development, and healthcare* (pp. 221–240). Hershey, PA: IGI Global. doi:10.4018/978-1-4666-3673-6.ch014

Heinrichs, W. L., Davies, D., & Davies, J. (2013). Virtual worlds in healthcare: Applications and implications. In S. Arnab, I. Dunwell, & K. Debattista (Eds.), *Serious games for healthcare: Applications and implications* (pp. 1–22). Hershey, PA: IGI Global. doi:10.4018/978-1-4666-1903-6.ch001

Hirata, M., Yanagisawa, T., Matsushita, K., Sugata, H., Kamitani, Y., & Suzuki, T. … Yoshimine, T. (2013). Brain–machine interface using brain surface electrodes: Real-time robotic control and a fully implantable wireless system. In J. Wu (Ed.), Technological advancements in biomedicine for healthcare applications (pp. 362-374). Hershey, PA: IGI Global. doi:10.4018/978-1-4666-2196-1.ch036

Hocine, N., & Gouaïch, A. (2013). Difficulty and scenario adaptation: An approach to customize therapeutic games. In S. Arnab, I. Dunwell, & K. Debattista (Eds.), *Serious games for healthcare: Applications and implications* (pp. 107–134). Hershey, PA: IGI Global. doi:10.4018/978-1-4666-1903-6.ch006

Hoonakker, P., Cartmill, R. S., Carayon, P., & Walker, J. M. (2013). Development and psychometric qualities of the SEIPS survey to evaluate CPOE/EHR implementation in ICUs. In J. Tan (Ed.), *Healthcare information technology innovation and sustainability: Frontiers and adoption* (pp. 161–179). Hershey, PA: IGI Global. doi:10.4018/978-1-4666-2797-0.ch010

Hoshi, K. (2013). Reframing dichotomies: Human experiential design of healthcare technologies. In I. Management Association (Ed.), User-driven healthcare: Concepts, methodologies, tools, and applications (pp. 1303-1331). Hershey, PA: IGI Global. doi:10.4018/978-1-4666-2770-3.ch065

Høstgaard, A. M. (2013). End-user participation in health IT development: The EUPHIT method. In I. Management Association (Ed.), User-driven healthcare: Concepts, methodologies, tools, and applications (pp. 608-629). Hershey, PA: IGI Global. doi:10.4018/978-1-4666-2770-3.ch030

Igrejas, G., Amaral, J. S., & Rodrigues, P. J. (2013). Fall detection systems to be used by elderly people. In M. Cruz-Cunha, I. Miranda, & P. Gonçalves (Eds.), *Handbook of research on ICTs for human-centered healthcare and social care services* (pp. 449–473). Hershey, PA: IGI Global. doi:10.4018/978-1-4666-3986-7.ch024

Inomata, C., & Nitta, S. (2013). Nursing in integrative medicine and nurses' engagement in caring-healing: A discussion based on the practice and study of music therapy and nursing care for patients with neurodegenerative disorders. In J. Wu (Ed.), *Technological advancements in biomedicine for healthcare applications* (pp. 235–239). Hershey, PA: IGI Global. doi:10.4018/978-1-4666-2196-1.ch025

Ishaq, G. M., Hussain, P. T., Iqbal, M. J., & Mushtaq, M. B. (2013). Risk-benefit analysis of combination vs. unopposed HRT in post-menopausal women. In I. Management Association (Ed.), Bioinformatics: Concepts, methodologies, tools, and applications (pp. 1424-1440). Hershey, PA: IGI Global. doi:10.4018/978-1-4666-3604-0.ch073

Iwaki, S. (2013). Multimodal neuroimaging to visualize human visual processing. In J. Wu (Ed.), *Biomedical engineering and cognitive neuroscience for healthcare: Interdisciplinary applications* (pp. 274–282). Hershey, PA: IGI Global. doi:10.4018/978-1-4666-2113-8.ch028

Ji, Z., Sugi, T., Goto, S., Wang, X., & Nakamura, M. (2013). Multi-channel template extraction for automatic EEG spike detection. In J. Wu (Ed.), *Biomedical engineering and cognitive neuroscience for healthcare: Interdisciplinary applications* (pp. 255–265). Hershey, PA: IGI Global. doi:10.4018/978-1-4666-2113-8.ch026

Jiang, Y., Wang, S., Tan, R., Ishida, K., Ando, T., & Fujie, M. G. (2013). Motor cortex activation during mental imagery of walking: An fNIRS study. In J. Wu (Ed.), *Biomedical engineering and cognitive neuroscience for healthcare: Interdisciplinary applications* (pp. 29–37). Hershey, PA: IGI Global. doi:10.4018/978-1-4666-2113-8.ch004

Johnson, K., & Tashiro, J. (2013). Interprofessional care and health care complexity: Factors shaping human resources effectiveness in health information management. In I. Management Association (Ed.), User-Driven Healthcare: Concepts, Methodologies, Tools, and Applications (pp. 1273-1302). Hershey, PA: IGI Global. doi:10.4018/978-1-4666-2770-3.ch064

Jose, J. (2013). Pharmacovigilance: Basic concepts and applications of pharmacoinformatics. In I. Management Association (Ed.), Bioinformatics: Concepts, methodologies, tools, and applications (pp. 1453-1473). Hershey, PA: IGI Global. doi:10.4018/978-1-4666-3604-0.ch075

Kalina, J., & Zvárová, J. (2013). Decision support systems in the process of improving patient safety. In A. Moumtzoglou & A. Kastania (Eds.), *E-health technologies and improving patient safety: Exploring organizational factors* (pp. 71–83). Hershey, PA: IGI Global. doi:10.4018/978-1-4666-2657-7.ch005

Kalina, J., & Zvárová, J. (2013). Decision support systems in the process of improving patient safety. In I. Management Association (Ed.), Bioinformatics: Concepts, methodologies, tools, and applications (pp. 1113-1125). Hershey, PA: IGI Global. doi:10.4018/978-1-4666-3604-0.ch057

Kamath, J. R., & Donahoe-Anshus, A. L. (2013). Electronic health record: Adoption, considerations and future direction. In I. Management Association (Ed.), User-driven healthcare: Concepts, methodologies, tools, and applications (pp. 34-56). Hershey, PA: IGI Global. doi:10.4018/978-1-4666-2770-3.ch003

Karamagkioli, K. Z., & Karamagioli, E. (2013). European e-health framework: Towards more "patient-friendly" healthcare services? In I. Management Association (Ed.), User-driven healthcare: Concepts, methodologies, tools, and applications (pp. 760-775). Hershey, PA: IGI Global. doi:10.4018/978-1-4666-2770-3.ch037

Kardaras, D. K., & Karakostas, B. (2013). Case studies in customization of e-health services. In I. Management Association (Ed.), User-driven healthcare: Concepts, methodologies, tools, and applications (pp. 1018-1036). Hershey, PA: IGI Global. doi:10.4018/978-1-4666-2770-3.ch051

Kastania, A. N. (2013). Evaluation considerations for e-health systems. In I. Management Association (Ed.), User-driven healthcare: Concepts, methodologies, tools, and applications (pp. 1126-1140). Hershey, PA: IGI Global. doi:10.4018/978-1-4666-2770-3.ch057

Kato, P. M. (2013). The role of the researcher in making serious games for health. In S. Arnab, I. Dunwell, & K. Debattista (Eds.), *Serious games for healthcare: Applications and implications* (pp. 213–231). Hershey, PA: IGI Global. doi:10.4018/978-1-4666-1903-6.ch010

Katsura, S. (2013). Preservation and reproduction of human motion based on a motion-copying system. In J. Wu (Ed.), *Technological advancements in biomedicine for healthcare applications* (pp. 375–384). Hershey, PA: IGI Global. doi:10.4018/978-1-4666-2196-1.ch037

Kikuchi, T. (2013). Human-friendly mechatronics systems with functional fluids and elastomers. In J. Wu (Ed.), *Technological advancements in biomedicine for healthcare applications* (pp. 94–101). Hershey, PA: IGI Global. doi:10.4018/978-1-4666-2196-1.ch010

Kimura, T., Miura, T., Shinohara, K., & Doi, S. (2013). Visual attention in 3-D space while moving forward. In J. Wu (Ed.), *Biomedical engineering and cognitive neuroscience for healthcare: Interdisciplinary applications* (pp. 81–88). Hershey, PA: IGI Global. doi:10.4018/978-1-4666-2113-8.ch009

Kldiashvili, E. (2013). Implementation of telecytology in Georgia. In V. Gulla, A. Mori, F. Gabbrielli, & P. Lanzafame (Eds.), *Telehealth networks for hospital services: New methodologies* (pp. 341–361). Hershey, PA: IGI Global. doi:10.4018/978-1-4666-2979-0.ch022

Kolovou, L. T., & Lymberopoulos, D. K. (2013). The concept of interoperability for AAL systems. In I. Management Association (Ed.), User-driven healthcare: Concepts, methodologies, tools, and applications (pp. 1364-1385). Hershey, PA: IGI Global. doi:10.4018/978-1-4666-2770-3.ch068

Koppar, A. R., & Sridhar, V. (2013). Malaria parasite detection: Automated method using microscope color image. In J. Rodrigues (Ed.), *Digital advances in medicine, e-health, and communication technologies* (pp. 289–300). Hershey, PA: IGI Global. doi:10.4018/978-1-4666-2794-9.ch016

Kotsonis, E., & Eliakis, S. (2013). Information security standards for health information systems: The implementer's approach. In I. Management Association (Ed.), User-driven healthcare: Concepts, methodologies, tools, and applications (pp. 225-257). Hershey, PA: IGI Global. doi:10.4018/978-1-4666-2770-3.ch013

Krishnaswamy, K., & Oates, T. (2014). Pathway to independence: Past, present, and beyond via robotics. In G. Kouroupetroglou (Ed.), *Disability informatics and web accessibility for motor limitations* (pp. 153–201). Hershey, PA: IGI Global. doi:10.4018/978-1-4666-4442-7.ch005

Kuehler, M., Schimke, N., & Hale, J. (2013). Privacy considerations for electronic health records. In I. Management Association (Ed.), User-driven healthcare: Concepts, methodologies, tools, and applications (pp. 1387-1402). Hershey, PA: IGI Global. doi:10.4018/978-1-4666-2770-3.ch069

Kurita, Y., Ikeda, A., Nagata, K., Okajima, M., & Ogasawara, T. (2013). Biomedical robotics for healthcare. In J. Wu (Ed.), *Technological advancements in biomedicine for healthcare applications* (pp. 160–169). Hershey, PA: IGI Global. doi:10.4018/978-1-4666-2196-1.ch017

Lakkaraju, S., & Lakkaraju, S. (2013). Mobile device application in healthcare. In S. Sarnikar, D. Bennett, & M. Gaynor (Eds.), *Cases on healthcare information technology for patient care management* (pp. 276–307). Hershey, PA: IGI Global. doi:10.4018/978-1-4666-2671-3.ch016

Laskowski, M. (2013). A prototype agent based model and machine learning hybrid system for healthcare decision support. In J. Rodrigues (Ed.), *Digital advances in medicine, e-health, and communication technologies* (pp. 230–253). Hershey, PA: IGI Global. doi:10.4018/978-1-4666-2794-9.ch013

Lee, T. (2014). Mobile healthcare computing in the cloud. In J. Rodrigues, K. Lin, & J. Lloret (Eds.), *Mobile networks and cloud computing convergence for progressive services and applications* (pp. 275–294). Hershey, PA: IGI Global. doi:10.4018/978-1-4666-4781-7.ch015

Lelardeux, C., Alvarez, J., Montaut, T., Galaup, M., & Lagarrigue, P. (2013). Healthcare games and the metaphoric approach. In S. Arnab, I. Dunwell, & K. Debattista (Eds.), *Serious games for healthcare: Applications and implications* (pp. 23–49). Hershey, PA: IGI Global. doi:10.4018/978-1-4666-1903-6.ch002

Lhotska, L., Bursa, M., Huptych, M., Chudacek, V., & Havlik, J. (2013). Interoperability of medical devices and information systems. In M. Cruz-Cunha, I. Miranda, & P. Gonçalves (Eds.), *Handbook of research on ICTs for human-centered healthcare and social care services* (pp. 749–762). Hershey, PA: IGI Global. doi:10.4018/978-1-4666-3986-7.ch039

Li, X., Lin, Z., & Wu, J. (2013). Language processing in the human brain of literate and illiterate subjects. In J. Wu (Ed.), *Biomedical engineering and cognitive neuroscience for healthcare: Interdisciplinary applications* (pp. 201–209). Hershey, PA: IGI Global. doi:10.4018/978-1-4666-2113-8.ch021

Liao, H. (2013). Biomedical information processing and visualization for minimally invasive neurosurgery. In J. Wu (Ed.), *Technological advancements in biomedicine for healthcare applications* (pp. 36–46). Hershey, PA: IGI Global. doi:10.4018/978-1-4666-2196-1.ch005

Libreri, C., & Graffigna, G. (2014). How web 2.0 shapes patient knowledge sharing: The case of diabetes in Italy. In C. El Morr (Ed.), *Research perspectives on the role of informatics in health policy and management* (pp. 238–260). Hershey, PA: IGI Global. doi:10.4018/978-1-4666-4321-5.ch014

Lin, C., Huang, Y., Li, C., & Jalleh, G. (2013). Key health information systems outsourcing issues from six hospital cases. In I. Management Association (Ed.), User-driven healthcare: Concepts, methodologies, tools, and applications (pp. 824-837). Hershey, PA: IGI Global. doi:10.4018/978-1-4666-2770-3.ch041

Lin, L., Chen, Y., Wu, J., & Tennyson, R. D. (2013). What skill/knowledge is important to a nursing professional? In P. Ordóñez de Pablos (Ed.), *Business, technology, and knowledge management in Asia: Trends and innovations* (pp. 234–249). Hershey, PA: IGI Global. doi:10.4018/978-1-4666-2652-2.ch018

Liu, G. (2014). Using case costing data and case mix for funding and benchmarking in rehabilitation hospitals. In C. El Morr (Ed.), *Research perspectives on the role of informatics in health policy and management* (pp. 62–78). Hershey, PA: IGI Global. doi:10.4018/978-1-4666-4321-5.ch005

Lixun, Z., Dapeng, B., & Lei, Y. (2013). Design of and experimentation with a walking assistance robot. In J. Wu (Ed.), *Technological advancements in biomedicine for healthcare applications* (pp. 123–127). Hershey, PA: IGI Global. doi:10.4018/978-1-4666-2196-1.ch013

Lui, K. (2013). The health informatics professional. In I. Management Association (Ed.), User-driven healthcare: Concepts, methodologies, tools, and applications (pp. 120-141). Hershey, PA: IGI Global. doi:10.4018/978-1-4666-2770-3.ch007

Ma, X., Chen, G., & Xiao, J. (2013). Understanding weight change behaviors through online social networks. In A. Gangopadhyay (Ed.), *Methods, models, and computation for medical informatics* (pp. 189–214). Hershey, PA: IGI Global. doi:10.4018/978-1-4666-2653-9.ch012

Makikawa, M., Okada, S., Fujiwara, Y., & Esaki, M. (2013). Sleep monitoring system equipped with a flexible non-contact ECG, respiration, and body motion sensor. In J. Wu (Ed.), *Technological advancements in biomedicine for healthcare applications* (pp. 287–297). Hershey, PA: IGI Global. doi:10.4018/978-1-4666-2196-1.ch030

Malindretos, G. (2013). Distribution and logistics outsourcing in the pharmaceutical sector. In D. Folinas (Ed.), *Outsourcing management for supply chain operations and logistics service* (pp. 202–222). Hershey, PA: IGI Global. doi:10.4018/978-1-4666-2008-7.ch012

Manvi, S. S., & B., M. R. (2013). A survey on health care services using wireless sensor networks. In M. Cruz-Cunha, I. Miranda, & P. Gonçalves (Eds.), *Handbook of research on ICTs for human-centered healthcare and social care services* (pp. 587-606). Hershey, PA: IGI Global. doi:10.4018/978-1-4666-3986-7.ch031

Marshall, S., & Hogan, J. (2013). The use of medical simulation to improve patient safety. In A. Moumtzoglou & A. Kastania (Eds.), *E-health technologies and improving patient safety: Exploring organizational factors* (pp. 155–172). Hershey, PA: IGI Global. doi:10.4018/978-1-4666-2657-7.ch011

Martin, J., & McKay, E. (2013). Mental health, post-secondary education, and information communications technology. In J. Lannon & E. Halpin (Eds.), *Human rights and information communication technologies: Trends and consequences of use* (pp. 196–213). Hershey, PA: IGI Global. doi:10.4018/978-1-4666-1918-0.ch012

Martin, J., & McKay, E. (2014). Mental health, post-secondary education, and information communications technology. In *Assistive technologies: Concepts, methodologies, tools, and applications* (pp. 1209–1226). Hershey, PA: IGI Global. doi:10.4018/978-1-4666-4422-9.ch063

Martin, V. (2013). Developing a library collection in bioinformatics: Support for an evolving profession. In I. Management Association (Ed.), Bioinformatics: Concepts, methodologies, tools, and applications (pp. 130-150). Hershey, PA: IGI Global. doi:10.4018/978-1-4666-3604-0.ch007

Masayuki, K., Eiji, K., Tetsuo, T., & Nozomu, M. (2013). Evaluation of olfactory impairment in Parkinson's disease using near-infrared spectroscopy. In J. Wu (Ed.), *Biomedical engineering and cognitive neuroscience for healthcare: Interdisciplinary applications* (pp. 293–302). Hershey, PA: IGI Global. doi:10.4018/978-1-4666-2113-8.ch030

Mazzanti, I., Maolo, A., & Antonicelli, R. (2013). E-health and telemedicine in the elderly: State of the art. In V. Gulla, A. Mori, F. Gabbrielli, & P. Lanzafame (Eds.), *Telehealth Networks for Hospital Services: New Methodologies* (pp. 33–43). Hershey, PA: IGI Global. doi:10.4018/978-1-4666-2979-0.ch003

Mazzanti, I., Maolo, A., & Antonicelli, R. (2014). E-health and telemedicine in the elderly: State of the art. In *Assistive technologies: Concepts, methodologies, tools, and applications* (pp. 693–704). Hershey, PA: IGI Global. doi:10.4018/978-1-4666-4422-9.ch034

McCrossan, B. A., & Casey, F. A. (2013). The role of telemedicine in paediatric cardiology. In V. Gulla, A. Mori, F. Gabbrielli, & P. Lanzafame (Eds.), *Telehealth networks for hospital services: New methodologies* (pp. 44–88). Hershey, PA: IGI Global. doi:10.4018/978-1-4666-2979-0.ch004

McGaha, J. (2013). Implementation issues on a national electronic health record network. In I. Management Association (Ed.), User-driven healthcare: Concepts, methodologies, tools, and applications (pp. 1236-1251). Hershey, PA: IGI Global. doi:10.4018/978-1-4666-2770-3.ch062

McGinnes, S., & Burke, M. (2013). Hoping for the best: A qualitative study of information technology in primary care. In M. Cruz-Cunha, I. Miranda, & P. Gonçalves (Eds.), *Handbook of research on ICTs and management systems for improving efficiency in healthcare and social care* (pp. 1088–1108). Hershey, PA: IGI Global. doi:10.4018/978-1-4666-3990-4.ch057

Medhekar, A., Wong, H. Y., & Hall, J. (2014). Innovation in medical tourism service marketing: A case of India. In A. Goyal (Ed.), *Innovations in services marketing and management: Strategies for emerging economies* (pp. 49–66). Hershey, PA: IGI Global. doi:10.4018/978-1-4666-4671-1.ch003

Medhekar, A., Wong, H. Y., & Hall, J. (2014). Medical tourism: A conceptual framework for an innovation in global healthcare provision. In A. Goyal (Ed.), *Innovations in services marketing and management: Strategies for emerging economies* (pp. 148–169). Hershey, PA: IGI Global. doi:10.4018/978-1-4666-4671-1.ch009

Menciassi, A., & Laschi, C. (2014). Biorobotics. In I. Management Association (Ed.), Robotics: Concepts, methodologies, tools, and applications (pp. 1613-1643). Hershey, PA: IGI Global. doi:10.4018/978-1-4666-4607-0.ch079

Mendes, D., & Rodrigues, I. P. (2013). A semantic web pragmatic approach to develop clinical ontologies, and thus semantic interoperability, based in HL7 v2.xml messaging. In R. Martinho, R. Rijo, M. Cruz-Cunha, & J. Varajão (Eds.), *Information systems and technologies for enhancing health and social care* (pp. 205–214). Hershey, PA: IGI Global. doi:10.4018/978-1-4666-3667-5.ch014

Mendoza-González, R., Martin, M. V., & Rodríguez-Martínez, L. C. (2013). Identifying the essential design requirements for usable e-health communities in mobile devices. In I. Management Association (Ed.), User-driven healthcare: Concepts, methodologies, tools, and applications (pp. 533-552). Hershey, PA: IGI Global. doi:10.4018/978-1-4666-2770-3.ch027

Mettler, T. (2013). Transformation of the hospital supply chain: How to measure the maturity of supplier relationship management systems in hospitals? In J. Tan (Ed.), *Healthcare information technology innovation and sustainability: Frontiers and adoption* (pp. 180–192). Hershey, PA: IGI Global. doi:10.4018/978-1-4666-2797-0.ch011

Miesenberger, K., Nussbaum, G., & Ossmann, R. (2014). AsTeRICS: A framework for including sensor technology into AT solutions for people with motor disabilities. In G. Kouroupetroglou (Ed.), *Assistive technologies and computer access for motor disabilities* (pp. 154–179). Hershey, PA: IGI Global. doi:10.4018/978-1-4666-4438-0.ch006

Miller, K., & Sankaranarayanan, S. (2013). Applications of policy based agents in wireless body sensor mesh networks for patient health monitoring. In J. Rodrigues (Ed.), *Digital advances in medicine, e-health, and communication technologies* (pp. 85–101). Hershey, PA: IGI Global. doi:10.4018/978-1-4666-2794-9.ch005

Mohammadian, M., & Jentzsch, R. (2013). User and data classification for a secure and practical approach for patient-doctor profiling using an RFID framework in hospital. In S. Sarnikar, D. Bennett, & M. Gaynor (Eds.), *Cases on healthcare information technology for patient care management* (pp. 224–253). Hershey, PA: IGI Global. doi:10.4018/978-1-4666-2671-3.ch014

Monguet, J. M., Huerta, E., Fernández, J., Ferruzca, M., & Badillo, S. (2013). E-health business models prototyping by incremental design. In I. Management Association (Ed.), User-driven healthcare: Concepts, methodologies, tools, and applications (pp. 776-790). Hershey, PA: IGI Global. doi:10.4018/978-1-4666-2770-3.ch038

Montazemi, A. R., Pittaway, J. J., & Keshavjee, K. (2013). State of IS integration in the context of patient-centered care: A network analysis and research directions. In J. Tan (Ed.), *Healthcare information technology innovation and sustainability: Frontiers and adoption* (pp. 127–144). Hershey, PA: IGI Global. doi:10.4018/978-1-4666-2797-0.ch008

Mori, A. R., Contenti, M., & Verbicaro, R. (2013). Policies on telemedicine-enhanced hospital services: Prioritization criteria for the interventions at regional level. In V. Gulla, A. Mori, F. Gabbrielli, & P. Lanzafame (Eds.), *Telehealth networks for hospital services: New methodologies* (pp. 1–14). Hershey, PA: IGI Global. doi:10.4018/978-1-4666-2979-0.ch001

Morita, A. (2013). The quantitative EEG change in Parkinson's disease. In J. Wu (Ed.), *Biomedical engineering and cognitive neuroscience for healthcare: Interdisciplinary applications* (pp. 225–234). Hershey, PA: IGI Global. doi:10.4018/978-1-4666-2113-8.ch023

Moromugi, S., & Ishimatsu, T. (2013). A strength training machine with a dynamic resistance control function based on muscle activity level. In J. Wu (Ed.), *Technological advancements in biomedicine for healthcare applications* (pp. 102–110). Hershey, PA: IGI Global. doi:10.4018/978-1-4666-2196-1.ch011

Morrow, D., & Chin, J. (2013). Technology as a bridge between health care systems and older adults. In R. Zheng, R. Hill, & M. Gardner (Eds.), *Engaging older adults with modern technology: Internet use and information access needs* (pp. 59–79). Hershey, PA: IGI Global. doi:10.4018/978-1-4666-1966-1.ch004

Morrow, D., & Chin, J. (2013). Technology as a bridge between health care systems and older adults. In I. Management Association (Ed.), User-driven healthcare: Concepts, methodologies, tools, and applications (pp. 99-119). Hershey, PA: IGI Global. doi:10.4018/978-1-4666-2770-3.ch006

Mostafa, R., Hasan, G. M., Kabir, A. A., & Rahman, M. A. (2013). Proposed framework for the deployment of telemedicine centers in rural Bangladesh. In J. Rodrigues (Ed.), *Digital advances in medicine, e-health, and communication technologies* (pp. 254–270). Hershey, PA: IGI Global. doi:10.4018/978-1-4666-2794-9.ch014

Motoi, K., Ogawa, M., Yamakoshi, T., & Yamakoshi, K. (2013). Fusion physiological sensing system for healthcare. In J. Wu (Ed.), *Technological advancements in biomedicine for healthcare applications* (pp. 298–313). Hershey, PA: IGI Global. doi:10.4018/978-1-4666-2196-1.ch031

Motorny, S. P. (2013). Big information technology bet of a small community hospital. In S. Sarnikar, D. Bennett, & M. Gaynor (Eds.), *Cases on healthcare information technology for patient care management* (pp. 70–94). Hershey, PA: IGI Global. doi:10.4018/978-1-4666-2671-3.ch004

Moumtzoglou, A. (2013). Health 2.0 and medicine 2.0: Safety, ownership and privacy issues. In I. Management Association (Ed.), User-driven healthcare: Concepts, methodologies, tools, and applications (pp. 1508-1522). Hershey, PA: IGI Global. doi:10.4018/978-1-4666-2770-3.ch075

Moumtzoglou, A. (2013). Risk perception as a patient safety dimension. In A. Moumtzoglou & A. Kastania (Eds.), *E-health technologies and improving patient safety: Exploring organizational factors* (pp. 285–299). Hershey, PA: IGI Global. doi:10.4018/978-1-4666-2657-7.ch017

Msanjila, S. S. (2013). Emerging ICT challenges on provision of online HIV/AIDS advisory services. In M. Cruz-Cunha, I. Miranda, & P. Gonçalves (Eds.), *Handbook of research on ICTs for human-centered healthcare and social care services* (pp. 248–269). Hershey, PA: IGI Global. doi:10.4018/978-1-4666-3986-7.ch013

Müller, A. (2013). Improving the identification of medication names by increasing phonological awareness via a language-teaching computer game (medicina). In S. Arnab, I. Dunwell, & K. Debattista (Eds.), *Serious games for healthcare: Applications and implications* (pp. 283–295). Hershey, PA: IGI Global. doi:10.4018/978-1-4666-1903-6.ch014

Murakami, S., Kim, H., Tan, J. K., Ishikawa, S., & Aoki, T. (2013). The development of a quantitative method for the detection of periarticular osteoporosis using density features within ROIs from computed radiography images of the hand. In J. Wu (Ed.), *Technological advancements in biomedicine for healthcare applications* (pp. 55–67). Hershey, PA: IGI Global. doi:10.4018/978-1-4666-2196-1.ch007

Nadathur, S. G., & Warren, J. R. (2013). Formal-transfer in and out of stroke care units: An analysis using Bayesian networks. In J. Tan (Ed.), *Healthcare information technology innovation and sustainability: Frontiers and adoption* (pp. 193–207). Hershey, PA: IGI Global. doi:10.4018/978-1-4666-2797-0.ch012

Naidoo, V., & Naidoo, Y. (2014). Home telecare, medical implant, and mobile technology: Evolutions in geriatric care. In C. El Morr (Ed.), *Research perspectives on the role of informatics in health policy and management* (pp. 222–237). Hershey, PA: IGI Global. doi:10.4018/978-1-4666-4321-5.ch013

Nakagawa, S. (2013). Bone-conducted ultrasonic perception: An elucidation of perception mechanisms and the development of a novel hearing aid for the profoundly deaf. In J. Wu (Ed.), *Technological advancements in biomedicine for healthcare applications* (pp. 148–159). Hershey, PA: IGI Global. doi:10.4018/978-1-4666-2196-1.ch016

Nakai, M., & Niinomi, M. (2013). Recent progress in mechanically biocompatible titanium-based materials. In J. Wu (Ed.), *Technological advancements in biomedicine for healthcare applications* (pp. 206–212). Hershey, PA: IGI Global. doi:10.4018/978-1-4666-2196-1.ch022

Nakakuki, T., & Okada-Hatakeyama, M. (2013). Methods for the analysis of intracellular signal transduction systems. In J. Wu (Ed.), *Technological advancements in biomedicine for healthcare applications* (pp. 347–353). Hershey, PA: IGI Global. doi:10.4018/978-1-4666-2196-1.ch034

Nalin, M., Verga, M., Sanna, A., & Saranummi, N. (2013). Directions for ICT research in disease prevention. In M. Cruz-Cunha, I. Miranda, & P. Gonçalves (Eds.), *Handbook of research on ICTs for human-centered healthcare and social care services* (pp. 229–247). Hershey, PA: IGI Global. doi:10.4018/978-1-4666-3986-7.ch012

Nap, H. H., & Diaz-Orueta, U. (2013). Rehabilitation gaming. In S. Arnab, I. Dunwell, & K. Debattista (Eds.), *Serious games for healthcare: Applications and implications* (pp. 50–75). Hershey, PA: IGI Global. doi:10.4018/978-1-4666-1903-6.ch003

Narushima, T., & Ueda, K. (2013). Calcium phosphate coating on titanium by RF magnetron sputtering. In J. Wu (Ed.), *Technological advancements in biomedicine for healthcare applications* (pp. 223–233). Hershey, PA: IGI Global. doi:10.4018/978-1-4666-2196-1.ch024

Nava-Muñoz, S., & Morán, A. L. (2013). A review of notifications systems in elder care environments: Challenges and opportunities. In M. Cruz-Cunha, I. Miranda, & P. Gonçalves (Eds.), *Handbook of research on ICTs for human-centered healthcare and social care services* (pp. 407–429). Hershey, PA: IGI Global. doi:10.4018/978-1-4666-3986-7.ch022

Nganji, J. T., & Nggada, S. H. (2014). Adoption of blended learning technologies in selected secondary schools in Cameroon and Nigeria: Challenges in disability inclusion. In N. Ololube (Ed.), *Advancing technology and educational development through blended learning in emerging economies* (pp. 159–173). Hershey, PA: IGI Global. doi:10.4018/978-1-4666-4574-5.ch009

Nikolov, S., Vera, J., & Wolkenhauer, O. (2013). Bifurcation analysis of a model accounting for the 14-3-3s signalling compartmentalisation. In I. Management Association (Ed.), Bioinformatics: Concepts, methodologies, tools, and applications (pp. 851-859). Hershey, PA: IGI Global. doi:10.4018/978-1-4666-3604-0.ch046

Nishiguchi, H. (2013). Description of and applications for a motion analysis method for upper limbs. In J. Wu (Ed.), *Technological advancements in biomedicine for healthcare applications* (pp. 1–10). Hershey, PA: IGI Global. doi:10.4018/978-1-4666-2196-1.ch001

Nokata, M. (2013). Small medical robot. In J. Wu (Ed.), *Technological advancements in biomedicine for healthcare applications* (pp. 170–179). Hershey, PA: IGI Global. doi:10.4018/978-1-4666-2196-1.ch018

Noritsugu, T. (2013). Wearable power assist robot driven with pneumatic rubber artificial muscles. In J. Wu (Ed.), *Technological advancements in biomedicine for healthcare applications* (pp. 139–147). Hershey, PA: IGI Global. doi:10.4018/978-1-4666-2196-1.ch015

Noteboom, C. (2013). Physician interaction with EHR: The importance of stakeholder identification and change management. In S. Sarnikar, D. Bennett, & M. Gaynor (Eds.), *Cases on healthcare information technology for patient care management* (pp. 95–112). Hershey, PA: IGI Global. doi:10.4018/978-1-4666-2671-3.ch005

O'Hanlon, S. (2013). Avoiding adverse consequences of e-health. In A. Moumtzoglou & A. Kastania (Eds.), *E-health technologies and improving patient safety: Exploring organizational factors* (pp. 13–26). Hershey, PA: IGI Global. doi:10.4018/978-1-4666-2657-7.ch002

Ogawa, K., Nishio, S., Minato, T., & Ishiguro, H. (2013). Android robots as telepresence media. In J. Wu (Ed.), *Biomedical engineering and cognitive neuroscience for healthcare: Interdisciplinary applications* (pp. 54–63). Hershey, PA: IGI Global. doi:10.4018/978-1-4666-2113-8.ch006

Ohashi, M., Sakimura, N., Fujimoto, M., Hori, M., & Kurata, N. (2013). Technical perspective of authentication policy extension for the adaptive social services and e-health care management. In M. Cruz-Cunha, I. Miranda, & P. Gonçalves (Eds.), *Handbook of research on ICTs for human-centered healthcare and social care services* (pp. 719–726). Hershey, PA: IGI Global. doi:10.4018/978-1-4666-3986-7.ch037

Ohta, Y., & Uchida, M. (2013). Non-contact pulse monitoring using live imaging. In J. Wu (Ed.), *Technological advancements in biomedicine for healthcare applications* (pp. 240–246). Hershey, PA: IGI Global. doi:10.4018/978-1-4666-2196-1.ch026

Ohuchida, K., & Hashizume, M. (2013). Biomedical robotics for healthcare. In J. Wu (Ed.), *Technological advancements in biomedicine for healthcare applications* (pp. 200–205). Hershey, PA: IGI Global. doi:10.4018/978-1-4666-2196-1.ch021

Oikonomou, D., Moulianitis, V., Lekkas, D., & Koutsabasis, P. (2013). DSS for health emergency response: A contextual, user-centred approach. In R. Biswas (Ed.), *Clinical solutions and medical progress through user-driven healthcare* (pp. 51–69). Hershey, PA: IGI Global. doi:10.4018/978-1-4666-1876-3.ch006

Okamoto, S., Hirotomi, T., Aoki, K., & Hosomi, Y. (2013). Evaluation of walking motions with the aid of walkers using acceleration sensors. In J. Wu (Ed.), *Biomedical engineering and cognitive neuroscience for healthcare: Interdisciplinary applications* (pp. 346–354). Hershey, PA: IGI Global. doi:10.4018/978-1-4666-2113-8.ch036

Okamura, H. (2013). Rehabilitation of elderly people with dementia. In J. Wu (Ed.), *Biomedical engineering and cognitive neuroscience for healthcare: Interdisciplinary applications* (pp. 235–242). Hershey, PA: IGI Global. doi:10.4018/978-1-4666-2113-8.ch024

Olvera-Lobo, M., & Gutiérrez-Artacho, J. (2013). Searching health information in question-answering systems. In M. Cruz-Cunha, I. Miranda, & P. Gonçalves (Eds.), *Handbook of research on ICTs for human-centered healthcare and social care services* (pp. 474–490). Hershey, PA: IGI Global. doi:10.4018/978-1-4666-3986-7.ch025

Padovani, E., Orelli, R. L., Agnoletti, V., & Buccioli, M. (2013). Low cost and human-centered innovations in healthcare services: A case of excellence in Italy. In S. Saeed & C. Reddick (Eds.), *Human-centered system design for electronic governance* (pp. 239–252). Hershey, PA: IGI Global. doi:10.4018/978-1-4666-3640-8.ch014

Paninchukunnath, A. (2014). Healthcare services delivery in India: special reference to mother and child health. In A. Goyal (Ed.), *Innovations in services marketing and management: Strategies for emerging economies* (pp. 170–189). Hershey, PA: IGI Global. doi:10.4018/978-1-4666-4671-1.ch010

Paparountas, T., Nikolaidou-Katsaridou, M. N., Rustici, G., & Aidinis, V. (2013). Data mining and meta-analysis on DNA microarray data. In I. Management Association (Ed.), Bioinformatics: Concepts, methodologies, tools, and applications (pp. 1196-1236). Hershey, PA: IGI Global. doi:10.4018/978-1-4666-3604-0.ch062

Parentela, G., Mancini, P., Naccarella, F., Feng, Z., & Rinaldi, G. (2013). Telemedicine, the European space agency, and the support to the african population for infectious disease problems: Potentiality and perspectives for Asia countries and China. In V. Gulla, A. Mori, F. Gabbrielli, & P. Lanzafame (Eds.), *Telehealth networks for hospital services: New methodologies* (pp. 89–96). Hershey, PA: IGI Global. doi:10.4018/978-1-4666-2979-0.ch005

Paterson, G. I., MacDonald, J. M., & Mensink, N. N. (2014). The administrative policy quandary in Canada's health service organizations. In C. El Morr (Ed.), *Research perspectives on the role of informatics in health policy and management* (pp. 116–134). Hershey, PA: IGI Global. doi:10.4018/978-1-4666-4321-5.ch008

Penchovsky, R. (2013). Engineering gene control circuits with allosteric ribozymes in human cells as a medicine of the future. In I. Management Association (Ed.), Bioinformatics: Concepts, methodologies, tools, and applications (pp. 860-883). Hershey, PA: IGI Global. doi:10.4018/978-1-4666-3604-0.ch047

Pereira, O. R., Caldeira, J. M., & Rodrigues, J. J. (2013). An advanced and secure symbian-based mobile approach for body sensor networks interaction. In J. Rodrigues (Ed.), *Digital advances in medicine, e-health, and communication technologies* (pp. 33–48). Hershey, PA: IGI Global. doi:10.4018/978-1-4666-2794-9.ch002

Petkovic, M., & Ibraimi, L. (2013). Privacy and security in e-health applications. In I. Management Association (Ed.), User-driven healthcare: Concepts, methodologies, tools, and applications (pp. 1141-1166). Hershey, PA: IGI Global. doi:10.4018/978-1-4666-2770-3.ch058

Peyton, L., & Hu, J. (2013). Identity management and audit trail support for privacy protection in e-health networks. In I. Management Association (Ed.), User-driven healthcare: Concepts, methodologies, tools, and applications (pp. 1112-1125). Hershey, PA: IGI Global. doi:10.4018/978-1-4666-2770-3.ch056

Pham, D. V., Halgamuge, M. N., Nirmalathas, T., & Moran, B. (2013). A centralized real-time e-healthcare system for remote detection and prediction of epileptic seizures. In I. Management Association (Ed.), User-driven healthcare: Concepts, methodologies, tools, and applications (pp. 326-356). Hershey, PA: IGI Global. doi:10.4018/978-1-4666-2770-3.ch017

Phua, C., Roy, P. C., Aloulou, H., Biswas, J., Tolstikov, A., & Foo, V. S. … Xu, D. (2014). State-of-the-art assistive technology for people with dementia. In Assistive technologies: Concepts, methodologies, tools, and applications (pp. 1606-1625). Hershey, PA: IGI Global. doi:10.4018/978-1-4666-4422-9.ch085

Pino, A. (2014). Augmentative and alternative communication systems for the motor disabled. In G. Kouroupetroglou (Ed.), *Disability informatics and web accessibility for motor limitations* (pp. 105–152). Hershey, PA: IGI Global. doi:10.4018/978-1-4666-4442-7.ch004

Portela, F., Cabral, A., Abelha, A., Salazar, M., Quintas, C., Machado, J., & Santos, M. F. et al. (2013). Knowledge acquisition process for intelligent decision support in critical health care. In R. Martinho, R. Rijo, M. Cruz-Cunha, & J. Varajão (Eds.), *Information systems and technologies for enhancing health and social care* (pp. 55–68). Hershey, PA: IGI Global. doi:10.4018/978-1-4666-3667-5.ch004

Previtali, P. (2013). Grid technology for archive solutions in health care organizations. In A. Moumtzoglou & A. Kastania (Eds.), *E-health technologies and improving patient safety: Exploring organizational factors* (pp. 148–154). Hershey, PA: IGI Global. doi:10.4018/978-1-4666-2657-7.ch010

Purkayastha, S. (2013). Design and implementation of mobile-based technology in strengthening health information system: Aligning mhealth solutions to infrastructures. In I. Management Association (Ed.), User-driven healthcare: Concepts, methodologies, tools, and applications (pp. 689-713). Hershey, PA: IGI Global. doi:10.4018/978-1-4666-2770-3.ch034

Qi, G., & Wu, J. (2013). Functional role of the left ventral occipito-temporal cortex in reading. In J. Wu (Ed.), *Biomedical engineering and cognitive neuroscience for healthcare: Interdisciplinary applications* (pp. 192–200). Hershey, PA: IGI Global. doi:10.4018/978-1-4666-2113-8.ch020

Queirós, A., Alvarelhão, J., Silva, A. G., Teixeira, A., & Pacheco da Rocha, N. (2013). A conceptual framework for the design and development of AAL services. In M. Cruz-Cunha, I. Miranda, & P. Gonçalves (Eds.), *Handbook of research on ICTs for human-centered healthcare and social care services* (pp. 568–586). Hershey, PA: IGI Global. doi:10.4018/978-1-4666-3986-7.ch030

Ravka, N. (2014). Informatics and health services: The potential benefits and challenges of electronic health records and personal electronic health records in patient care, cost control, and health research – An overview. In C. El Morr (Ed.), *Research perspectives on the role of informatics in health policy and management* (pp. 89–114). Hershey, PA: IGI Global. doi:10.4018/978-1-4666-4321-5.ch007

Reibling, N., & Wendt, C. (2013). Regulating patients' access to healthcare services. In M. Merviö (Ed.), *Healthcare management and economics: Perspectives on public and private administration* (pp. 53–68). Hershey, PA: IGI Global. doi:10.4018/978-1-4666-3982-9.ch005

Reis, C. I., Freire, C. S., Fernández, J., & Monguet, J. M. (2013). Patient centered design: Challenges and lessons learned from working with health professionals and schizophrenic patients in e-therapy contexts. In R. Martinho, R. Rijo, M. Cruz-Cunha, & J. Varajão (Eds.), *Information systems and technologies for enhancing health and social care* (pp. 120–135). Hershey, PA: IGI Global. doi:10.4018/978-1-4666-3667-5.ch008

Remmers, H., & Hülsken-Giesler, M. (2013). e-Health technologies in home care nursing: Recent survey results and subsequent ethical issues. In I. Management Association (Ed.), User-driven healthcare: Concepts, methodologies, tools, and applications (pp. 396-420). Hershey, PA: IGI Global. doi:10.4018/978-1-4666-2770-3.ch020

Ricketts, M. (2014). Making health information personal: How anecdotes bring concepts to life. In S. Hai-Jew (Ed.), *Packaging digital information for enhanced learning and analysis: Data visualization, spatialization, and multidimensionality* (pp. 1–36). Hershey, PA: IGI Global. doi:10.4018/978-1-4666-4462-5.ch001

Rocha, Á. (2013). Evolution of information systems and technologies maturity in healthcare. In J. Tan (Ed.), *Healthcare information technology innovation and sustainability: Frontiers and adoption* (pp. 238–246). Hershey, PA: IGI Global. doi:10.4018/978-1-4666-2797-0.ch015

Rodríguez-Gómez, D., & Gairín, J. (2014). Communities of practice in the Catalan public administration: Promoting their improvement. In Y. Al-Bastaki & A. Shajera (Eds.), *Building a competitive public sector with knowledge management strategy* (pp. 383–402). Hershey, PA: IGI Global. doi:10.4018/978-1-4666-4434-2.ch018

Rodríguez-Solano, C., Lezcano, L., & Sicilia, M. (2013). Automated generation of SNOMED CT subsets from clinical guidelines. In R. Martinho, R. Rijo, M. Cruz-Cunha, & J. Varajão (Eds.), *Information systems and technologies for enhancing health and social care* (pp. 190–204). Hershey, PA: IGI Global. doi:10.4018/978-1-4666-3667-5.ch013

Rosu, S. M., & Dragoi, G. (2014). E-health sites development using open source software and OMT methodology as support for family doctors' activities: A Romanian case study. In M. Cruz-Cunha, F. Moreira, & J. Varajão (Eds.), *Handbook of research on enterprise 2.0: Technological, social, and organizational dimensions* (pp. 72–88). Hershey, PA: IGI Global. doi:10.4018/978-1-4666-4373-4.ch004

Roy, N., Das, S. K., & Julien, C. (2013). Resolving and mediating ambiguous contexts in pervasive environments. In I. Management Association (Ed.), User-driven healthcare: Concepts, methodologies, tools, and applications (pp. 630-654). Hershey, PA: IGI Global. doi:10.4018/978-1-4666-2770-3.ch031

Russo, M. R. (2014). Emergency management professional development: Linking information communication technology and social communication skills to enhance a sense of community and social justice in the 21st century. In I. Management Association (Ed.), Crisis management: Concepts, methodologies, tools and applications (pp. 651-665). Hershey, PA: IGI Global. doi:10.4018/978-1-4666-4707-7.ch031

Sabone, M. B., Mogobe, K. D., & Sabone, T. G. (2013). ICTS and their role in health promotion: A preliminary situation analysis in selected botswana rural communities. In I. Management Association (Ed.), User-driven healthcare: Concepts, methodologies, tools, and applications (pp. 211-224). Hershey, PA: IGI Global. doi:10.4018/978-1-4666-2770-3.ch012

Saha, P. (2014). Systemic enterprise architecture as future: Tackling complexity in governments in the cusp of change. In P. Saha (Ed.), *A systemic perspective to managing complexity with enterprise architecture* (pp. 1–70). Hershey, PA: IGI Global. doi:10.4018/978-1-4666-4518-9.ch001

Saijo, Y. (2013). Biomedical application of multimodal ultrasound microscope. In J. Wu (Ed.), *Technological advancements in biomedicine for healthcare applications* (pp. 27–35). Hershey, PA: IGI Global. doi:10.4018/978-1-4666-2196-1.ch004

Santos, M., Bastião, L., Costa, C., Silva, A., & Rocha, N. (2013). Clinical data mining in small hospital PACS: Contributions for radiology department improvement. In R. Martinho, R. Rijo, M. Cruz-Cunha, & J. Varajão (Eds.), *Information systems and technologies for enhancing health and social care* (pp. 236–251). Hershey, PA: IGI Global. doi:10.4018/978-1-4666-3667-5.ch016

Santos, M. F., Portela, F., Miranda, M., Machado, J., Abelha, A., Silva, Á., & Rua, F. (2013). Grid data mining strategies for outcome prediction in distributed intensive care units. In R. Martinho, R. Rijo, M. Cruz-Cunha, & J. Varajão (Eds.), *Information systems and technologies for enhancing health and social care* (pp. 87–101). Hershey, PA: IGI Global. doi:10.4018/978-1-4666-3667-5.ch006

Santos, R. J., Bernardino, J., & Vieira, M. (2013). A hypotension surveillance and prediction system for critical care. In M. Cruz-Cunha, I. Miranda, & P. Gonçalves (Eds.), *Handbook of research on ICTs and management systems for improving efficiency in healthcare and social care* (pp. 341–355). Hershey, PA: IGI Global. doi:10.4018/978-1-4666-3990-4.ch017

Sanz, P. R., Mezcua, B. R., & Pena, J. M. (2013). ICTs for orientation and mobility for blind people: A state of the art. In M. Cruz-Cunha, I. Miranda, & P. Gonçalves (Eds.), *Handbook of research on ICTs for human-centered healthcare and social care services* (pp. 646–669). Hershey, PA: IGI Global. doi:10.4018/978-1-4666-3986-7.ch034

Sarabdeen, J. (2013). Legal issues in e-healthcare systems. In I. Management Association (Ed.), User-driven healthcare: Concepts, methodologies, tools, and applications (pp. 1194-1219). Hershey, PA: IGI Global. doi:10.4018/978-1-4666-2770-3.ch060

Sarbadhikari, S. N. (2013). Unlearning and relearning in online health education. In I. Management Association (Ed.), User-driven healthcare: Concepts, methodologies, tools, and applications (pp. 1348-1363). Hershey, PA: IGI Global. doi:10.4018/978-1-4666-2770-3.ch067

Sasayama, T., Hamada, S., & Kobayashi, T. (2013). Application of prewhitening beamformer with linear constraints for correlated EEG signal source estimation. In J. Wu (Ed.), *Biomedical engineering and cognitive neuroscience for healthcare: Interdisciplinary applications* (pp. 243–254). Hershey, PA: IGI Global. doi:10.4018/978-1-4666-2113-8.ch025

Sato, T., & Minato, K. (2013). Differences in analysis methods of the human uncinate fasciculus using diffusion tensor MRI. In J. Wu (Ed.), *Biomedical engineering and cognitive neuroscience for healthcare: Interdisciplinary applications* (pp. 162–170). Hershey, PA: IGI Global. doi:10.4018/978-1-4666-2113-8.ch017

Satoh, J. (2013). Molecular network analysis of target RNAs and interacting proteins of TDP-43, a causative gene for the neurodegenerative diseases ALS/FTLD. In I. Management Association (Ed.), Bioinformatics: Concepts, methodologies, tools, and applications (pp. 964-985). Hershey, PA: IGI Global. doi:10.4018/978-1-4666-3604-0.ch052

Satoh, J. (2013). Molecular network analysis of target RNAs and interacting proteins of TDP-43, a causative gene for the neurodegenerative diseases ALS/FTLD. In J. Wu (Ed.), *Technological advancements in biomedicine for healthcare applications* (pp. 314–335). Hershey, PA: IGI Global. doi:10.4018/978-1-4666-2196-1.ch032

Schafer, S. B. (2013). Fostering psychological coherence: With ICTs. In M. Cruz-Cunha, I. Miranda, & P. Gonçalves (Eds.), *Handbook of research on ICTs for human-centered healthcare and social care services* (pp. 29–47). Hershey, PA: IGI Global. doi:10.4018/978-1-4666-3986-7.ch002

Schmeida, M., & McNeal, R. (2013). Bridging the inequality gap to accessing medicare and medicaid information online: An empirical analysis of e-government success 2002 through 2010. In J. Gil-Garcia (Ed.), *E-government success around the world: Cases, empirical studies, and practical recommendations* (pp. 60–78). Hershey, PA: IGI Global. doi:10.4018/978-1-4666-4173-0.ch004

Scholl, J. C., & Olaniran, B. A. (2013). ICT use and multidisciplinary healthcare teams. In M. Cruz-Cunha, I. Miranda, & P. Gonçalves (Eds.), *Handbook of research on ICTs for human-centered healthcare and social care services* (pp. 627–645). Hershey, PA: IGI Global. doi:10.4018/978-1-4666-3986-7.ch033

Serenko, N. (2013). The impact of genetic testing and genetic information on ethical, legal and social issues in North America: The framework. In I. Management Association (Ed.), Bioinformatics: Concepts, methodologies, tools, and applications (pp. 1317-1333). Hershey, PA: IGI Global. doi:10.4018/978-1-4666-3604-0.ch067

Serrano, M., Elmisery, A., Foghlú, M. Ó., Donnelly, W., Storni, C., & Fernström, M. (2013). Pervasive computing support in the transition towards personalised health systems. In J. Rodrigues (Ed.), *Digital advances in medicine, e-health, and communication technologies* (pp. 49–64). Hershey, PA: IGI Global. doi:10.4018/978-1-4666-2794-9.ch003

Shaw, V., & Braa, J. (2013). "Developed in the south": An evolutionary and prototyping approach to developing scalable and sustainable health information systems. In I. Management Association (Ed.), User-driven healthcare: Concepts, methodologies, tools, and applications (pp. 583-607). Hershey, PA: IGI Global. doi:10.4018/978-1-4666-2770-3.ch029

Shi, J., Upadhyaya, S., & Erdem, E. (2013). Health information exchange for improving the efficiency and quality of healthcare delivery. In I. Management Association (Ed.), User-driven healthcare: Concepts, methodologies, tools, and applications (pp. 714-736). Hershey, PA: IGI Global. doi:10.4018/978-1-4666-2770-3.ch035

Shibata, T. (2013). A human-like cognitive computer based on a psychologically inspired VLSI brain model. In J. Wu (Ed.), *Technological advancements in biomedicine for healthcare applications* (pp. 247–266). Hershey, PA: IGI Global. doi:10.4018/978-1-4666-2196-1.ch027

Shimada, S. (2013). Self-body recognition and its impairment. In J. Wu (Ed.), *Biomedical engineering and cognitive neuroscience for healthcare: Interdisciplinary applications* (pp. 156–161). Hershey, PA: IGI Global. doi:10.4018/978-1-4666-2113-8.ch016

Shimogonya, Y., Ishikawa, T., Yamaguchi, T., Kumamaru, H., & Itoh, K. (2013). Computational study of the hemodynamics of cerebral aneurysm initiation. In J. Wu (Ed.), *Technological advancements in biomedicine for healthcare applications* (pp. 267–277). Hershey, PA: IGI Global. doi:10.4018/978-1-4666-2196-1.ch028

Shimonomura, K. (2013). A neuromorphic robot vision system to predict the response of visual neurons. In J. Wu (Ed.), *Technological advancements in biomedicine for healthcare applications* (pp. 193–199). Hershey, PA: IGI Global. doi:10.4018/978-1-4666-2196-1.ch020

Shrestha, S. (2013). Clinical decision support system for diabetes prevention: An illustrative case. In S. Sarnikar, D. Bennett, & M. Gaynor (Eds.), *Cases on healthcare information technology for patient care management* (pp. 308–329). Hershey, PA: IGI Global. doi:10.4018/978-1-4666-2671-3.ch017

Siddiqui, Z. S., & Jonas-Dwyer, D. R. (2013). Mobile learning in health professions education: A systematic review. In J. Keengwe (Ed.), *Pedagogical applications and social effects of mobile technology integration* (pp. 193–205). Hershey, PA: IGI Global. doi:10.4018/978-1-4666-2985-1.ch011

Silvana de Rosa, A., Fino, E., & Bocci, E. (2014). Addressing healthcare on-line demand and supply relating to mental illness: Knowledge sharing about psychiatry and psychoanalysis through social networks in Italy and France. In A. Kapoor & C. Kulshrestha (Eds.), *Dynamics of competitive advantage and consumer perception in social marketing* (pp. 16–55). Hershey, PA: IGI Global. doi:10.4018/978-1-4666-4430-4.ch002

Siqueira, S. R., Rocha, E. C., & Nery, M. S. (2013). Brazilian occupational therapy perspective about digital games as an inclusive resource to disabled people in schools. In I. Management Association (Ed.), User-driven healthcare: Concepts, methodologies, tools, and applications (pp. 918-937). Hershey, PA: IGI Global. doi:10.4018/978-1-4666-2770-3.ch046

Sliedrecht, S., & Kotzé, E. (2013). Patients with a spinal cord injury inform and co-construct services at a spinal cord rehabilitation unit. In I. Management Association (Ed.), User-driven healthcare: Concepts, methodologies, tools, and applications (pp. 1054-1072). Hershey, PA: IGI Global. doi:10.4018/978-1-4666-2770-3.ch053

Smedberg, Å. (2013). E-health communities for learning healthy habits: How to consider quality and usability. In I. Management Association (Ed.), User-driven healthcare: Concepts, methodologies, tools, and applications (pp. 310-325). Hershey, PA: IGI Global. doi:10.4018/978-1-4666-2770-3.ch016

Smedberg, Å., & Sandmark, H. (2013). Dynamic stress management: Self-help through holistic system design. In I. Management Association (Ed.), User-driven healthcare: Concepts, methodologies, tools, and applications (pp. 1469-1486). Hershey, PA: IGI Global. doi:10.4018/978-1-4666-2770-3.ch073

Sobol, M., & Prater, E. (2013). Adoption, usage and efficiency: Benchmarking healthcare IT in private practices. In J. Tan (Ed.), *Healthcare information technology innovation and sustainability: Frontiers and adoption* (pp. 145–159). Hershey, PA: IGI Global. doi:10.4018/978-1-4666-2797-0.ch009

Sobrinho, Á. A., Dias da Silva, L., Melo de Medeiros, L., & Pinheiro, M. E. (2013). A mobile assistant to aid early detection of chronic kidney disease. In R. Martinho, R. Rijo, M. Cruz-Cunha, & J. Varajão (Eds.), *Information systems and technologies for enhancing health and social care* (pp. 309–323). Hershey, PA: IGI Global. doi:10.4018/978-1-4666-3667-5.ch020

Soomlek, C., & Benedicenti, L. (2013). Agent-based wellness indicator. In V. Gulla, A. Mori, F. Gabbrielli, & P. Lanzafame (Eds.), *Telehealth networks for hospital services: New methodologies* (pp. 300–330). Hershey, PA: IGI Global. doi:10.4018/978-1-4666-2979-0.ch020

Spadaro, L., Timpano, F., Marino, S., & Bramanti, P. (2013). Telemedicine and Alzheimer disease: ICT-based services for people with Alzheimer disease and their caregivers. In V. Gulla, A. Mori, F. Gabbrielli, & P. Lanzafame (Eds.), *Telehealth networks for hospital services: New methodologies* (pp. 191–206). Hershey, PA: IGI Global. doi:10.4018/978-1-4666-2979-0.ch013

Springer, J. A., Beever, J., Morar, N., Sprague, J. E., & Kane, M. D. (2013). Ethics, privacy, and the future of genetic information in healthcare information assurance and security. In I. Management Association (Ed.), Bioinformatics: Concepts, methodologies, tools, and applications (pp. 1405-1423). Hershey, PA: IGI Global. doi:10.4018/978-1-4666-3604-0.ch072

Stachura, M. E., Wood, J., Angjellari-Dajci, F., Grayson, J., Astapova, E. V., Tung, H., . . . Lawless, W. (2013). Representing organizational conservation of information: A review of telemedicine and e-health in Georgia. In I. Management Association (Ed.), User-driven healthcare: Concepts, methodologies, tools, and applications (pp. 1220-1235). Hershey, PA: IGI Global. doi:10.4018/978-1-4666-2770-3.ch061

Stefaniak, J. E. (2013). Resuscitating team roles within wayburn health system. In A. Ritzhaupt & S. Kumar (Eds.), *Cases on educational technology implementation for facilitating learning* (pp. 130–145). Hershey, PA: IGI Global. doi:10.4018/978-1-4666-3676-7.ch008

Sugiura, M. (2013). A cognitive neuroscience approach to self and mental health. In J. Wu (Ed.), *Biomedical engineering and cognitive neuroscience for healthcare: Interdisciplinary applications* (pp. 1–10). Hershey, PA: IGI Global. doi:10.4018/978-1-4666-2113-8.ch001

Supnithi, T., Buranarach, M., Thatphithakkul, N., Junsirimongkol, B., Wongrochananan, S., Kulnawan, N., & Jiamjarasrangsi, W. (2014). A self-management service framework to support chronic disease patients' self-management. In M. Kosaka & K. Shirahada (Eds.), *Progressive trends in knowledge and system-based science for service innovation* (pp. 425–450). Hershey, PA: IGI Global. doi:10.4018/978-1-4666-4663-6.ch023

Takahashi, K., & Watanabe, K. (2013). Crossmodal interactions in visual competition. In J. Wu (Ed.), *Biomedical engineering and cognitive neuroscience for healthcare: Interdisciplinary applications* (pp. 64–72). Hershey, PA: IGI Global. doi:10.4018/978-1-4666-2113-8.ch007

Tamiya, T., Kawanishi, M., Miyake, K., Kawai, N., & Guo, S. (2013). Neurosurgical operations using navigation microscope integration system. In J. Wu (Ed.), *Technological advancements in biomedicine for healthcare applications* (pp. 128–138). Hershey, PA: IGI Global. doi:10.4018/978-1-4666-2196-1.ch014

Tan, R., Wang, S., Jiang, Y., Ishida, K., & Fujie, M. G. (2013). Motion control of an omni-directional walker for walking support. In J. Wu (Ed.), *Biomedical engineering and cognitive neuroscience for healthcare: Interdisciplinary applications* (pp. 20–28). Hershey, PA: IGI Global. doi:10.4018/978-1-4666-2113-8.ch003

Tanaka, H., & Furutani, M. (2013). Sleep management promotes healthy lifestyle, mental health, QOL, and a healthy brain. In J. Wu (Ed.), *Biomedical engineering and cognitive neuroscience for healthcare: Interdisciplinary applications* (pp. 211–224). Hershey, PA: IGI Global. doi:10.4018/978-1-4666-2113-8.ch022

Tang, C., & Carpendale, S. (2013). Human-centered design for health information technology: A qualitative approach. In I. Management Association (Ed.), User-driven healthcare: Concepts, methodologies, tools, and applications (pp. 158-179). Hershey, PA: IGI Global. doi:10.4018/978-1-4666-2770-3.ch009

Tang, X., Gao, Y., Yang, W., Zhang, M., & Wu, J. (2013). Audiovisual integration of natural auditory and visual stimuli in the real-world situation. In J. Wu (Ed.), *Biomedical engineering and cognitive neuroscience for healthcare: Interdisciplinary applications* (pp. 337–344). Hershey, PA: IGI Global. doi:10.4018/978-1-4666-2113-8.ch035

Targowski, A. (2013). Well-being, wisdom, health, and IT: From the big-picture to the small-picture. In M. Cruz-Cunha, I. Miranda, & P. Gonçalves (Eds.), *Handbook of research on ICTs for human-centered healthcare and social care services* (pp. 1–28). Hershey, PA: IGI Global. doi:10.4018/978-1-4666-3986-7.ch001

Tayabali, S., & Martin, C. M. (2013). The need to transform the core values of medical care and health organizations. In R. Biswas (Ed.), *Clinical solutions and medical progress through user-driven healthcare* (pp. 85–92). Hershey, PA: IGI Global. doi:10.4018/978-1-4666-1876-3.ch009

Taylor, B. W. (2014). Decision-making and decision support in acute care. In C. El Morr (Ed.), *Research perspectives on the role of informatics in health policy and management* (pp. 1–18). Hershey, PA: IGI Global. doi:10.4018/978-1-4666-4321-5.ch001

Teixeira, C., Pinto, J. S., Ferreira, F., Oliveira, A., Teixeira, A., & Pereira, C. (2013). Cloud computing enhanced service development architecture for the living usability lab. In R. Martinho, R. Rijo, M. Cruz-Cunha, & J. Varajão (Eds.), *Information systems and technologies for enhancing health and social care* (pp. 33–53). Hershey, PA: IGI Global. doi:10.4018/978-1-4666-3667-5.ch003

Teixeira, L., Saavedra, V., Ferreira, C., & Santos, B. S. (2013). The role of ICTs in the management of rare chronic diseases: The case of hemophilia. In M. Cruz-Cunha, I. Miranda, & P. Gonçalves (Eds.), *Handbook of research on ICTs and management systems for improving efficiency in healthcare and social care* (pp. 635–649). Hershey, PA: IGI Global. doi:10.4018/978-1-4666-3990-4.ch033

Teoh, S. Y., Singh, M., & Chong, J. (2013). An overview of e-health development in Australia. In I. Management Association (Ed.), User-driven healthcare: Concepts, methodologies, tools, and applications (pp. 901-917). Hershey, PA: IGI Global. doi:10.4018/978-1-4666-2770-3.ch045

Tiwari, S., & Srivastava, R. (2014). Research and developments in medical image reconstruction methods and its applications. In R. Srivastava, S. Singh, & K. Shukla (Eds.), *Research developments in computer vision and image processing: Methodologies and applications* (pp. 274–312). Hershey, PA: IGI Global. doi:10.4018/978-1-4666-4558-5.ch014

Tobolcea, I. (2013). The psychosocial impact of ICT efficiency on speech disorders-treatment. In M. Cruz-Cunha, I. Miranda, & P. Gonçalves (Eds.), *Handbook of research on ICTs for human-centered healthcare and social care services* (pp. 70–92). Hershey, PA: IGI Global. doi:10.4018/978-1-4666-3986-7.ch004

Toda, T., Chen, P., Ozaki, S., Fujita, K., & Ideguchi, N. (2013). A simple web-based image database system for facilitating medical care in dermatological clinics. In I. Management Association (Ed.), User-driven healthcare: Concepts, methodologies, tools, and applications (pp. 502-513). Hershey, PA: IGI Global. doi:10.4018/978-1-4666-2770-3.ch025

Toda, T., Chen, P., Ozaki, S., Fujita, K., & Ideguchi, N. (2013). A simple web-based image database system for facilitating medical care in dermatological clinics. In J. Wu (Ed.), *Technological advancements in biomedicine for healthcare applications* (pp. 385–397). Hershey, PA: IGI Global. doi:10.4018/978-1-4666-2196-1.ch038

Trudeau, S. (2013). CoRDS registry: An HIT case study concerning setup and maintenance of a disease registry. In S. Sarnikar, D. Bennett, & M. Gaynor (Eds.), *Cases on healthcare information technology for patient care management* (pp. 197–207). Hershey, PA: IGI Global. doi:10.4018/978-1-4666-2671-3.ch012

Tseng, R., & Yi-Luen Do, E. (2013). The role of information and computer technology for children with autism spectrum disorder and the facial expression wonderland (FEW). In A. Gangopadhyay (Ed.), *Methods, models, and computation for medical informatics* (pp. 98–116). Hershey, PA: IGI Global. doi:10.4018/978-1-4666-2653-9.ch006

Uchitomi, H., Suzuki, K., Nishi, T., Hove, M. J., Miyake, Y., Orimo, S., & Wada, Y. (2013). Gait rhythm of Parkinson's disease patients and an interpersonal synchrony emulation system based on cooperative gait. In J. Wu (Ed.), *Biomedical engineering and cognitive neuroscience for healthcare: Interdisciplinary applications* (pp. 38–53). Hershey, PA: IGI Global. doi:10.4018/978-1-4666-2113-8.ch005

Usher, W., & San Too, L. (2013). E-health knowledge management by australian university students. In I. Management Association (Ed.), User-driven healthcare: Concepts, methodologies, tools, and applications (pp. 938-953). Hershey, PA: IGI Global. doi:10.4018/978-1-4666-2770-3.ch047

Van Genderen, E. (2014). Intensive care. In V. Jham & S. Puri (Eds.), *Cases on consumer-centric marketing management* (pp. 53–67). Hershey, PA: IGI Global. doi:10.4018/978-1-4666-4357-4.ch006

Van Leuven, N., Newton, D., Leuenberger, D. Z., & Esteves, T. (2014). Reaching citizen 2.0: How government uses social media to send public messages during times of calm and times of crisis. In I. Management Association (Ed.), Crisis management: Concepts, methodologies, tools and applications (pp. 839-857). Hershey, PA: IGI Global. doi:10.4018/978-1-4666-4707-7.ch041

Vasudevan, V., & Rao, H. (2013). E-discovery and health care IT: An investigation. In I. Management Association (Ed.), User-driven healthcare: Concepts, methodologies, tools, and applications (pp. 1622-1635). Hershey, PA: IGI Global. doi:10.4018/978-1-4666-2770-3.ch080

Vat, K. H. (2013). Conceiving community knowledge records as e-governance concerns in wired healthcare provision. In I. Management Association (Ed.), User-driven healthcare: Concepts, methodologies, tools, and applications (pp. 1093-1111). Hershey, PA: IGI Global. doi:10.4018/978-1-4666-2770-3.ch055

Venkatasubramanian, K. K., Nabar, S., Gupta, S. K., & Poovendran, R. (2013). Cyber physical security solutions for pervasive health monitoring systems. In I. Management Association (Ed.), User-driven healthcare: Concepts, methodologies, tools, and applications (pp. 447-465). Hershey, PA: IGI Global. doi:10.4018/978-1-4666-2770-3.ch022

Victan, H. (2013). Emerging trends in user-driven healthcare: Negotiating disclosure in online health community organizations. In I. Management Association (Ed.), User-driven healthcare: Concepts, methodologies, tools, and applications (pp. 1589-1606). Hershey, PA: IGI Global. doi:10.4018/978-1-4666-2770-3.ch078

Vidal, B., Pereira, J. M., & Santos, G. (2013). SimBody: An interactive simulator for health education. In S. Arnab, I. Dunwell, & K. Debattista (Eds.), *Serious games for healthcare: Applications and implications* (pp. 265–282). Hershey, PA: IGI Global. doi:10.4018/978-1-4666-1903-6.ch013

Vivekananda-Schmidt, P. (2013). Ethics in the design of serious games for healthcare and medicine. In S. Arnab, I. Dunwell, & K. Debattista (Eds.), *Serious games for healthcare: Applications and implications* (pp. 91–106). Hershey, PA: IGI Global. doi:10.4018/978-1-4666-1903-6.ch005

Wahbeh, A. (2013). Application of handheld computing and mobile phones in diabetes self-care. In S. Sarnikar, D. Bennett, & M. Gaynor (Eds.), *Cases on healthcare information technology for patient care management* (pp. 254–275). Hershey, PA: IGI Global. doi:10.4018/978-1-4666-2671-3.ch015

Waidyanatha, N., & Dekker, S. (2013). The RTBP – Collective intelligence driving health for the user. In R. Biswas (Ed.), *Clinical solutions and medical progress through user-driven healthcare* (pp. 70–78). Hershey, PA: IGI Global. doi:10.4018/978-1-4666-1876-3.ch007

Waidyanatha, N., Dubrawski, A. M. G., & Gow, G. (2013). Affordable system for rapid detection and mitigation of emerging diseases. In J. Rodrigues (Ed.), *Digital advances in medicine, e-health, and communication technologies* (pp. 271–288). Hershey, PA: IGI Global. doi:10.4018/978-1-4666-2794-9.ch015

Walker, D. (2013). How would a ban on prescriber-identifying information impact pharmaceutical marketing? In M. Merviö (Ed.), *Healthcare management and economics: Perspectives on public and private administration* (pp. 141–153). Hershey, PA: IGI Global. doi:10.4018/978-1-4666-3982-9.ch011

Wang, B., Yan, T., & Wu, J. (2013). Neuronal function in the cortical face perception network. In J. Wu (Ed.), *Biomedical engineering and cognitive neuroscience for healthcare: Interdisciplinary applications* (pp. 171–182). Hershey, PA: IGI Global. doi:10.4018/978-1-4666-2113-8.ch018

Wang, Y., & Wang, Q. (2013). Evaluating the IEEE 802.15.6 2.4GHz WBAN proposal on medical multi-parameter monitoring under WiFi/bluetooth interference. In J. Rodrigues (Ed.), *Digital advances in medicine, e-health, and communication technologies* (pp. 312–325). Hershey, PA: IGI Global. doi:10.4018/978-1-4666-2794-9.ch018

Watanabe, T., & Miura, N. (2013). Functional electrical stimulation (FES) control for restoration and rehabilitation of motor function. In J. Wu (Ed.), *Technological advancements in biomedicine for healthcare applications* (pp. 80–93). Hershey, PA: IGI Global. doi:10.4018/978-1-4666-2196-1.ch009

Watanabe, Y., Tanaka, H., & Hirata, K. (2013). Evaluation of cognitive function in migraine patients: A study using event-related potentials. In J. Wu (Ed.), *Biomedical engineering and cognitive neuroscience for healthcare: Interdisciplinary applications* (pp. 303–310). Hershey, PA: IGI Global. doi:10.4018/978-1-4666-2113-8.ch031

Watfa, M. K., Kaur, M., & Daruwala, R. F. (2013). RFID applications in e-healthcare. In I. Management Association (Ed.), User-driven healthcare: Concepts, methodologies, tools, and applications (pp. 259-287). Hershey, PA: IGI Global. doi:10.4018/978-1-4666-2770-3.ch014

Wesorick, B. (2013). Essential steps for successful implementation of the EHR to achieve sustainable, safe, quality care. In A. Moumtzoglou & A. Kastania (Eds.), *E-health technologies and improving patient safety: Exploring organizational factors* (pp. 27–55). Hershey, PA: IGI Global. doi:10.4018/978-1-4666-2657-7.ch003

Whitaker, R. (2013). Securing health-effective medicine in practice: A critical perspective on user-driven healthcare. In R. Biswas (Ed.), *Clinical solutions and medical progress through user-driven healthcare* (pp. 35–50). Hershey, PA: IGI Global. doi:10.4018/978-1-4666-1876-3.ch005

Wickramasinghe, N., Troshani, I., Hill, S. R., Hague, W., & Goldberg, S. (2013). A transaction cost assessment of a pervasive technology solution for gestational diabetes. In J. Tan (Ed.), *Healthcare information technology innovation and sustainability: Frontiers and adoption* (pp. 109–126). Hershey, PA: IGI Global. doi:10.4018/978-1-4666-2797-0.ch007

Wilkowska, W., & Ziefle, M. (2013). User diversity as a challenge for the integration of medical technology into future smart home environments. In I. Management Association (Ed.), User-driven healthcare: Concepts, methodologies, tools, and applications (pp. 553-582). Hershey, PA: IGI Global. doi:10.4018/978-1-4666-2770-3.ch028

Willis, E., Wang, Y., & Rodgers, S. (2013). Online health communities and health literacy: Applying a framework for understanding domains of health literacy. In I. Management Association (Ed.), User-driven healthcare: Concepts, methodologies, tools, and applications (pp. 180-196). Hershey, PA: IGI Global. doi:10.4018/978-1-4666-2770-3.ch010

Wu, Q., Li, C., Takahashi, S., & Wu, J. (2013). Visual-tactile bottom-up and top-down attention. In J. Wu (Ed.), *Biomedical engineering and cognitive neuroscience for healthcare: Interdisciplinary applications* (pp. 183–191). Hershey, PA: IGI Global. doi:10.4018/978-1-4666-2113-8.ch019

Yamaguchi, S., Onoda, K., & Abe, S. (2013). Feedback-related negativity and its clinical implications. In J. Wu (Ed.), *Biomedical engineering and cognitive neuroscience for healthcare: Interdisciplinary applications* (pp. 283–292). Hershey, PA: IGI Global. doi:10.4018/978-1-4666-2113-8.ch029

Yan, B., Lei, Y., Tong, L., & Chen, K. (2013). Functional neuroimaging of acupuncture: A systematic review. In J. Wu (Ed.), *Biomedical engineering and cognitive neuroscience for healthcare: Interdisciplinary applications* (pp. 142–155). Hershey, PA: IGI Global. doi:10.4018/978-1-4666-2113-8.ch015

Yang, J. (2014). Towards healthy public policy: GIS and food systems analysis. In C. El Morr (Ed.), *Research perspectives on the role of informatics in health policy and management* (pp. 135–152). Hershey, PA: IGI Global. doi:10.4018/978-1-4666-4321-5.ch009

Yang, J., Li, Q., Gao, Y., & Wu, J. (2013). Temporal dependency of multisensory audiovisual integration. In J. Wu (Ed.), *Biomedical engineering and cognitive neuroscience for healthcare: Interdisciplinary applications* (pp. 320–326). Hershey, PA: IGI Global. doi:10.4018/978-1-4666-2113-8.ch033

Yang, J. J., Liu, J. F., Kurokawa, T., Kitamura, N., Yasuda, K., & Gong, J. P. (2013). Tough double-network hydrogels as scaffolds for tissue engineering: Cell behavior in vitro and in vivo test. In J. Wu (Ed.), *Technological advancements in biomedicine for healthcare applications* (pp. 213–222). Hershey, PA: IGI Global. doi:10.4018/978-1-4666-2196-1.ch023

Yang, W., Gao, Y., & Wu, J. (2013). Effects of selective and divided attention on audiovisual interaction. In J. Wu (Ed.), *Biomedical engineering and cognitive neuroscience for healthcare: Interdisciplinary applications* (pp. 311–319). Hershey, PA: IGI Global. doi:10.4018/978-1-4666-2113-8.ch032

Yano, Y. (2013). An EMG control system for an ultrasonic motor using a PSoC microcomputer. In J. Wu (Ed.), *Technological advancements in biomedicine for healthcare applications* (pp. 11–17). Hershey, PA: IGI Global. doi:10.4018/978-1-4666-2196-1.ch002

Yap, K. Y. (2013). The evolving role of pharmacoinformatics in targeting drug-related problems in clinical oncology practice. In I. Management Association (Ed.), User-driven healthcare: Concepts, methodologies, tools, and applications (pp. 1541-1588). Hershey, PA: IGI Global. doi:10.4018/978-1-4666-2770-3.ch077

Yokoi, H., Kato, R., Mori, T., Yamamura, O., & Kubota, M. (2013). Functional electrical stimulation based on interference-driven PWM signals for neuro-rehabilitation. In J. Wu (Ed.), *Technological advancements in biomedicine for healthcare applications* (pp. 180–192). Hershey, PA: IGI Global. doi:10.4018/978-1-4666-2196-1.ch019

York, A. M., & Nordengren, F. R. (2013). E-learning and web 2.0 case study: The role of gender in contemporary models of health care leadership. In H. Yang & S. Wang (Eds.), *Cases on formal and informal e-learning environments: Opportunities and practices* (pp. 292–313). Hershey, PA: IGI Global. doi:10.4018/978-1-4666-1930-2.ch016

Yu, W. D., & Bhagwat, R. (2013). Modeling emergency and telemedicine health support system: A service oriented architecture approach using cloud computing. In J. Rodrigues (Ed.), *Digital advances in medicine, e-health, and communication technologies* (pp. 187–213). Hershey, PA: IGI Global. doi:10.4018/978-1-4666-2794-9.ch011

Yu, Y., Yang, J., & Wu, J. (2013). Cognitive functions and neuronal mechanisms of tactile working memory. In J. Wu (Ed.), *Biomedical engineering and cognitive neuroscience for healthcare: Interdisciplinary applications* (pp. 89–98). Hershey, PA: IGI Global. doi:10.4018/978-1-4666-2113-8.ch010

Zaheer, S. (2014). Implementation of evidence-based practice and the PARIHS framework. In C. El Morr (Ed.), *Research perspectives on the role of informatics in health policy and management* (pp. 19–36). Hershey, PA: IGI Global. doi:10.4018/978-1-4666-4321-5.ch002

Zalzala, A., Chia, S., Zalzala, L., Sahu, S., Vaghasiya, S., & Karimi, A. (2013). Rural e-health infrastructure development. In I. Management Association (Ed.), User-driven healthcare: Concepts, methodologies, tools, and applications (pp. 870-900). Hershey, PA: IGI Global. doi:10.4018/978-1-4666-2770-3.ch044

Zapirain, B. G., & Zorrilla, A. M. (2013). Independent living support for disabled and elderly people using cell phones. In M. Cruz-Cunha, I. Miranda, & P. Gonçalves (Eds.), *Handbook of research on ICTs for human-centered healthcare and social care services* (pp. 379–397). Hershey, PA: IGI Global. doi:10.4018/978-1-4666-3986-7.ch020

Zgodavová, K., & Bourek, A. (2013). Potential of web based learning in managing for the sustained success of a healthcare organization based on IMPROHEALTH® project. In I. Management Association (Ed.), User-driven healthcare: Concepts, methodologies, tools, and applications (pp. 1523-1540). Hershey, PA: IGI Global. doi:10.4018/978-1-4666-2770-3.ch076

Zhao, X., Zuo, M. J., & Moghaddass, R. (2013). Generating indicators for diagnosis of fault levels by integrating information from two or more sensors. In I. Management Association (Ed.), User-driven healthcare: Concepts, methodologies, tools, and applications (pp. 288-309). Hershey, PA: IGI Global. doi:10.4018/978-1-4666-2770-3.ch015

Zhou, X., & Ren, X. (2013). Speed-accuracy tradeoff models of target-based and trajectory-based movements. In J. Wu (Ed.), *Biomedical engineering and cognitive neuroscience for healthcare: Interdisciplinary applications* (pp. 355–368). Hershey, PA: IGI Global. doi:10.4018/978-1-4666-2113-8.ch037

Zouag, N., & Driouchi, A. (2014). Trends and prospects of the Moroccan health system: 2010-2030. In A. Driouchi (Ed.), *Labor and health economics in the mediterranean region: Migration and mobility of medical doctors* (pp. 314–336). Hershey, PA: IGI Global. doi:10.4018/978-1-4666-4723-7.ch013

Zvikhachevskaya, A., & Mihaylova, L. (2013). Advanced video distribution for wireless e-healthcare systems. In I. Management Association (Ed.), User-driven healthcare: Concepts, methodologies, tools, and applications (pp. 421-446). Hershey, PA: IGI Global. doi:10.4018/978-1-4666-2770-3.ch021

Compilation of References

Aalto, A. M., Uutela, A., & Aro, A. R. (1997). Health related quality of life among insulin-dependent diabetics: Disease-related and psychosocial correlates. *Patient Education and Counseling*, *30*(3), 215–225. doi:10.1016/S0738-3991(96)00963-9 PMID:9104378

Aas, I. H. (2013). Improving patient safety with telemedicine: Exploring organizational factors. In A. Moumtzoglou & A. Kastania (Eds.), *E-health technologies and improving patient safety: Exploring organizational factors* (pp. 56–70). Hershey, PA: IGI Global. doi:10.4018/978-1-4666-2657-7.ch004

Abera, M., Tesfaye, M., Belachew, T., & Hanlon, C. (2014). *Perceived challenges and opportunities arising from integration of mental health into primary care: A cross-sectional survey of primary health care workers in south-west Ethiopia*. BioMed Central Ltd.

Aboelfotoh, M. H., Martin, P., & Hassanein, H. (2013). Ubiquitous multimedia data access in electronic health care systems. In D. Tjondronegoro (Ed.), *Tools for mobile multimedia programming and development* (pp. 191–227). Hershey, PA: IGI Global. doi:10.4018/978-1-4666-4054-2.ch011

Abreu, J. F., Almeida, P., & Silva, T. (2013). iNeighbour TV: A social TV application to promote wellness of senior citizens. In R. Martinho, R. Rijo, M. Cruz-Cunha, & J. Varajão (Eds.), Information systems and technologies for enhancing health and social care (pp. 1-19). Hershey, PA: IGI Global. doi:10.4018/978-1-4666-3667-5.ch001

Aceti, V., & Luppicini, R. (2013). Exploring the effect of mhealth technologies on communication and information sharing in a pediatric critical care unit: A case study. In J. Tan (Ed.), *Healthcare information technology innovation and sustainability: Frontiers and adoption* (pp. 88–108). Hershey, PA: IGI Global. doi:10.4018/978-1-4666-2797-0.ch006

Adami, I., Antona, M., & Stephanidis, C. (2014). Ambient assisted living for people with motor impairments. In G. Kouroupetroglou (Ed.), *Disability informatics and web accessibility for motor limitations* (pp. 76–104). Hershey, PA: IGI Global. doi:10.4018/978-1-4666-4442-7.ch003

Adelman, M. B., & Albrecht, T. L. (1987). *Communicating social support*. Sage Publications.

Adeyemo, O. (2013). The nationwide health information network: A biometric approach to prevent medical identity theft. In I. Management Association (Ed.), User-driven healthcare: Concepts, methodologies, tools, and applications (pp. 1636-1649). Hershey, PA: IGI Global. doi:10.4018/978-1-4666-2770-3.ch081

Åkerberg, A., Lindén, M., & Folke, M. (2013). Pedometer cell phone applications and future trends in measuring physical activity. In R. Martinho, R. Rijo, M. Cruz-Cunha, & J. Varajão (Eds.), *Information systems and technologies for enhancing health and social care* (pp. 324–339). Hershey, PA: IGI Global. doi:10.4018/978-1-4666-3667-5.ch021

Al Hamouche, V. (2014). Making quality control decisions in radiology department: A decision support system for radiographers' performance appraisal using PACS. In C. El Morr (Ed.), *Research perspectives on the role of informatics in health policy and management* (pp. 48–61). Hershey, PA: IGI Global. doi:10.4018/978-1-4666-4321-5.ch004

Albrecht, T. L., & Adelman, M. B. (1984). Social support and life stress. *Human Communication Research, 11*(1), 3–32. doi:10.1111/j.1468-2958.1984.tb00036.x

Albrecht, T. L., & Halsey, J. (1992). Mutual support in mixed-status relationships. *Journal of Social and Personal Relationships, 9*(2), 237–252. doi:10.1177/0265407592092005

Albuquerque, C. (2013). The study of social needs as a strategic tool for the innovation of the social care sector: The contribution of new technologies. In M. Cruz-Cunha, I. Miranda, & P. Gonçalves (Eds.), *Handbook of research on ICTs for human-centered healthcare and social care services* (pp. 347–365). Hershey, PA: IGI Global. doi:10.4018/978-1-4666-3986-7.ch018

Alexandrou, D. A., & Pardalis, K. V. (2013). SEMantic PATHways: Modeling, executing, and monitoring intra-organizational healthcare business processes towards personalized treatment. In A. Moumtzoglou & A. Kastania (Eds.), *E-health technologies and improving patient safety: Exploring organizational factors* (pp. 98–123). Hershey, PA: IGI Global. doi:10.4018/978-1-4666-2657-7.ch007

Algarín, A. D., Demurjian, S. A., Ziminski, T. B., Sánchez, Y. K., & Kuykendall, R. (2014). Securing XML with role-based access control: Case study in health care. In A. Ruiz-Martinez, R. Marin-Lopez, & F. Pereniguez-Garcia (Eds.), *Architectures and protocols for secure information technology infrastructures* (pp. 334–365). Hershey, PA: IGI Global. doi:10.4018/978-1-4666-4514-1.ch013

Alhaqbani, B., & Fidge, C. (2013). A medical data trustworthiness assessment model. In I. Management Association (Ed.), User-driven healthcare: Concepts, methodologies, tools, and applications (pp. 1425-1445). Hershey, PA: IGI Global. doi:10.4018/978-1-4666-2770-3.ch071

Al-Khudairy, S. (2014). Caring for our aging population: Using CPOE and telehomecare systems as a response to health policy concerns. In C. El Morr (Ed.), *Research perspectives on the role of informatics in health policy and management* (pp. 153–166). Hershey, PA: IGI Global. doi:10.4018/978-1-4666-4321-5.ch010

Almeida, L., Menezes, P., & Dias, J. (2013). Augmented reality framework for the socialization between elderly people. In M. Cruz-Cunha, I. Miranda, & P. Gonçalves (Eds.), *Handbook of research on ICTs for human-centered healthcare and social care services* (pp. 430–448). Hershey, PA: IGI Global. doi:10.4018/978-1-4666-3986-7.ch023

Altimier, L. (2004). Communicating with the next generation. *Newborn and Infant Nursing Reviews; NAINR*, *4*(1), 2–3. doi:10.1053/j.nainr.2003.10.001

Alvarez-Jimenez, M., Alcazar-Corcoles, M. A., González-Blanch, C., Bendall, S., McGorry, P. D., & Gleeson, J. F. (2014). Online, social media and mobile technologies for psychosis treatment: A systematic review on novel user-led interventions. *Schizophrenia Research*, *156*(1), 96–106. doi:10.1016/j.schres.2014.03.021 PMID:24746468

Alvidrez, J. (1999). Ethnic Variations in Mental Health Attitudes and Service Use Among Low-Income African American, Latina, and European American Young Women. *Community Mental Health Journal*, *35*(6), 515–530. doi:10.1023/A:1018759201290 PMID:10863988

Ambrosini, A., & Stanghellini, G. (2012). Myths of motherhood: The role of culture in the development of postpartum depression. *Annali dell'Istituto Superiore di Sanita*, *48*(3), 277–286. doi:10.4415/ANN_12_03_08 PMID:23007052

Amer, M. B., Amawi, M., & El-Khatib, H. (2013). A novel neural fuzzy approach for diagnosis of potassium disturbances. In J. Tan (Ed.), *Healthcare information technology innovation and sustainability: Frontiers and adoption* (pp. 208–218). Hershey, PA: IGI Global. doi:10.4018/978-1-4666-2797-0.ch013

Ammaniti, M., & Trentini, C. (2009). How new knowledge about parenting reveals the neurobiological implications of intersubjectivity: A conceptual synthesis of recent research. *Psychoanalytic Dialogues*, *19*(5), 537–555. doi:10.1080/10481880903231951

Andersen, S. T., & Jansen, A. (2013). Innovation in ICT-based health care provision. In J. Tan (Ed.), *Healthcare information technology innovation and sustainability: Frontiers and adoption* (pp. 58–72). Hershey, PA: IGI Global. doi:10.4018/978-1-4666-2797-0.ch004

Anderson, J., & Rainie, L. (2010). *Millennials will make online sharing in networks a lifelong habit.* Pew Research. Retrieved from Pewinternet. org website: http://pewresearch. org/millennials

Anderson, J., & Rainie, L. (2012). *Millennials will benefit and suffer due to their hyperconnected lives.* Washington, DC: Pew Research Center.

Anderson, O. A. (2007). Linking work stress, parental self-efficacy, ineffective parenting, and youth problem behavior. *Journal of Family Studies*, *13*(1), 119–120.

Aneshensel, C. S., & Stone, J. D. (1982). Stress and depression: A test of the buffering model of social support. *Archives of General Psychiatry*, *39*(12), 1392–1396. doi:10.1001/archpsyc.1982.04290120028005 PMID:7149899

Angjellari-Dajci, F., Lawless, W. F., Stachura, M. E., Wood, E. A., & DiBattisto, C. (2013). Economic evaluations for service delivery in autism spectrum disorders: benefit-cost analysis for emerging telehealth systems. In M. Cruz-Cunha, I. Miranda, & P. Gonçalves (Eds.), *Handbook of research on ICTs and management systems for improving efficiency in healthcare and social care* (pp. 16–42). Hershey, PA: IGI Global. doi:10.4018/978-1-4666-3990-4.ch002

Archibald, D., MacDonald, C. J., Hogue, R., & Mercer, J. (2013). Accessing knowledge from the bedside: Introducing the tablet computer to clinical teaching. In C. Rückemann (Ed.), *Integrated information and computing systems for natural, spatial, and social sciences* (pp. 96–109). Hershey, PA: IGI Global. doi:10.4018/978-1-4666-2190-9.ch005

Archondakis, S. (2013). Static telecytological applications for proficiency testing. In V. Gulla, A. Mori, F. Gabbrielli, & P. Lanzafame (Eds.), *Telehealth networks for hospital services: New methodologies* (pp. 228–239). Hershey, PA: IGI Global. doi:10.4018/978-1-4666-2979-0.ch015

Arling, P. A., Doebbeling, B. N., & Fox, R. L. (2013). Improving the implementation of evidence-based practice and information systems in healthcare: A social network approach. In J. Tan (Ed.), *Healthcare information technology innovation and sustainability: Frontiers and adoption* (pp. 247–270). Hershey, PA: IGI Global. doi:10.4018/978-1-4666-2797-0.ch016

Arriaga, P., Esteves, F., & Fernandes, S. (2013). Playing for better or for worse?: Health and social outcomes with electronic gaming. In M. Cruz-Cunha, I. Miranda, & P. Gonçalves (Eds.), *Handbook of research on ICTs for human-centered healthcare and social care services* (pp. 48–69). Hershey, PA: IGI Global. doi:10.4018/978-1-4666-3986-7.ch003

Arslan, P. (2014). Collaborative participation in personalized health through mobile diaries. In K. Rızvanoğlu & G. Çetin (Eds.), *Research and design innovations for mobile user experience* (pp. 150–181). Hershey, PA: IGI Global. doi:10.4018/978-1-4666-4446-5.ch009

Assis-Hassid, S., Reychav, I., Pliskin, J. S., & Heart, T. H. (2013). The effects of electronic medical record (EMR) use in primary care on the physician-patient relationship. In M. Cruz-Cunha, I. Miranda, & P. Gonçalves (Eds.), *Handbook of research on ICTs for human-centered healthcare and social care services* (pp. 130–150). Hershey, PA: IGI Global. doi:10.4018/978-1-4666-3986-7.ch007

Attard, A., & Coulson, N. S. (2012). A thematic analysis of patient communication in Parkinson's disease online support group discussion forums. *Computers in Human Behavior*, *28*(2), 500–506. doi:10.1016/j.chb.2011.10.022

Au, J. S., Yip, P. S., Chan, C. L., & Law, Y. W. (2004). Newspaper reporting of suicide cases in Hong Kong. *Crisis*, *25*(4), 161–168. doi:10.1027/0227-5910.25.4.161 PMID:15580851

Ayvaz, T. (2016, January 29). *İnternet ve Sosyal Medya Kullanıcı İstatistikleri 2016*. Retrieved from http://www.dijitalajanslar.com/internet-ve-sosyal-medya-kullanici-istatistikleri-2016/

Azar, A. T. (2013). Overview of biomedical engineering. In I. Management Association (Ed.), Bioinformatics: Concepts, methodologies, tools, and applications (pp. 1-28). Hershey, PA: IGI Global. doi:10.4018/978-1-4666-3604-0.ch001

Azar, A. T., & Eljamel, M. S. (2014). Medical robotics. In I. Management Association (Ed.), Robotics: Concepts, methodologies, tools, and applications (pp. 1116-1147). Hershey, PA: IGI Global. doi:10.4018/978-1-4666-4607-0.ch054

Baker, F., Denniston, M., Haffer, S. C., & Liberatos, P. (2009). Change in health-related quality of life of newly diagnosed cancer patients, cancer survivors, and controls. *Cancer*, *115*(13), 3024–3033. doi:10.1002/cncr.24330 PMID:19402049

Baladrón, C., Aguiar, J. M., Calavia, L., Carro, B., & Sánchez-Esguevillas, A. (2014). Learning on the move in the web 2.0: New initiatives in m-learning. In *K-12 education: Concepts, methodologies, tools, and applications* (pp. 1693–1714). Hershey, PA: IGI Global. doi:10.4018/978-1-4666-4502-8.ch097

Ballantine, P. W., & Stephenson, R. J. (2011). Help me, I'm fat! Social support in online weight loss networks. *Journal of Consumer Behaviour*, *10*(6), 332–337. doi:10.1002/cb.374

Bambina, A. (2007). *Online social support: the interplay of social networks and computer-mediated communication*. Cambria Press.

Barak, A., Boniel-Nissim, M., & Suler, J. (2008). Fostering empowerment in online support groups. *Computers in Human Behavior*, *24*(5), 1867–1883. doi:10.1016/j.chb.2008.02.004

Baron, E., Hanlon, C., Mall, S., Honikman, S., Breuer, E., Kathree, T., ... Tomlinson, M. (2016). *Maternal mental health in primary care in five low- and middle-income countries: A situational analysis*. BioMed Central Ltd.

Barraclough, B., Shepherd, D., & Jennings, C. (1977). Do newspaper reports of coroners' inquests incite people to commit suicide? *The British Journal of Psychiatry*, *131*(5), 528–532. doi:10.1192/bjp.131.5.528 PMID:588871

Barrera, M. (2000). Social support research in community psychology. In J. Rappaport & E. Seidman (Eds.), *Handbook of Community Psychology* (pp. 215–245). New York: Kluwer Academic/Plenum. doi:10.1007/978-1-4615-4193-6_10

Bartholomew, M. K., Schoppe-Sullivan, S. J., Glassman, M., Kamp Dush, C. M., & Sullivan, J. M. (2012). New parents' Facebook use at the transition to parenthood. *Family Relations*, *61*(3), 455–469. doi:10.1111/j.1741-3729.2012.00708.x PMID:23671354

Batenburg, A., & Das, E. (2015). Virtual Support Communities and Psychological Well-Being: The Role of Optimistic and Pessimistic Social Comparison Strategies. *Journal of Computer-Mediated Communication*, *20*(6), 585–600. doi:10.1111/jcc4.12131

Bauer, K. A. (2013). Caught in the web: The internet and the demise of medical privacy. In I. Management Association (Ed.), User-driven healthcare: Concepts, methodologies, tools, and applications (pp. 1252-1272). Hershey, PA: IGI Global. doi:10.4018/978-1-4666-2770-3.ch063

Bayer, J. B., Ellison, N. B., Schoenebeck, S. Y., & Falk, E. B. (2016). Sharing the small moments: Ephermeral social interaction on Snapchat. *Information Communication and Society*, *19*(17), 956–977. doi:10.1080/1369118X.2015.1084349

Bell Canada. (2017). *Let's Talk results and impact*. Retrieved from: http://letstalk.bell.ca/en/results-impact/

Belsis, P., Skourlas, C., & Gritzalis, S. (2013). Secure electronic healthcare records management in wireless environments. In M. Khosrow-Pour (Ed.), *Interdisciplinary advances in information technology research* (pp. 202–219). Hershey, PA: IGI Global. doi:10.4018/978-1-4666-3625-5.ch015

Bender, J. L., Katz, J., Ferris, L. E., Oh, H., & Jadad, A. R. (2013). What is the role of online support from the perspective of facilitators of face-to-face support groups? A multi-method study of the use of breast cancer online communities. *Patient Education and Counseling*, *93*(3), 472–479. doi:10.1016/j.pec.2013.07.009 PMID:23928354

Bender, T. (1978). *Community and social change in America*. New Brunswick, NJ: Rutgers University Press.

Benito, R. V., Vega-Colado, C., Coco, M. B., Cuadrado, R., Torres-Zafra, J. C., Sánchez-Pena, J. M., & López-Miguel, A. et al. (2013). New electro-optic and display technology for visually disabled people. In M. Cruz-Cunha, I. Miranda, & P. Gonçalves (Eds.), *Handbook of research on ICTs for human-centered healthcare and social care services* (pp. 687–718). Hershey, PA: IGI Global. doi:10.4018/978-1-4666-3986-7.ch036

Bergenti, F., Poggi, A., & Tomaiuolo, M. (2013). Using multi-agent systems to support e-health services. In M. Cruz-Cunha, I. Miranda, & P. Gonçalves (Eds.), *Handbook of research on ICTs for human-centered healthcare and social care services* (pp. 549–567). Hershey, PA: IGI Global. doi:10.4018/978-1-4666-3986-7.ch029

Berger, J., & Milkman, K. L. (2012). What makes online content viral? *JMR, Journal of Marketing Research*, *49*(2), 192–205. doi:10.1509/jmr.10.0353

Berger, M., Wagner, T. H., & Baker, L. C. (2005). Internet use and stigmatized illness. *Social Science & Medicine*, *61*(1), 1821–1827. doi:10.1016/j.socscimed.2005.03.025 PMID:16029778

Berkman, L. F., & Syme, S. L. (1979). Social networks, host resistance, and mortality: A nine-year follow-up study of Alameda County residents. *American Journal of Epidemiology*, *109*(2), 186–204. doi:10.1093/oxfordjournals.aje.a112674 PMID:425958

Berler, A., & Apostolakis, I. (2014). Normalizing cross-border healthcare in Europe via new e-prescription paradigms. In C. El Morr (Ed.), *Research perspectives on the role of informatics in health policy and management* (pp. 168–208). Hershey, PA: IGI Global. doi:10.4018/978-1-4666-4321-5.ch011

Berman, A. L. (1988). Fictional depiction of suicide in television films and imitation effects. *The American Journal of Psychiatry*, *145*(8), 982–986. doi:10.1176/ajp.145.8.982 PMID:3394883

Bernardi, R. (2013). Information technology and resistance to public sector reforms: A case study in Kenya. In I. Management Association (Ed.), User-driven healthcare: Concepts, methodologies, tools, and applications (pp. 14-33). Hershey, PA: IGI Global. doi:10.4018/978-1-4666-2770-3.ch002

Bernhard, S., Al Zoukra, K., & Schtte, C. (2013). From non-invasive hemodynamic measurements towards patient-specific cardiovascular diagnosis. In *Data mining: Concepts, methodologies, tools, and applications* (pp. 2069–2093). Hershey, PA: IGI Global. doi:10.4018/978-1-4666-2455-9.ch106

Bert, F., Gualano, M. R., Brusaferro, S., De Vito, E., De Waure, C., La Torre, G., & Torregrossa, M. V. et al. (2013). Pregnancy e-health: A multicenter Italian cross-sectional study on Internet use and decision-making among pregnant women. *Journal of Epidemiology and Community Health*, *0*, 1–6. PMID:24072743

Bessiere, K., Pressman, S., Kiesler, S., & Kraut, R. (2010). Effects of internet use on health and depression: A longitudinal study. *Journal of Medical Internet Research*, *12*(1), e6. doi:10.2196/jmir.1149 PMID:20228047

Best, C., O'Neill, B., & Gillespie, A. (2013). Assistive technology for cognition: Enabling activities of daily living. In M. Cruz-Cunha, I. Miranda, & P. Gonçalves (Eds.), *Handbook of research on ICTs for human-centered healthcare and social care services* (pp. 112–129). Hershey, PA: IGI Global. doi:10.4018/978-1-4666-3986-7.ch006

Bevan, J. L., Sparks, L., Ernst, J., Francies, J., & Santora, N. (2013). Healthcare Reform Information Sources in Relation to Information Quality, Information-Seeking, and Uncertainty. In R. Ahmed & B. R. Bates (Eds.), *Health Communication and Mass Media – An Integrated Approach to Policy and Practice* (pp. 19–34). New York, NY: Routledge.

Bhattacharya, P., Asanga, A. P., & Biswas, R. (2013). Stomodeum to proctodeum: Email narratives on clinical problem solving in gastroenterology. In I. Management Association (Ed.), User-driven healthcare: Concepts, methodologies, tools, and applications (pp. 1073-1091). Hershey, PA: IGI Global. doi:10.4018/978-1-4666-2770-3.ch054

Bibring, G. L. (1959). Some considerations of the psychological processes in pregnancy. *The Psychoanalytic Study of the Child*, *14*, 113–121.

Blair-Loy, M. (2009). *Competing devotions: Career and family among women executives*. Cambridge, MA: Harvard University Press.

Bland, H. W., Melton, B. F., Welle, P., & Bigham, L. (2012). Stress tolerance: New challenges for millennial college students. *College Student Journal*, *46*(2), 362.

Blease, C. (2016). In defense of utility: The medical humanities and medical education. *Medical Humanities*, *42*(2), 103–108. doi:10.1136/medhum-2015-010827 PMID:26842744

Boboc, C., & Ţiţan, E. (2014). Migration of medical doctors, health, medical education, and employment in eastern and central Europe. In A. Driouchi (Ed.), *Labor and health economics in the Mediterranean region: Migration and mobility of medical doctors* (pp. 158–191). Hershey, PA: IGI Global. doi:10.4018/978-1-4666-4723-7.ch007

Bodie, G. D., & Burleson, B. R. (2008). Explaining variations in the effects of supportive messages a dual-process framework. *Annals of the International Communication Association, 32*(1), 355–398. doi:10.1080/23808985.2008.11679082

Bollen, K. A., & Phillips, D. P. (1982). Imitative suicides: A national study of the effects of television news stories. *American Sociological Review, 47*(6), 802–809. doi:10.2307/2095217

Bolton, R. N., Parasuraman, A., Hoefnagels, A., Migchels, N., Kabadayi, S., Gruber, T., & Solnet, D. (2013). Understanding Generation Y and their use of social media: A review and research agenda. *Journal of Service Management, 24*(3), 245–267. doi:10.1108/09564231311326987

Botella, C., Baños, R. M., Etchemendy, E., Castilla, D., García-Palacios, A., & Alcañiz, M. (2013). An e-health system for promoting wellbeing in the elderly: The butler system. In I. Management Association (Ed.), User-driven healthcare: Concepts, methodologies, tools, and applications (pp. 838-852). Hershey, PA: IGI Global. doi:10.4018/978-1-4666-2770-3.ch042

Boulos, M. N. K., Brewer, A. C., Karimkhani, C., Buller, D. B., & Dellavalle, R. P. (2014). Mobile medical and health apps: State of the art, concerns, regulatory control and certification. *Online Journal of Public Health Informatics, 5*(3). PMID:24683442

Bourdieu, P. (1980). "Structures, Habitus, Practices," and "Belief and the Body. In *The Logic of Practice*. Stanford, CA: Stanford University Press.

Boyd, D. (2015). *It's complicated: The social lives of networked teens*. Yale University Press.

Boyes, M. E., & Cluver, L. D. (2015). Relationships between familial HIV/AIDS and symptoms of anxiety and depression: The mediating effect of bullying victimization in a prospective sample of South African children and adolescents. *Journal of Youth and Adolescence, 44*(4), 847–859. doi:10.1007/s10964-014-0146-3 PMID:24996836

Bradai, N., Chaari, L., & Kamoun, L. (2013). A comprehensive overview of wireless body area networks (WBAN). In J. Rodrigues (Ed.), *Digital advances in medicine, e-health, and communication technologies* (pp. 1–32). Hershey, PA: IGI Global. doi:10.4018/978-1-4666-2794-9.ch001

Brady, E., & Guerin, S. (2010). "Not the romantic, all happy, coochy coo experience": A qualitative analysis of interactions on an Irish parenting web site. *Family Relations, 59*(1), 14–27. doi:10.1111/j.1741-3729.2009.00582.x

Brashers, D. E., Goldsmith, D. J., & Hsieh, E. (2002). Information seeking and avoiding in health contexts. *Human Communication Research, 28*(2), 258–271. doi:10.1111/j.1468-2958.2002.tb00807.x

Braun, V., & Clarke, V. (2006). Using thematic analysis in psychology. *Qualitative Research in Psychology, 3*(2), 77–101. doi:10.1191/1478088706qp063oa

Braun, V., & Clarke, V. (2013). Successful qualitative research: A practical guide for beginners. *Sage (Atlanta, Ga.).*

Brown, M. (2013). Will comparative effectiveness research lead to healthcare rationing? In I. Management Association (Ed.), User-driven healthcare: Concepts, methodologies, tools, and applications (pp. 1487-1507). Hershey, PA: IGI Global. doi:10.4018/978-1-4666-2770-3.ch074

Brown, I. (2010). Ambivalence of the motherhood experience. In A. O'Reilly (Ed.), *Twenty-first-century motherhood: Experience, identity, policy, agency* (pp. 121–139). New York, NY: Columbia University Press.

Brown, K. E., Bayley, J., & Newby, K. (2013). Serious game for relationships and sex education: Application of an intervention mapping approach to development. In S. Arnab, I. Dunwell, & K. Debattista (Eds.), *Serious games for healthcare: Applications and implications* (pp. 135–166). Hershey, PA: IGI Global. doi:10.4018/978-1-4666-1903-6.ch007

Burlamaqui, A. M., Azevedo, S. O., Silva, I. R., Silva, S. R., Souto da Silva, G. H., & Benjamim, X. C. … Felix de Castro, A. (2013). Low cost t-health and t-social with ginga: Experience with mime TV, ImFine, and iFunnyCube interactive TV programs. In M. Cruz-Cunha, I. Miranda, & P. Gonçalves (Eds.), Handbook of research on ICTs for human-centered healthcare and social care services (pp. 303-318). Hershey, PA: IGI Global. doi:10.4018/978-1-4666-3986-7.ch015

Burleson, B. R. (2010). Explaining recipient responses to supportive messages. *New directions in interpersonal communication research*, 159-179.

Burns, J., Blanchard, M., & Metcalf, A. (2013). Bridging the digital divide in Australia: The potential implications for the mental health of young people experiencing marginalisation. In *Digital literacy: Concepts, methodologies, tools, and applications* (pp. 772–793). Hershey, PA: IGI Global. doi:10.4018/978-1-4666-1852-7.ch040

Buunk, B. P., Collins, R. L., Taylor, S. E., VanYperen, N. W., & Dakof, G. A. (1990). The affective consequences of social comparison: Either direction has its ups and downs. *Journal of Personality and Social Psychology, 59*(6), 1238–1249. doi:10.1037/0022-3514.59.6.1238 PMID:2283590

Buyurgan, N., Rardin, R. L., Jayaraman, R., Varghese, V. M., & Burbano, A. (2013). A novel GS1 data standard adoption roadmap for healthcare providers. In J. Tan (Ed.), *Healthcare information technology innovation and sustainability: Frontiers and adoption* (pp. 41–57). Hershey, PA: IGI Global. doi:10.4018/978-1-4666-2797-0.ch003

Cabrita, M. D., & Cabrita, M. (2014). Applying social marketing to healthcare: Challenges and opportunities. In A. Kapoor & C. Kulshrestha (Eds.), *Dynamics of competitive advantage and consumer perception in social marketing* (pp. 78–97). Hershey, PA: IGI Global. doi:10.4018/978-1-4666-4430-4.ch004

Cadei, L., & Simeone, D. (2011). Tra il chiaro e lo scuro. Riflessioni pedagogiche sul ruolo dell'ecografia ostetrica nel processo di transizione alla genitorialità. In E. Catarsi & J. P. Pourtois (Eds.), *Educazione familiare e servizi per l'infanzia. Education familiare et services pour l'enfance* (pp. 184–187). Firenze: University Press.

Cahn, D., & Cahn, J. (2016). *When Millennials Rule: The Reshaping of America.* Simon and Schuster.

Calhoun, C. J. (1980). Community: Toward a variable conceptualization for comparative research. *Social History*, *5*(1), 105–129. doi:10.1080/03071028008567472

Callison-Burch, V., Guadagno, J., & Davis, A. (2016, March 1). Building a safer community with new suicide prevention tools. *Facebook Newsroom.* Retrieved from: http://newsroom.fb.com/news/2017/03/building-a-safer-community-with-new-suicide-prevention-tools/

Cameron, C., Ashbury, F. D., & Iverson, D. C. (1997). Perspectives on Reach to Recovery and CanSurmount: informing the evaluation model. Cancer prevention & control: CPC= Prevention & controle en cancerologie. *PCC, 1*(2), 102–107. PMID:9765731

Campbell-Grossman, C. K., Hudson, D. B., Keating-Lefler, R., & Heusinkvelt, S. (2009). New mothers network the provision of social support to single, low-income, African American mothers via e-mail messages. *Journal of Family Nursing*, *15*(2), 220–236. doi:10.1177/1074840708323048 PMID:19211545

Campbell, H. S., Phaneuf, M. R., & Deane, K. (2004). Cancer peer support programs—do they work? *Patient Education and Counseling*, *55*(1), 3–15. doi:10.1016/j.pec.2003.10.001 PMID:15476984

Campbell, K., & Wright, K. B. (2002). Online support groups: An investigation of relationships among source credibility, dimensions of relational communication, and perceptions of emotional support. *Communication Research Reports*, *19*(2), 183–193. doi:10.1080/08824090209384846

Caplan, S. E., & Turner, J. S. (2007). Bringing theory to research on computer-mediated comforting communication. *Computers in Human Behavior*, *23*(2), 985–998. doi:10.1016/j.chb.2005.08.003

Caputo, J. D. (1997). *Deconstruction in a nutshell.* New York, NY: Fordham University Press.

Carr, N. G. (2011). *The shallows: What the Internet is doing to our brains*. New York, NY: Norton.

Carroll, J. M., & Rosson, M. B. (2013). Community networks: Infrastructure and models for therapeutic support. In M. Cruz-Cunha, I. Miranda, & P. Gonçalves (Eds.), *Handbook of research on ICTs for human-centered healthcare and social care services* (pp. 187–207). Hershey, PA: IGI Global. doi:10.4018/978-1-4666-3986-7.ch010

Castiglioni, I., Gilardi, M. C., & Gallivanone, F. (2013). E-health decision support systems for the diagnosis of dementia diseases. In A. Moumtzoglou & A. Kastania (Eds.), *E-health technologies and improving patient safety: Exploring organizational factors* (pp. 84–97). Hershey, PA: IGI Global. doi:10.4018/978-1-4666-2657-7.ch006

Catley, C., Smith, K., McGregor, C., James, A., & Eklund, J. M. (2013). A framework for multidimensional real-time data analysis: A case study for the detection of apnoea of prematurity. In A. Gangopadhyay (Ed.), *Methods, models, and computation for medical informatics* (pp. 16–35). Hershey, PA: IGI Global. doi:10.4018/978-1-4666-2653-9.ch002

Chaari, L., & Kamoun, L. (2013). QoS concepts and architecture over wireless body area networks for healthcare applications. In J. Rodrigues (Ed.), *Digital advances in medicine, e-health, and communication technologies* (pp. 114–130). Hershey, PA: IGI Global. doi:10.4018/978-1-4666-2794-9.ch007

Chamberlin, B., Maloney, A., Gallagher, R. R., & Garza, M. L. (2013). Active video games: Potential for increased activity, suggestions for use, and guidelines for implementation. In S. Arnab, I. Dunwell, & K. Debattista (Eds.), *Serious games for healthcare: Applications and implications* (pp. 191–212). Hershey, PA: IGI Global. doi:10.4018/978-1-4666-1903-6.ch009

Chang, R., Pimentel, S., & Svistunov, A. (2011). Sentiment analysis of occupy wall street tweets. In *CS 229*. Machine Learning Final Projects.

Charisi, A., Korvesis, P., & Megalooikonomou, V. (2013). Similarity searching of medical image data in distributed systems: Facilitating telemedicine applications. In A. Gangopadhyay (Ed.), *Methods, models, and computation for medical informatics* (pp. 58–77). Hershey, PA: IGI Global. doi:10.4018/978-1-4666-2653-9.ch004

Chastian, J. (2013). *Shock! Millennials pass on Obamacare*. National Center for Policy Analysis.

Chattopadhyay, A., Malhotra, K., & Chatterjee, S. (2013). Ethical guidelines for the quality assessment of healthcare. In I. Management Association (Ed.), User-driven healthcare: Concepts, methodologies, tools, and applications (pp. 1332-1347). Hershey, PA: IGI Global. doi:10.4018/978-1-4666-2770-3.ch066

Chatwin, J. (2006). Patient narratives: A micro-interactional analysis. *Communication & Medicine*, *3*(2), 113–123.

Chen, J. Y., Xu, H., Shi, P., Culbertson, A., & Meslin, E. M. (2013). Ethics and privacy considerations for systems biology applications in predictive and personalized medicine. In I. Management Association (Ed.), Bioinformatics: Concepts, methodologies, tools, and applications (pp. 1378-1404). Hershey, PA: IGI Global. doi:10.4018/978-1-4666-3604-0.ch071

Cheng, B., Stanley, R. J., De, S., Antani, S., & Thoma, G. R. (2013). Automatic detection of arrow annotation overlays in biomedical images. In J. Tan (Ed.), *Healthcare information technology innovation and sustainability: Frontiers and adoption* (pp. 219–236). Hershey, PA: IGI Global. doi:10.4018/978-1-4666-2797-0.ch014

Chen, W., & Choi, A. S. K. (2011). Internet and social support among Chinese migrants in Singapore. *New Media & Society*, *13*(7), 1067–1084. doi:10.1177/1461444810396311

Chen, Y. (2013). Construction of digital statistical atlases of the liver and their applications to computer-aided diagnosis. In J. Wu (Ed.), *Technological advancements in biomedicine for healthcare applications* (pp. 68–79). Hershey, PA: IGI Global. doi:10.4018/978-1-4666-2196-1.ch008

Cherian, E. J., & Ryan, T. W. (2014). Incongruent needs: Why differences in the iron-triangle of priorities make health information technology adoption and use difficult. In C. El Morr (Ed.), *Research perspectives on the role of informatics in health policy and management* (pp. 209–221). Hershey, PA: IGI Global. doi:10.4018/978-1-4666-4321-5.ch012

Chodorow, N. J. (2003). "Too late": Ambivalence about motherhood, choice, and time. *Journal of the American Psychoanalytic Association, 51*(4), 1181–1198. doi:10.1177/00030651030510040701 PMID:14713010

Chodorow, N. J., & Contratto, S. (1989). The Fantasy of the Perfect Mother. In N. J. Chodorow (Ed.), *Feminism and Psychoanalytic Theory* (pp. 79–96). New Haven: Yale University Press.

Choudhury, M. D., Gamon, M., Counts, S., & Horvitz, E. (2013). Predicting Depression via Social Media. In E. Kiciman, N. B. Ellison, B. Hogan, P. Resnick, & I. Soboroff (Eds.), *ICWSM. The AAAI Press.*

Chou, W. Y., Hunt, Y. M., Beckjord, E. B., Moser, R. P., & Hesse, B. W. (2009). Social Media Use in the United States: Implications for Health Communication. *Journal of Medical Internet Research, 11*(4), e48. doi:10.2196/jmir.1249 PMID:19945947

Chowdhry, N., Ashraf, A., Chowdhry, B., Baloch, A., Ansari, A., & De Meer, H. (2013). Grid for post operative care through wireless sensor networks. In I. Management Association (Ed.), User-driven healthcare: Concepts, methodologies, tools, and applications (pp. 514-531). Hershey, PA: IGI Global. doi:10.4018/978-1-4666-2770-3.ch026

Chun, S. A., Kwon, J. H., & Lee, H. (2013). Social credential-based role recommendation and patient privacy control in medical emergency. In A. Gangopadhyay (Ed.), *Methods, models, and computation for medical informatics* (pp. 215–237). Hershey, PA: IGI Global. doi:10.4018/978-1-4666-2653-9.ch013

Ciot, M., Sonderegger, M., & Ruths, D. (2013, October). *Gender inference of Twitter users in non-English contexts*. EMNLP.

Çobaner, A. A. (2017). *Social Support Through Digital Media? Breast Cancer Groups on Facebook.* Manuscript in preparation.

Cohen, J. F., Bancilhon, J., & Sergay, S. (2013). An empirical study of patient willingness to use self-service technologies in the healthcare context. In M. Cruz-Cunha, I. Miranda, & P. Gonçalves (Eds.), *Handbook of research on ICTs and management systems for improving efficiency in healthcare and social care* (pp. 378–395). Hershey, PA: IGI Global. doi:10.4018/978-1-4666-3990-4.ch019

Colineau, N., & Paris, C. (2010). Talking about your health to strangers: Understanding the use of online social networks by patients. *New Review of Hypermedia and Multimedia, 16*(1-2), 141–160. doi:10.1080/13614568.2010.496131

Constantinides, P. (2013). The development of a regional health information infrastructure in Greece. In I. Management Association (Ed.), User-driven healthcare: Concepts, methodologies, tools, and applications (pp. 992-1017). Hershey, PA: IGI Global. doi:10.4018/978-1-4666-2770-3.ch050

Constantinides, P. (2013). The development of the English national health information infrastructure. In I. Management Association (Ed.), User-driven healthcare: Concepts, methodologies, tools, and applications (pp. 968-991). Hershey, PA: IGI Global. doi:10.4018/978-1-4666-2770-3.ch049

Correa, T., Hinsley, A. W., & De Zúñiga, H. G. (2010). Who interacts on the Web?: The intersection of users' personality and social media use. *Computers in Human Behavior*, *26*(2), 247–253. doi:10.1016/j.chb.2009.09.003

Corrigan, D., Hederman, L., Khan, H., Taweel, A., Kostopoulou, O., & Delaney, B. (2013). An ontology-driven approach to clinical evidence modelling implementing clinical prediction rules. In A. Moumtzoglou & A. Kastania (Eds.), *E-health technologies and improving patient safety: Exploring organizational factors* (pp. 257–284). Hershey, PA: IGI Global. doi:10.4018/978-1-4666-2657-7.ch016

Corritore, C. L., Kracher, B., Wiedenbeck, S., & Marble, R. (2013). Foundations of trust for e-health. In I. Management Association (Ed.), User-driven healthcare: Concepts, methodologies, tools, and applications (pp. 1167-1193). Hershey, PA: IGI Global. doi:10.4018/978-1-4666-2770-3.ch059

Costa, Â., Andrade, F., & Novais, P. (2013). Privacy and data protection towards elderly healthcare. In M. Cruz-Cunha, I. Miranda, & P. Gonçalves (Eds.), *Handbook of research on ICTs for human-centered healthcare and social care services* (pp. 330–346). Hershey, PA: IGI Global. doi:10.4018/978-1-4666-3986-7.ch017

Costigan, C. L., Cox, M. J., & Cauce, A. M. (2003). Work-parenting linkages among dual-earner couples at the transition to parenthood. *Journal of Family Psychology*, *17*(3), 397–408. doi:10.1037/0893-3200.17.3.397 PMID:14562463

Cotten, S. R., & Gupta, S. S. (2004). Characteristics of online and offline health information seekers and factors that discriminate between them. *Social Science & Medicine*, *59*(9), 1795–1806. doi:10.1016/j.socscimed.2004.02.020 PMID:15312915

Coughlan, J., & Brinkman, W. (2013). Design considerations for delivering e-learning to surgical trainees. In J. Rodrigues (Ed.), *Digital advances in medicine, e-health, and communication technologies* (pp. 341–350). Hershey, PA: IGI Global. doi:10.4018/978-1-4666-2794-9.ch020

Coulson, N. S. (2005). Receiving social support online: An analysis of a computer-mediated support group for individuals living with irritable bowel syndrome. *Cyberpsychology & Behavior*, *8*(6), 580–584. doi:10.1089/cpb.2005.8.580 PMID:16332169

Coulson, N. S., Buchanan, H., & Aubeeluck, A. (2007). Social support in cyberspace: A content analysis of communication within a Huntington's disease online support group. *Patient Education and Counseling*, *68*(2), 173–178. doi:10.1016/j.pec.2007.06.002 PMID:17629440

Coulson, N., & Knibb, R. (2007). Coping with food allergy: Exploring the role of the online support group. *Cyberpsychology & Behavior, 10*(1), 145–148. doi:10.1089/cpb.2006.9978 PMID:17305463

Cowan, M. (2010). Millennial transformation for primary care. *Military Medicine, 175*(6), 379–381. doi:10.7205/MILMED-D-10-00184 PMID:20572466

Crouter, A. C., & Bumpus, M. F. (2001). Linking parents' work stress to children's and adolescents' psychological adjustment. *Current Directions in Psychological Science, 10*(5), 156–159. doi:10.1111/1467-8721.00138

Culnan, M. J., & Markus, M. L. (1987). Information technologies. Handbook of organizational communication: An interdisciplinary perspective, 420-443.

Custers, K., & Van den Bulck, J. (2009). Viewership of pro-anorexia websites in seventh, ninth and eleventh graders. *European Eating Disorders Review, 17*(3), 214–219. doi:10.1002/erv.910 PMID:19142974

D'Abundo, M. L. (2013). Electronic health record implementation in the United States healthcare industry: Making the process of change manageable. In I. Management Association (Ed.), User-driven healthcare: Concepts, methodologies, tools, and applications (pp. 382-395). Hershey, PA: IGI Global. doi:10.4018/978-1-4666-2770-3.ch019

D'Abundo, M. L. (2013). Electronic health record implementation in the United States healthcare industry: Making the process of change manageable. In V. Wang (Ed.), *Handbook of research on technologies for improving the 21st century workforce: Tools for lifelong learning* (pp. 272–286). Hershey, PA: IGI Global. doi:10.4018/978-1-4666-2181-7.ch018

D'Andrea, A., Ferri, F., & Grifoni, P. (2013). RFID technologies in the health sector. In A. Moumtzoglou & A. Kastania (Eds.), *E-health technologies and improving patient safety: Exploring organizational factors* (pp. 140–147). Hershey, PA: IGI Global. doi:10.4018/978-1-4666-2657-7.ch009

D'Astolfo, C. (2014). Investing in a "rehabilitation model" to improve the decision-making process in long-term care. In C. El Morr (Ed.), *Research perspectives on the role of informatics in health policy and management* (pp. 37–47). Hershey, PA: IGI Global. doi:10.4018/978-1-4666-4321-5.ch003

Dahlberg, L. (2001). The Internet and democratic discourse: Exploring the prospects of online deliberative forums extending the public sphere. *Information Communication and Society, 4*(4), 615–633. doi:10.1080/13691180110097030

Daniel, V. M. (2013). Genomics and genetic engineering: Playing God? In I. Management Association (Ed.), Bioinformatics: Concepts, methodologies, tools, and applications (pp. 249-267). Hershey, PA: IGI Global. doi:10.4018/978-1-4666-3604-0.ch013

Dasgupta, S. S. (2013). Cyber capability framework: A tool to evaluate ICT for development projects. In M. Cruz-Cunha, I. Miranda, & P. Gonçalves (Eds.), *Handbook of research on ICTs for human-centered healthcare and social care services* (pp. 399–406). Hershey, PA: IGI Global. doi:10.4018/978-1-4666-3986-7.ch021

Davey, Z., Schifano, F., Corazza, O., & Deluca, P. (2012). e-Psychonauts: Conducting research in online drug forum communities. *Journal of Mental Health (Abingdon, England)*, *21*(4), 386–394. doi:10.3109/09638237.2012.682265 PMID:22823094

Davis, J. J. (2010). The effect of placement and modality on the recall of information from pharmaceutical web sites. *Journal of Medical Marketing*, *10*(2), 99–114. doi:10.1057/jmm.2009.42

Davis, S. A. (2013). Global telemedicine and ehealth: Advances for future healthcare – Using a systems approach to integrate healthcare functions. In V. Gulla, A. Mori, F. Gabbrielli, & P. Lanzafame (Eds.), *Telehealth networks for hospital services: New methodologies* (pp. 15–32). Hershey, PA: IGI Global. doi:10.4018/978-1-4666-2979-0.ch002

De André, F. (1971). Il medico. In *Non al denaro, non all'amore, né al cielo* [CD]. Milano, Italy: Produttori Associati.

De Choudhury, M., Gamon, M., Counts, S., & Horvitz, E. (2013). Predicting depression via social media. *Microsoft Research & the Association for the Advancement of Artificial Intelligence*. Retrieved from: https://www.microsoft.com/en-us/research/wp- content/uploads/2016/02/icwsm_13.pdf

DeAndrea, D. C. (2015). Testing the proclaimed affordances of online support groups in a nationally representative sample of adults seeking mental health assistance. *Journal of Health Communication*, *20*(2), 147–156. doi:10.1080/10810730.2014.914606 PMID:25116383

Deave, T., Johnson, D., & Ingram, J. (2008) Transition to parenthood: The needs of parents in pregnancy and early parenthood. *BioMed Central pregnancy and Childbirth*, *8*(30), 1-11.

Delbene, R. (2011, January 01). Patients' narratives of chronic illnesses and the notion of biographical disruption. *Communication & Medicine*, *8*(1), 17–27. doi:10.1558/cam.v8i1.17 PMID:22616353

Deng, J., Hu, J., Wu, W., Dong, B., & Wu, H. (2010). Subjective well-being, social support, and age-related functioning among the very old in China. *International Journal of Geriatric Psychiatry*, *25*(7), 697–703. doi:10.1002/gps.2410 PMID:20033902

Deng, M., Petkovic, M., Nalin, M., & Baroni, I. (2013). Home healthcare in cloud computing. In M. Cruz-Cunha, I. Miranda, & P. Gonçalves (Eds.), *Handbook of research on ICTs and management systems for improving efficiency in healthcare and social care* (pp. 614–634). Hershey, PA: IGI Global. doi:10.4018/978-1-4666-3990-4.ch032

Dennis, C. L. (2010). Postpartum depression peer support: Maternal perceptions from a randomized controlled trial. *International Journal of Nursing Studies*, *47*(5), 560–568. doi:10.1016/j.ijnurstu.2009.10.015 PMID:19962699

Dennis, C. L., Hodnett, E., Kenton, L., Weston, J., Zupancic, J., Stewart, D. E., & Kiss, A. (2009). Effect of peer support on prevention of postnatal depression among high risk women: Multisite randomised controlled trial. *British Medical Journal, 338*, 280–284. PMID:19147637

Depression Understood. (2017). Retrieved from http://www.depression-understood.org/

DeVany, M., Knobloch-Ludwig, K., Penticoff, M., Assimacopoulos, A., & Speedie, S. (2013). Telehealth implementation: The voice of experience. In S. Sarnikar, D. Bennett, & M. Gaynor (Eds.), *Cases on healthcare information technology for patient care management* (pp. 126–139). Hershey, PA: IGI Global. doi:10.4018/978-1-4666-2671-3.ch008

Devisch, I., & Vanheule, S. (2014). Singularity and medicine: Is there a place for heteronomy in medical ethics? *Journal of Evaluation in Clinical Practice, 20*(6), 965–969. doi:10.1111/jep.12110 PMID:24387804

Diala, C. C. (2001). Racial/ethnic differences in attitudes toward seeking professional mental health services. *American Journal of Public Health, 91*, 5. PMID:11344893

Diclegis. (2017). Retrieved from https://www.diclegis.com/en/diclegis/what-is-diclegis

Diesing, G. (2016). Milleniala: Who they are, what they want, & why you need them. *Hospitals & Health Networks, 90*(11), 22.

Ding, W., Qiu, P., Liu, Y., & Feng, W. (2013). Current omics technologies in biomarker discovery. In I. Management Association (Ed.), Bioinformatics: Concepts, methodologies, tools, and applications (pp. 465-497). Hershey, PA: IGI Global. doi:10.4018/978-1-4666-3604-0.ch027

Dingli, A., Abela, C., & D'Ambrogio, I. (2013). PINATA: Taking e-health a step forward. In A. Moumtzoglou & A. Kastania (Eds.), *E-health technologies and improving patient safety: Exploring organizational factors* (pp. 173–195). Hershey, PA: IGI Global. doi:10.4018/978-1-4666-2657-7.ch012

Dogra, D. P., Nandam, K., Majumdar, A. K., Sural, S., Mukhopadhyay, J., Majumdar, B., & Mukherjee, S. et al. (2013). A tool for automatic hammersmith infant neurological examination. In J. Rodrigues (Ed.), *Digital advances in medicine, e-health, and communication technologies* (pp. 301–311). Hershey, PA: IGI Global. doi:10.4018/978-1-4666-2794-9.ch017

Donatone, B. (2014). A prescription for helping millennials grow up. *The Washington Post.*

Doyle, J., Bertolotto, M., & Wilson, D. (2013). Towards multimodal mobile GIS for the elderly. In *Digital literacy: Concepts, methodologies, tools, and applications* (pp. 590–609). Hershey, PA: IGI Global. doi:10.4018/978-1-4666-1852-7.ch031

Dragoni, A. F. (2013). Health services through digital terrestrial television. In V. Gulla, A. Mori, F. Gabbrielli, & P. Lanzafame (Eds.), *Telehealth networks for hospital services: New methodologies* (pp. 207–227). Hershey, PA: IGI Global. doi:10.4018/978-1-4666-2979-0.ch014

Dragoni, A. F. (2013). Virtual carer: A first prototype. In V. Gulla, A. Mori, F. Gabbrielli, & P. Lanzafame (Eds.), *Telehealth networks for hospital services: New methodologies* (pp. 290–299). Hershey, PA: IGI Global. doi:10.4018/978-1-4666-2979-0.ch019

Drentea, P., & Moren-Cross, J. L. (2005). Social capital and social support on the web: The case of an internet mother site. *Sociology of Health & Illness*, *27*(7), 920–943. doi:10.1111/j.1467-9566.2005.00464.x PMID:16313523

Driouchi, A. (2014). Introduction to labor and health economics: Mobility of medical doctors in the Mediterranean region. In A. Driouchi (Ed.), *Labor and health economics in the Mediterranean region: Migration and mobility of medical doctors* (pp. 1–22). Hershey, PA: IGI Global. doi:10.4018/978-1-4666-4723-7.ch001

Driouchi, A. (2014). Medical knowledge, north-south cooperation, and mobility of medical doctors. In A. Driouchi (Ed.), *Labor and health economics in the Mediterranean region: Migration and mobility of medical doctors* (pp. 376–395). Hershey, PA: IGI Global. doi:10.4018/978-1-4666-4723-7.ch015

Driouchi, A. (2014). Skilled human resources in the health sectors and impacts of new health technologies on health workforce in developing economies. In A. Driouchi (Ed.), *Labor and health economics in the Mediterranean region: Migration and mobility of medical doctors* (pp. 23–50). Hershey, PA: IGI Global. doi:10.4018/978-1-4666-4723-7.ch002

du Pré, A. (2005). *Communicating about health: Current issues and perspectives* (2nd ed.). New York: Oxford University Press.

Duam, M. (2015). Millennial self-esteem or narcissism? *Newsday.*

Duan, X., Wang, X., & Huang, Q. (2013). Medical manipulators for surgical applications. In J. Wu (Ed.), *Technological advancements in biomedicine for healthcare applications* (pp. 111–122). Hershey, PA: IGI Global. doi:10.4018/978-1-4666-2196-1.ch012

Dugdale, A. (2013). Australian patient organizations: Using digital technologies to engage health citizen communities in health policy. In I. Management Association (Ed.), User-driven healthcare: Concepts, methodologies, tools, and applications (pp. 853-869). Hershey, PA: IGI Global. doi:10.4018/978-1-4666-2770-3.ch043

Duncan, B., Hart, G., Scoular, A., & Bigrigg, A. (2001). Qualitative analysis of psychosocial impact of diagnosis of Chlamydia trachomatis: Implications for screening. *BMJ (Clinical Research Ed.)*, *322*(7280), 195–199. doi:10.1136/bmj.322.7280.195 PMID:11159612

Dunkerley, B. (2014, August 15). Josh Gracin posts suicide note on Facebook. *Rolling Stone.* Retrieved from: http://www.rollingstone.com/music/news/josh-gracin-posts-suicide-note-on-facebook-20140815

Dunne, Á., Lawlor, M. A., & Rowley, J. (2010). Young people's use of online social networking sites–a uses and gratifications perspective. *Journal of Research in Interactive Marketing*, *4*(1), 46–58. doi:10.1108/17505931011033551

Dunwell, I., & Jarvis, S. (2013). A serious game for on-the-ward infection control awareness training: Ward off infection. In S. Arnab, I. Dunwell, & K. Debattista (Eds.), *Serious games for healthcare: Applications and implications* (pp. 233–246). Hershey, PA: IGI Global. doi:10.4018/978-1-4666-1903-6.ch011

Durant, K. T., McCray, A. T., & Safran, C. (2013). Identifying temporal changes and topics that promote growth within online communities: A prospective study of six online cancer forums. In A. Gangopadhyay (Ed.), *Methods, models, and computation for medical informatics* (pp. 78–97). Hershey, PA: IGI Global. doi:10.4018/978-1-4666-2653-9.ch005

Eichhorn, K. C. (2008). Soliciting and providing support over the Internet: An investigation of online eating disorder groups. *Journal of Computer-Mediated Communication, 14*(1), 67–78. doi:10.1111/j.1083-6101.2008.01431.x

Eisenlauer, V. (2014). Facebook: A multimodal discourse analysis of (semi-)automated communicative modes. In C. Maier & S. Norris (Eds.), Interactions, Images and Texts: A Reader of Multimodality (pp. 309-317). Berlin: de Gruyter.

El-Farargy, N. (2013). Refresher training in clinical psychology supervision: A blended learning approach. In A. Benson, J. Moore, & S. Williams van Rooij (Eds.), *Cases on educational technology planning, design, and implementation: A project management perspective* (pp. 295–317). Hershey, PA: IGI Global. doi:10.4018/978-1-4666-4237-9.ch016

Elkin, N. (2008). *How America searches: Health and wellness.* Retrieved from http://www.rx-edge.com/research%20pdfs/How_America_Searches_Health_and_Wellness.pdf

Ellison, N. B., Steinfield, C., & Lampe, C. (2007). The benefits of Facebook "friends": Social capital and college students' use of online social network sites. *Journal of Computer-Mediated Communication, 12*(4), 1143–1168. doi:10.1111/j.1083-6101.2007.00367.x

Enquist, H. (2013). From idea to use: lessons learned from a participatory ICT healthcare case study. In I. Management Association (Ed.), User-driven healthcare: Concepts, methodologies, tools, and applications (pp. 1037-1053). Hershey, PA: IGI Global. doi:10.4018/978-1-4666-2770-3.ch052

Ervin, K. (2014). Legal and ethical considerations in the implementation of electronic health records. In J. Krueger (Ed.), *Cases on electronic records and resource management implementation in diverse environments* (pp. 193–210). Hershey, PA: IGI Global. doi:10.4018/978-1-4666-4466-3.ch012

Escayola, J., Trigo, J., Martínez, I., Martínez-Espronceda, M., Aragüés, A., Sancho, D., . . . García, J. (2013). Overview of the ISO/IEEE11073 family of standards and their applications to health monitoring. In I. Management Association (Ed.), User-driven healthcare: Concepts, methodologies, tools, and applications (pp. 357-381). Hershey, PA: IGI Global. doi:10.4018/978-1-4666-2770-3.ch018

Etzersdorfer, E., & Sonneck, G. (1998). Preventing suicide by influencing mass-media reporting: The Viennese experience 1980-1996. *Archives of Suicide Research*, *4*(1), 67–74. doi:10.1080/13811119808258290

Eysenbach, G. (2003). The impact of the Internet on cancer outcomes. *CA: a Cancer Journal for Clinicians*, *53*(6), 356–371. doi:10.3322/canjclin.53.6.356 PMID:15224975

Facebook Newsroom. (2017). *Company info*. Retrieved from: http://newsroom.fb.com/company-info/

Facelli, J. C., Hurdle, J. F., & Mitchell, J. A. (2013). Medical informatics and bioinformatics. In I. Management Association (Ed.), Bioinformatics: Concepts, methodologies, tools, and applications (pp. 195-221). Hershey, PA: IGI Global. doi:10.4018/978-1-4666-3604-0.ch010

Faith, J., Thorburn, S., & Sinky, T. H. (2016). Exploring healthcare experiences among online interactive weight loss forum users. *Computers in Human Behavior*, *57*, 326–333. doi:10.1016/j.chb.2015.12.048

Fakhar, A. (2014). Beyond brain drain: A case study of the benefits of cooperation on medical immigration. In A. Driouchi (Ed.), *Labor and health economics in the Mediterranean region: Migration and mobility of medical doctors* (pp. 294–313). Hershey, PA: IGI Global. doi:10.4018/978-1-4666-4723-7.ch012

Falan, S. L., Han, B., Zoeller, L. H., Tarn, J. M., & Roach, D. M. (2013). Sustaining healthcare through waste elimination: A taxonomic analysis with case illustrations. In J. Tan (Ed.), *Healthcare information technology innovation and sustainability: Frontiers and adoption* (pp. 18–39). Hershey, PA: IGI Global. doi:10.4018/978-1-4666-2797-0.ch002

Fanning, J., Mullen, S. P., & McAuley, E. (2012). Increasing physical activity with mobile devices: A meta-analysis. *Journal of Medical Internet Research*, *14*(6), e161. doi:10.2196/jmir.2171 PMID:23171838

Farinha, C., & Mira da Silva, M. (2013). Identifying requirements for healthcare information systems with focus groups. In M. Cruz-Cunha, I. Miranda, & P. Gonçalves (Eds.), *Handbook of research on ICTs for human-centered healthcare and social care services* (pp. 491–510). Hershey, PA: IGI Global. doi:10.4018/978-1-4666-3986-7.ch026

Farris, R., Chong, F., & Danning, D. (2002). Generation Y: Purchasing power and implications for marketing. *Academy of Marketing Studies Journal*, *6*(1-2), 89.

Faw, L. (2012). Why Millennials are Spending More than They Earn, And Parents are Footing the Bill. *Forbes*. Retrieved from http://www.forbes.com/sites/larissafaw/2012/05/18/why-millennials-are-spending-more-than-they-earn/

Federal Trade Commission. (2015). *The FTC's endorsement guides: What people are asking*. Retrieved from https://www.ftc.gov/system/files/documents/plain-language/pdf-0205-endorsement-guides-faqs_0.pdf

Fekete, S., & Schmidtke, A. (1995). The impact of mass media and reports on suicide and attitudes toward self-destruction. In B. L. Mishara (Ed.), *The Impact of Suicide* (pp. 142–155). New York: Springer Publishing Company.

Fernando, J. (2013). The protocols of privileged information handling in an e-health context: Australia. In I. Management Association (Ed.), User-driven healthcare: Concepts, methodologies, tools, and applications (pp. 737-759). Hershey, PA: IGI Global. doi:10.4018/978-1-4666-2770-3.ch036

Ferraro, F., & Nunziante Cesàro, A. (1985). *Lo spazio cavo e il corpo saturato. La gravidanza come "agire" tra fusione e separazione*. Milano: Franco Angeli Editore.

Ferreira, L., Teixeira, A., & Cunha, J. P. (2013). Medical information extraction in European Portuguese. In M. Cruz-Cunha, I. Miranda, & P. Gonçalves (Eds.), *Handbook of research on ICTs for human-centered healthcare and social care services* (pp. 607–626). Hershey, PA: IGI Global. doi:10.4018/978-1-4666-3986-7.ch032

Festinger, L. (1954). A theory of social comparison processes. *Human Relations*, *7*(2), 117–140. doi:10.1177/001872675400700202

Finn, J. (1999). An exploration of helping processes in an online self-help group focusing on issues of disability. *Health & Social Work*, *24*(3), 220–231. doi:10.1093/hsw/24.3.220 PMID:10505283

Fitzpatrick, J. (2013). An exploration of the experiences of migrant women: Implications for policy development of effective user driven health care delivery systems. In I. Management Association (Ed.), User-driven healthcare: Concepts, methodologies, tools, and applications (pp. 954-967). Hershey, PA: IGI Global. doi:10.4018/978-1-4666-2770-3.ch048

Fitzpatrick, J., & Ako, W. (2013). Developing community ontologies in user driven healthcare. In I. Management Association (Ed.), User-driven healthcare: Concepts, methodologies, tools, and applications (pp. 655-672). Hershey, PA: IGI Global. doi:10.4018/978-1-4666-2770-3.ch032

Flores, A. E., Win, K. T., & Susilo, W. (2013). Secure exchange of electronic health records. In I. Management Association (Ed.), IT policy and ethics: Concepts, methodologies, tools, and applications (pp. 1059-1079). Hershey, PA: IGI Global. doi:10.4018/978-1-4666-2919-6.ch048

Flores, A. E., Win, K. T., & Susilo, W. (2013). Secure exchange of electronic health records. In I. Management Association (Ed.), User-driven healthcare: Concepts, methodologies, tools, and applications (pp. 1403-1424). Hershey, PA: IGI Global. doi:10.4018/978-1-4666-2770-3.ch070

Fogel, J., Albert, S. M., Schnabel, F., Ditkoff, B.A., &Neugut, A. I. (2002). Use of the Internet by Women with Breast Cancer. *Journal of Medical Internet Research*, *4*(2).

Fogel, J., Albert, S. M., Schnabel, F., Ann Ditkoff, B., & Neugut, A. I. (2003). Racial/ethnic differences and potential psychological benefits in use of the internet by women with breast cancer. *Psycho-Oncology*, *12*(2), 107–117. doi:10.1002/pon.617 PMID:12619143

Food and Drug Administration. (2015a). *Warning letter*. Retrieved from https://www.fda.gov/downloads/Drugs/GuidanceComplianceRegulatoryInformation/EnforcementActivitiesbyFDA/WarningLettersandNoticeofViolationLetterstoPharmaceuticalCompanies/UCM457961.pdf

Food and Drug Administration. (2015b). *Incorrect reminder ad*. Retrieved from https://www.fda.gov/Drugs/ResourcesForYou/Consumers/PrescriptionDrugAdvertising/ucm082287.htm

Forrestal, E. J., Cellucci, L. W., Zeng, X., Kennedy, M. H., & Smith, D. (2013). Health information technology collaboration in community health centers: The community partners HealthNet, Inc. In S. Sarnikar, D. Bennett, & M. Gaynor (Eds.), *Cases on healthcare information technology for patient care management* (pp. 171–196). Hershey, PA: IGI Global. doi:10.4018/978-1-4666-2671-3.ch011

Fox, S. (2011). *Pew Internet & American Life Project: Health Topics*. Retrieved March 11, 2011 from http://www.perwinternet.org/Reports/2011/HealthTopics.aspx

Fox, S., & Duggan, M. (2013). *Health online 2013*. Washington, DC: Pew Internet & American Life Project.

Frederico, C. (2013). Nutrition games. In S. Arnab, I. Dunwell, & K. Debattista (Eds.), *Serious games for healthcare: Applications and implications* (pp. 167–190). Hershey, PA: IGI Global. doi:10.4018/978-1-4666-1903-6.ch008

Freitas, L., Pereira, R. T., Pereira, H. G., Martini, R., Mozzaquatro, B. A., Kasper, J., & Librelotto, G. (2013). Ontological representation and an architecture for homecare pervasive systems. In R. Martinho, R. Rijo, M. Cruz-Cunha, & J. Varajão (Eds.), *Information systems and technologies for enhancing health and social care* (pp. 215–234). Hershey, PA: IGI Global. doi:10.4018/978-1-4666-3667-5.ch015

Frigo, C. A., & Pavan, E. E. (2014). Prosthetic and orthotic devices. In *Assistive technologies: Concepts, methodologies, tools, and applications* (pp. 549–613). Hershey, PA: IGI Global. doi:10.4018/978-1-4666-4422-9.ch028

Frost, J. H., & Massagli, M. H. (2008). Social uses of personal health information within PatientsLikeMe, an online patient community: What can happen when patients have access to one another's data. *Journal of Medical Internet Research*, *10*(3), e15. doi:10.2196/jmir.1053 PMID:18504244

Fukami, T., & Wu, J. (2013). Image fusion method and the efficacy of multimodal cardiac images. In J. Wu (Ed.), *Technological advancements in biomedicine for healthcare applications* (pp. 47–54). Hershey, PA: IGI Global. doi:10.4018/978-1-4666-2196-1.ch006

Fukunishi, I., Horikawa, N., Yamazaki, T., Shirasaka, K., Kanno, K., & Akimoto, M. (1998). Perception and utilization of social support in diabetic control. *Diabetes Research and Clinical Practice*, *41*(3), 207–211. doi:10.1016/S0168-8227(98)00083-7 PMID:9829351

Furchtgott-Roth, D., & Meyer, J. (2015). *Disinherited: How Washington is Betraying America's Young*. Encounter Books.

Furdu, I., & Patrut, B. (2013). ICT applications and solutions in healthcare: Present and perspectives. In M. Cruz-Cunha, I. Miranda, & P. Gonçalves (Eds.), *Handbook of research on ICTs and management systems for improving efficiency in healthcare and social care* (pp. 559–576). Hershey, PA: IGI Global. doi:10.4018/978-1-4666-3990-4.ch029

Gabbrielli, F. (2013). Telemedicine R&D influencing incoming strategies and organization models. In V. Gulla, A. Mori, F. Gabbrielli, & P. Lanzafame (Eds.), *Telehealth networks for hospital services: New methodologies* (pp. 250–264). Hershey, PA: IGI Global. doi:10.4018/978-1-4666-2979-0.ch017

Gaivéo, J. M. (2013). Security of ICTs supporting healthcare activities. In M. Cruz-Cunha, I. Miranda, & P. Gonçalves (Eds.), *Handbook of research on ICTs for human-centered healthcare and social care services* (pp. 208–228). Hershey, PA: IGI Global. doi:10.4018/978-1-4666-3986-7.ch011

Gallant, M. P. (2003). The influence of social support on chronic illness self-management: A review and directions for research. *Health Education & Behavior*, *30*(2), 170–195. doi:10.1177/1090198102251030 PMID:12693522

Gallo, C. (2013). A multichannel framework for multimedia content deployment in e-health environments. In M. Cruz-Cunha, I. Miranda, & P. Gonçalves (Eds.), *Handbook of research on ICTs and management systems for improving efficiency in healthcare and social care* (pp. 872–891). Hershey, PA: IGI Global. doi:10.4018/978-1-4666-3990-4.ch045

Gao, Y., Yang, W., Yang, J., Satoshi, T., & Wu, J. (2013). Neural mechanisms of audiovisual integration in integrated processing for verbal perception and spatial factors. In J. Wu (Ed.), *Biomedical engineering and cognitive neuroscience for healthcare: Interdisciplinary applications* (pp. 327–336). Hershey, PA: IGI Global. doi:10.4018/978-1-4666-2113-8.ch034

Garden, R. (2015). Who speaks for whom? Health humanities and the ethics of representation. *Medical Humanities*. PMID:25795700

Garzo, A., Carmien, S. P., & Madina, X. (2013). Mapping input technology to ability. In I. Management Association (Ed.), User-driven healthcare: Concepts, methodologies, tools, and applications (pp. 480-501). Hershey, PA: IGI Global. doi:10.4018/978-1-4666-2770-3.ch024

Gass, E., & Bezold, M. P. (2013). Generation Y, shifting funding structures, and health care reform: Reconceiving the public health paradigm through social work. *Social Work in Public Health*, *28*(7), 685–693. doi:10.1080/19371918.2011.619460 PMID:24074132

Gatzidis, C. (2013). First-person shooter game engines and healthcare: An examination of the current state of the art and future potential. In S. Arnab, I. Dunwell, & K. Debattista (Eds.), *Serious Games for Healthcare: Applications and Implications* (pp. 76–89). Hershey, PA: IGI Global. doi:10.4018/978-1-4666-1903-6.ch004

Gaughan, M. (2013). The hybridized nature of America's health care system: Medicare as a case of both market and public failure. In M. Merviö (Ed.), *Healthcare management and economics: Perspectives on public and private administration* (pp. 154–164). Hershey, PA: IGI Global. doi:10.4018/978-1-4666-3982-9.ch012

Gavgani, V. Z. (2013). Ubiquitous information therapy service through social networking libraries: An operational web 2.0 service model. In I. Management Association (Ed.), User-driven healthcare: Concepts, methodologies, tools, and applications (pp. 673-688). Hershey, PA: IGI Global. doi:10.4018/978-1-4666-2770-3.ch033

Gavgani, V. Z. (2013). Information therapy (ix) service and patients' preference. In A. Gangopadhyay (Ed.), *Methods, models, and computation for medical informatics* (pp. 117–125). Hershey, PA: IGI Global. doi:10.4018/978-1-4666-2653-9.ch007

Germaine-McDaniel, N. S. (2013). The emerging hispanic use of online health information in the United States: Cultural convergence or dissociation? In I. Management Association (Ed.), User-driven healthcare: Concepts, methodologies, tools, and applications (pp. 1607-1621). Hershey, PA: IGI Global. doi:10.4018/978-1-4666-2770-3.ch079

Gholson, J., & Tennyson, H. (2013). One system of care, one electronic chart. In S. Sarnikar, D. Bennett, & M. Gaynor (Eds.), *Cases on healthcare information technology for patient care management* (pp. 55–69). Hershey, PA: IGI Global. doi:10.4018/978-1-4666-2671-3.ch003

Ghose, T. (2013,). Study shows rise in teenage narcissism and sense of entitlement (posted 2013-05-06 22:14:52): A new study reinforces observations about millenials as lazy and materialistic. *The Washington Post.*

Ghosh, B. (2013). Healthcare systems using clinical data: Addressing data interoperability challenges. In S. Sarnikar, D. Bennett, & M. Gaynor (Eds.), *Cases on healthcare information technology for patient care management* (pp. 208–223). Hershey, PA: IGI Global. doi:10.4018/978-1-4666-2671-3.ch013

Gibson, L., Sloan, D., & Moncur, W. (2013). E-health and digital inclusion. In I. Management Association (Ed.), User-driven healthcare: Concepts, methodologies, tools, and applications (pp. 197-210). Hershey, PA: IGI Global. doi:10.4018/978-1-4666-2770-3.ch011

Gibson, L., & Hanson, V. L. (2013). Digital motherhood: How does technology help new mothers? In J. A. Konstan, & K. Höök (Eds.), *Proceedings of the SIGCHI conference on human factors in computing systems* (pp. 313-322). ACM. doi:10.1145/2470654.2470700

Gillespie, N. (2014). Millennials are selfish and entitled, and helicopter parents are to blame. *Time Magazine.*

Gillies, A. C., & Howard, J. (2013). Information as change agent or barrier in health care reform? In J. Tan (Ed.), *Healthcare information technology innovation and sustainability: Frontiers and adoption* (pp. 1–17). Hershey, PA: IGI Global. doi:10.4018/978-1-4666-2797-0.ch001

Glass, G. V., & Hopkins, K. D. (1996). *Statistical Methods in Education and Psychology* (3rd ed.). Needham Heights, MA: Pearson.

Global Diabetes Community. (2016). *Guide to HbA1c*. Retrieved March 15, 2016, from http://www.diabetes.co.uk/what-is-hba1c.html

Glusker, A., & Hoelscher, E. (2014). Transitioning from print to online-only resources: The experience of a medium-sized healthcare organization library. In J. Krueger (Ed.), *Cases on electronic records and resource management implementation in diverse environments* (pp. 226–242). Hershey, PA: IGI Global. doi:10.4018/978-1-4666-4466-3.ch014

Goffman, E. (1981). Footing. In *Forms of talk. Philadelphia: University of Pennsylvania Press*. Abingdon, UK: Routledge.

Gofuku, A., Fukumori, S., & Sato, K. (2013). A mirror visual feedback therapy system applying virtual reality technology. In J. Wu (Ed.), *Biomedical engineering and cognitive neuroscience for healthcare: Interdisciplinary applications* (pp. 73–80). Hershey, PA: IGI Global. doi:10.4018/978-1-4666-2113-8.ch008

Goldsmith, D. J., & Albrecht, T. L. (2011). Social support, social networks, and health. The Routledge handbook of health communication, 335-348.

Gomes, C., Sperandio, F., Peles, A., Borges, J., Brito, A. C., & Almada-Lobo, B. (2013). An operating theater planning decision support system. In R. Martinho, R. Rijo, M. Cruz-Cunha, & J. Varajão (Eds.), *Information systems and technologies for enhancing health and social care* (pp. 69–86). Hershey, PA: IGI Global. doi:10.4018/978-1-4666-3667-5.ch005

Gonzales, A. L., & Hancock, J. T. (2011). Mirror, mirror on my Facebook wall: Effects of exposure to Facebook on self-esteem. *Cyberpsychology, Behavior, and Social Networking*, *14*(1-2), 79–83. doi:10.1089/cyber.2009.0411 PMID:21329447

Gould, M., Jamieson, P., & Romer, D. (2003). Media contagion and the young. *The American Behavioral Scientist*, *46*(9), 1269–1284. doi:10.1177/0002764202250670

Granovetter, M. S. (1973). The strength of weak ties. *American Journal of Sociology*, *78*(6), 1360–1380. doi:10.1086/225469

Greenberger, E., O'neil, R., & Nagel, S. K. (1994). Linking workplace and homeplace: Relations between the nature of adults' work and their parenting behaviors. *Developmental Psychology*, *30*(6), 990–1002. doi:10.1037/0012-1649.30.6.990

Greene, J. A., Choudhry, N. K., Kilabuk, E., & Shrank, W. H. (2010). Online social networking by patients with diabetes: A qualitative evaluation of communication with Facebook. *Journal of General Internal Medicine*, *26*(3), 287–292. doi:10.1007/s11606-010-1526-3 PMID:20945113

Green-Hamann, S., Campbell Eichhorn, K., & Sherblom, J. C. (2011). An exploration of why people participate in Second Life social support groups. *Journal of Computer-Mediated Communication*, *16*(4), 465–491. doi:10.1111/j.1083-6101.2011.01543.x

Green-Hamann, S., & Sherblom, J. C. (2014). *The influences of optimal matching and social capital on communicating support. Journal of Health Communication*. doi:10.1080/10810730.2013.864734

Grienenberger, J., & Slade, A. (2002). Maternal reflective functioning, mother-infant affective communication, and infant attachment: Implications for psychodynamic treatment with children and families. *Psychologist-Psychoanalyst*, *22*(3), 1–8.

Grissom, T. E., DuKatz, A., Kordylewski, H. A., & Dutton, R. P. (2013). Bring out your data: The evolution of the national anesthesia clinical outcomes registry (NACOR). In A. Gangopadhyay (Ed.), *Methods, models, and computation for medical informatics* (pp. 126–145). Hershey, PA: IGI Global. doi:10.4018/978-1-4666-2653-9.ch008

Gudes, O., Kendall, E., Yigitcanlar, T., Han, J. H., & Pathak, V. (2013). Developing a competitive city through healthy decision-making. In I. Management Association (Ed.), User-driven healthcare: Concepts, methodologies, tools, and applications (pp. 808-822). Hershey, PA: IGI Global. doi:10.4018/978-1-4666-2770-3.ch040

Guendouzi, J. (2006). "The guilt thing": Balancing domestic and professional roles. *Journal of Marriage and the Family*, *68*(4), 901–909. doi:10.1111/j.1741-3737.2006.00303.x

Gugerty, B., & Maranda, M. J. (2013). The promises and challenges of health information technology. In I. Management Association (Ed.), User-driven healthcare: Concepts, methodologies, tools, and applications (pp. 57-76). Hershey, PA: IGI Global. doi:10.4018/978-1-4666-2770-3.ch004

Guggenheim, L., Jang, S. M., Bae, S. Y., & Neuman, W. R. (2015). The dynamics of issue frame competition in traditional and social media. *The Annals of the American Academy of Political and Social Science*, *659*(1), 207–224. doi:10.1177/0002716215570549

Guimarães, C., Antunes, D. R., García, L. S., & Fernandes, S. (2013). Information challenges of the deaf in their health and social care needs. In M. Cruz-Cunha, I. Miranda, & P. Gonçalves (Eds.), *Handbook of research on ICTs for human-centered healthcare and social care services* (pp. 93–111). Hershey, PA: IGI Global. doi:10.4018/978-1-4666-3986-7.ch005

Guinalíu, M., Marta, J., & Subero, J. M. (2013). Social networks as a tool to improve the life quality of chronic patients and their relatives. In M. Cruz-Cunha, I. Miranda, & P. Gonçalves (Eds.), *Handbook of research on ICTs for human-centered healthcare and social care services* (pp. 172–186). Hershey, PA: IGI Global. doi:10.4018/978-1-4666-3986-7.ch009

Gullà, V. (2013). Leading the technological innovation in healthcare systems: The telematic medicine approach. In V. Gulla, A. Mori, F. Gabbrielli, & P. Lanzafame (Eds.), *Telehealth networks for hospital services: New methodologies* (pp. 134–153). Hershey, PA: IGI Global. doi:10.4018/978-1-4666-2979-0.ch009

Gullà, V., & Cancellotti, C. (2013). Telemedicine in emergency: A first aid hospital network experience. In V. Gulla, A. Mori, F. Gabbrielli, & P. Lanzafame (Eds.), *Telehealth networks for hospital services: New methodologies* (pp. 240–248). Hershey, PA: IGI Global. doi:10.4018/978-1-4666-2979-0.ch016

Gunnell. (1994). Reporting suicide: The effect of media coverage on patterns of self harm. *British Medical Journal, 308*, 1446-47.

Guo, M., Yu, Y., Yang, J., & Wu, J. (2013). The crossmodal between the visual and tactile for motion perception. In J. Wu (Ed.), *Biomedical engineering and cognitive neuroscience for healthcare: Interdisciplinary applications* (pp. 99–108). Hershey, PA: IGI Global. doi:10.4018/978-1-4666-2113-8.ch011

Guo, Y., & Goh, D. H. L. (2014). "I Have AIDS": Content analysis of postings in HIV/AIDS support group on a Chinese microblog. *Computers in Human Behavior, 34*, 219–226. doi:10.1016/j.chb.2014.02.003

Gutt, C. N., Oniu, T., Schemmer, P., Mehrabi, A., & Büchler, M. W. (2004). Fewer adhesions induced by laparoscopic surgery?. *Surgical Endoscopy and Other Interventional Techniques, 18*(6), 898-906.

Habib, M. K. (2014). Web-based multi-user distributed and collaborative environment supporting emergency and relief activities. In I. Management Association (Ed.), Crisis management: Concepts, methodologies, tools and applications (pp. 425-445). Hershey, PA: IGI Global. doi:10.4018/978-1-4666-4707-7.ch019

Hafeez-Baig, A., & Gururajan, R. (2013). Phenomena of adoption of wireless handheld devices: A case of healthcare setting. In H. Muga & K. Thomas (Eds.), *Cases on the diffusion and adoption of sustainable development practices* (pp. 20–43). Hershey, PA: IGI Global. doi:10.4018/978-1-4666-2842-7.ch002

Haida, M. (2013). Implications of NIRS brain signals. In J. Wu (Ed.), *Biomedical engineering and cognitive neuroscience for healthcare: Interdisciplinary applications* (pp. 120–128). Hershey, PA: IGI Global. doi:10.4018/978-1-4666-2113-8.ch013

Hall, W., & Irvine, V. (2009). E-communication among mothers of infants and toddlers in a community-based cohort: A content analysis. *Journal of Advanced Nursing, 65*(1), 175–183. doi:10.1111/j.1365-2648.2008.04856.x PMID:19016925

Hammer, L., & Thompson, C. A. (2003) Work-family role conflict. In *An encyclopedia entry for the Sloan Work and Family Research Network*. Retrieved March 18, 2017, from www.bc.edu/wfnetwork

Han, D., & Braun, K. L. (2013). Promoting active ageing through technology training in Korea. In *Digital literacy: Concepts, methodologies, tools, and applications* (pp. 572–589). Hershey, PA: IGI Global. doi:10.4018/978-1-4666-1852-7.ch030

Haniff, D. (2013). Usability engineering and e-health. In I. Management Association (Ed.), User-driven healthcare: Concepts, methodologies, tools, and applications (pp. 1446-1468). Hershey, PA: IGI Global. doi:10.4018/978-1-4666-2770-3.ch072

Han, J. Y., Kim, J. H., Yoon, H. J., Shim, M., McTavish, F. M., & Gustafson, D. H. (2012). Social and psychological determinants of levels of engagement with an online breast cancer support group: Posters, lurkers, and nonusers. *Journal of Health Communication*, *17*(3), 356–371. doi:10.1080/10810730.2011.585696 PMID:22085215

Hareva, D. H., Okada, H., & Oka, H. (2013). Ecological momentary assessment using a mobile phone. In J. Wu (Ed.), *Technological advancements in biomedicine for healthcare applications* (pp. 398–407). Hershey, PA: IGI Global. doi:10.4018/978-1-4666-2196-1.ch039

Harnett, B. (2013). Patient centered medicine and technology adaptation. In I. Management Association (Ed.), User-driven healthcare: Concepts, methodologies, tools, and applications (pp. 77-98). Hershey, PA: IGI Global. doi:10.4018/978-1-4666-2770-3.ch005

Hassan, R. (1995). Effects of newspaper stories on the incidence of suicide in Australia: A research note. *The Australian and New Zealand Journal of Psychiatry*, *29*(3), 480–483. doi:10.3109/00048679509064957 PMID:8573052

Hatton, J. D., Schmidt, T. M., & Jelen, J. (2013). Adoption of electronic health care records: Physician heuristics and hesitancy. In R. Martinho, R. Rijo, M. Cruz-Cunha, & J. Varajão (Eds.), *Information systems and technologies for enhancing health and social care* (pp. 148–165). Hershey, PA: IGI Global. doi:10.4018/978-1-4666-3667-5.ch010

Hawton, K., & Williams, K. (2002). Influences of the media on suicide. *British Medical Journal*, *352*(7377), 1374–1375. doi:10.1136/bmj.325.7377.1374 PMID:12480830

Hays, S. (1996). *Cultural Contradictions of Motherhood.* New Haven, CT: Yale University Press.

Heinrichs, L., Fellander-Tsai, L., & Davies, D. (2013). Clinical virtual worlds: The wider implications for professional development in healthcare. In K. Bredl & W. Bösche (Eds.), *Serious games and virtual worlds in education, professional development, and healthcare* (pp. 221–240). Hershey, PA: IGI Global. doi:10.4018/978-1-4666-3673-6.ch014

Heinrichs, W. L., Davies, D., & Davies, J. (2013). Virtual worlds in healthcare: Applications and implications. In S. Arnab, I. Dunwell, & K. Debattista (Eds.), *Serious games for healthcare: Applications and implications* (pp. 1–22). Hershey, PA: IGI Global. doi:10.4018/978-1-4666-1903-6.ch001

Heinze, J. E., Kruger, D. J., Reischl, T. M., Cupal, S., & Zimmerman, M. A. (2015). Relationships among disease, social support, and perceived health: A lifespan approach. *American Journal of Community Psychology*, *56*(3-4), 268–279. doi:10.1007/s10464-015-9758-3 PMID:26462808

Helgeson, V. S., & Gottlieb, B. H. (2000). Support groups. *Social support measurement and intervention: A guide for health and social scientists*, 221-245.

Hempler, N. F., Ekholm, O., & Willaing, I. (2013). Differences in social relations between persons with type 2 diabetes and the general population. *Scandinavian Journal of Public Health*, *41*(4), 340–343. PMID:23554389

Henry, S. L., Rook, K. S., Stephens, M. A., & Franks, M. M. (2013). Spousal undermining of older diabetic patients' disease management. *Journal of Health Psychology, 18*(12), 1550–1561. doi:10.1177/1359105312465913 PMID:23325381

Herek, G., & Glunt, E. K. (1988). An epidemic of stigma: Public reactions to AIDS. *The American Psychologist, 43*(11), 886–891. doi:10.1037/0003-066X.43.11.886 PMID:3063145

Heteronomous. (2017). In *Oxford Dictionary*. Retrieved from https://en.oxforddictionaries.com/definition/heteronomous

Hewlett, S. A. (2002). *Creating a Life. Professional Women and the Quest for Children.* New York: Talk Miramax Books.

Himelboim, I., & Han, J. Y. (2014). Cancer talk on Twitter: Community structure and information sources in breast and prostate cancer social networks. *Journal of Health Communication, 19*(2), 210–225. doi:10.1080/10810730.2013.811321 PMID:24111482

Hirata, M., Yanagisawa, T., Matsushita, K., Sugata, H., Kamitani, Y., & Suzuki, T. … Yoshimine, T. (2013). Brain–machine interface using brain surface electrodes: Real-time robotic control and a fully implantable wireless system. In J. Wu (Ed.), Technological advancements in biomedicine for healthcare applications (pp. 362-374). Hershey, PA: IGI Global. doi:10.4018/978-1-4666-2196-1.ch036

Hlebec, V., Manfreda, K. L., & Vehovar, V. (2006). The social support networks of internet users. *New Media & Society, 8*(1), 9–32. doi:10.1177/1461444806058166

Ho, K. K. (2016, January 31). *Let's talk about how my job at Bell gave me mental health issues and no benefits*. Retrieved from: http://www.canadalandshow.com/lets-talk-about-how-my-job-bell-gave-me-mental-health-issues-and-no-benefits/

Hocine, N., & Gouaïch, A. (2013). Difficulty and scenario adaptation: An approach to customize therapeutic games. In S. Arnab, I. Dunwell, & K. Debattista (Eds.), *Serious games for healthcare: Applications and implications* (pp. 107–134). Hershey, PA: IGI Global. doi:10.4018/978-1-4666-1903-6.ch006

Holbrey, S., & Coulson, N. S. (2013). A qualitative investigation of the impact of peer to peer online support for women living with polycystic ovary syndrome. *BMC Women's Health, 13*(1), 51. doi:10.1186/1472-6874-13-51 PMID:24341398

Hong, Y., Pena-Purcell, N. C., & Ory, M. G. (2012). Outcomes of online support and resources for cancer survivors: A systematic literature review. *Patient Education and Counseling, 86*(3), 288–296. doi:10.1016/j.pec.2011.06.014 PMID:21798685

Hooley, T., Wellens, J., & Marriott, J. (2011). *What is Online research?: Using the Internet for social science research.* A&C Black.

Hoonakker, P., Cartmill, R. S., Carayon, P., & Walker, J. M. (2013). Development and psychometric qualities of the SEIPS survey to evaluate CPOE/EHR implementation in ICUs. In J. Tan (Ed.), *Healthcare information technology innovation and sustainability: Frontiers and adoption* (pp. 161–179). Hershey, PA: IGI Global. doi:10.4018/978-1-4666-2797-0.ch010

Hoshi, K. (2013). Reframing dichotomies: Human experiential design of healthcare technologies. In I. Management Association (Ed.), User-driven healthcare: Concepts, methodologies, tools, and applications (pp. 1303-1331). Hershey, PA: IGI Global. doi:10.4018/978-1-4666-2770-3.ch065

Høstgaard, A. M. (2013). End-user participation in health IT development: The EUPHIT method. In I. Management Association (Ed.), User-driven healthcare: Concepts, methodologies, tools, and applications (pp. 608-629). Hershey, PA: IGI Global. doi:10.4018/978-1-4666-2770-3.ch030

House, J. S. (1981). *Work Stress and Social Support*. Addison-Wesley Publishing Co.

House, J. S., & Kahn, R. L. (1985). Measures and concepts of social support. In S. Cohen & L. Syme (Eds.), *Social Support and Health* (pp. 83–108). Orlando, FL: Academic Press.

Houston, T. K., Cooper, L. A., & Ford, D. E. (2002). Internet support groups for depression: A 1-year prospective cohort study. *The American Journal of Psychiatry*, *159*(12), 2062–2068. doi:10.1176/appi.ajp.159.12.2062 PMID:12450957

Høybye, M. T., Johansen, C., & Tjørnhøj-Thomsen, T. (2005). Online interaction. Effects of storytelling in an internet breast cancer support group. *Psycho-Oncology*, *14*(3), 211–220. doi:10.1002/pon.837 PMID:15386774

Huang, F. Y. (1997). Health insurance coverage of the children of immigrants in the United States. *Maternal and Child Health Journal*, *1*(2), 69–80. doi:10.1023/A:1026266205885 PMID:10728229

Hughes, D. J., Rowe, M., Batey, M., & Lee, A. (2012). A tale of two sites: Twitter vs. Facebook and the personality predictors of social media usage. *Computers in Human Behavior*, *28*(2), 561–569. doi:10.1016/j.chb.2011.11.001

Hughes, S., & Cohen, D. (2011). Can online consumers contribute to drug knowledge? A mixed-methods comparison of consumer-generated and professionally controlled psychotropic medication information on the Internet. *Journal of Medical Internet Research*, *13*(3), e53. doi:10.2196/jmir.1716 PMID:21807607

Huh, J., Liu, L. S., Neogi, T., Inkpen, K., & Pratt, W. (2014). Health vlogs as social support for chronic illness management. *ACM Transactions on Computer-Human Interaction*, *21*(4), 1–31. doi:10.1145/2630067 PMID:26146474

Hu, Y. (2015). Health communication research in the digital age: A systematic review. *Journal of Communication in Healthcare*, *8*(4), 260–288. doi:10.1080/17538068.2015.1107308

Igrejas, G., Amaral, J. S., & Rodrigues, P. J. (2013). Fall detection systems to be used by elderly people. In M. Cruz-Cunha, I. Miranda, & P. Gonçalves (Eds.), *Handbook of research on ICTs for human-centered healthcare and social care services* (pp. 449–473). Hershey, PA: IGI Global. doi:10.4018/978-1-4666-3986-7.ch024

Influencers. (2017). In *Business Dictionary*. Retrieved from http://www.businessdictionary.com/definition/influencers.html

Inomata, C., & Nitta, S. (2013). Nursing in integrative medicine and nurses' engagement in caring-healing: A discussion based on the practice and study of music therapy and nursing care for patients with neurodegenerative disorders. In J. Wu (Ed.), *Technological advancements in biomedicine for healthcare applications* (pp. 235–239). Hershey, PA: IGI Global. doi:10.4018/978-1-4666-2196-1.ch025

Ishaq, G. M., Hussain, P. T., Iqbal, M. J., & Mushtaq, M. B. (2013). Risk-benefit analysis of combination vs. unopposed HRT in post-menopausal women. In I. Management Association (Ed.), Bioinformatics: Concepts, methodologies, tools, and applications (pp. 1424-1440). Hershey, PA: IGI Global. doi:10.4018/978-1-4666-3604-0.ch073

Ivanoff, S. D., & Hultberg, J. (2006). Understanding the multiple realities of everyday life: Basic assumptions in focus-group methodology. *Scandinavian Journal of Occupational Therapy*, *13*(2), 125–132. doi:10.1080/11038120600691082 PMID:16856469

Iwaki, S. (2013). Multimodal neuroimaging to visualize human visual processing. In J. Wu (Ed.), *Biomedical engineering and cognitive neuroscience for healthcare: Interdisciplinary applications* (pp. 274–282). Hershey, PA: IGI Global. doi:10.4018/978-1-4666-2113-8.ch028

Jang, J., Dworkin, J., & Connell, J. (2012). Babycenter. com: New parent behavior in an online community. The Forum for Family and Consumer Issues.

Jiang, Y., Wang, S., Tan, R., Ishida, K., Ando, T., & Fujie, M. G. (2013). Motor cortex activation during mental imagery of walking: An fNIRS study. In J. Wu (Ed.), *Biomedical engineering and cognitive neuroscience for healthcare: Interdisciplinary applications* (pp. 29–37). Hershey, PA: IGI Global. doi:10.4018/978-1-4666-2113-8.ch004

Jirasevijinda, T. (2015). Reaching into our doctor's bag of tricks to help patients navigate health information technology. *Journal of Communication in Healthcare*, *8*(4), 255–257. doi:10.1080/17538068.2015.1126052

Ji, Z., Sugi, T., Goto, S., Wang, X., & Nakamura, M. (2013). Multi-channel template extraction for automatic EEG spike detection. In J. Wu (Ed.), *Biomedical engineering and cognitive neuroscience for healthcare: Interdisciplinary applications* (pp. 255–265). Hershey, PA: IGI Global. doi:10.4018/978-1-4666-2113-8.ch026

Johnson, K., & Tashiro, J. (2013). Interprofessional care and health care complexity: Factors shaping human resources effectiveness in health information management. In I. Management Association (Ed.), User-Driven Healthcare: Concepts, Methodologies, Tools, and Applications (pp. 1273-1302). Hershey, PA: IGI Global. doi:10.4018/978-1-4666-2770-3.ch064

Johnston, A. C., Worrell, J. L., Di Gangi, P. M., & Wasko, M. (2013). Online health communities: An assessment of the influence of participation on patient empowerment outcomes. *Information Technology & People*, *26*(2), 213–235. doi:10.1108/ITP-02-2013-0040

Jomhari, N., Gonzalez, V. M., & Kurniawan, S. H. (2009). See the apple of my eye: Baby storytelling in social space. In *Proceedings of the 23rd British HCI Group Annual Conference on People and Computers: Celebrating People and Technology* (pp. 238-243). British Computer Society.

Jones, C., & Czerniewicz, L. (2010). Describing or debunking? The net generation and digital natives. *Journal of Computer Assisted Learning*, *26*(5), 317–320. doi:10.1111/j.1365-2729.2010.00379.x

Jones, C., & Healing, G. (2010). Net generation students: Agency and choice and the new technologies. *Journal of Computer Assisted Learning*, *26*(5), 344–356. doi:10.1111/j.1365-2729.2010.00370.x

Jordan, C. J. (2010). Evolution of autism support and understanding via the World Wide Web. *Intellectual and Developmental Disabilities*, *48*(3), 220–227. doi:10.1352/1934-9556-48.3.220 PMID:20597733

Jose, J. (2013). Pharmacovigilance: Basic concepts and applications of pharmacoinformatics. In I. Management Association (Ed.), Bioinformatics: Concepts, methodologies, tools, and applications (pp. 1453-1473). Hershey, PA: IGI Global. doi:10.4018/978-1-4666-3604-0.ch075

Kale, M., Schwendig, L. W., Culberstone, V., Cady, P. S., Sharp, W., & Adamick, B. (1996). Monitoring the regulatory process of prescribed drug advertisement. *The Journal of Pharmacy & Law*, *229*, 229–243.

Kalina, J., & Zvárová, J. (2013). Decision support systems in the process of improving patient safety. In I. Management Association (Ed.), Bioinformatics: Concepts, methodologies, tools, and applications (pp. 1113-1125). Hershey, PA: IGI Global. doi:10.4018/978-1-4666-3604-0.ch057

Kalina, J., & Zvárová, J. (2013). Decision support systems in the process of improving patient safety. In A. Moumtzoglou & A. Kastania (Eds.), *E-health technologies and improving patient safety: Exploring organizational factors* (pp. 71–83). Hershey, PA: IGI Global. doi:10.4018/978-1-4666-2657-7.ch005

Kamath, J. R., & Donahoe-Anshus, A. L. (2013). Electronic health record: Adoption, considerations and future direction. In I. Management Association (Ed.), User-driven healthcare: Concepts, methodologies, tools, and applications (pp. 34-56). Hershey, PA: IGI Global. doi:10.4018/978-1-4666-2770-3.ch003

Kant, I. (1997). *Critique of practical reason*. Cambridge, UK: Cambridge University Press. doi:10.1017/CBO9780511809576

Karamagkioli, K. Z., & Karamagioli, E. (2013). European e-health framework: Towards more "patient-friendly" healthcare services? In I. Management Association (Ed.), User-driven healthcare: Concepts, methodologies, tools, and applications (pp. 760-775). Hershey, PA: IGI Global. doi:10.4018/978-1-4666-2770-3.ch037

Kardaras, D. K., & Karakostas, B. (2013). Case studies in customization of e-health services. In I. Management Association (Ed.), User-driven healthcare: Concepts, methodologies, tools, and applications (pp. 1018-1036). Hershey, PA: IGI Global. doi:10.4018/978-1-4666-2770-3.ch051

Kardashian, K. [kimkardashian]. (2015, August 7). Post [Instagram page]. Retrieved from https://www.instagram.com/p/7B07j_uSww/?taken-by=kimkardashian

Kardashian, K. [kimkardashian]. (2016, August 27). Post [Instagram page]. Retrieved from https://www.instagram.com/p/BJbEC96h3a5/?taken-by=kimkardashian&hl=it

Karnieli-Miller, O., Vu, T. R., Holtman, M. C., Clyman, S. G., & Inui, T. S. (2010). Medical students' professionalism narratives: A window on the informal and hidden curriculum. *Academic Medicine*, *85*(1), 124–133. doi:10.1097/ACM.0b013e3181c42896 PMID:20042838

Kastania, A. N. (2013). Evaluation considerations for e-health systems. In I. Management Association (Ed.), User-driven healthcare: Concepts, methodologies, tools, and applications (pp. 1126-1140). Hershey, PA: IGI Global. doi:10.4018/978-1-4666-2770-3.ch057

Kato, P. M. (2013). The role of the researcher in making serious games for health. In S. Arnab, I. Dunwell, & K. Debattista (Eds.), *Serious games for healthcare: Applications and implications* (pp. 213–231). Hershey, PA: IGI Global. doi:10.4018/978-1-4666-1903-6.ch010

Katsura, S. (2013). Preservation and reproduction of human motion based on a motion-copying system. In J. Wu (Ed.), *Technological advancements in biomedicine for healthcare applications* (pp. 375–384). Hershey, PA: IGI Global. doi:10.4018/978-1-4666-2196-1.ch037

Kelly, K., Slade, A., & Grienenberger, J. F. (2005). Maternal reflective functioning, mother–infant affective communication, and infant attachment: Exploring the link between mental states and observed caregiving behavior in the intergenerational transmission of attachment. *Attachment & Human Development*, *7*(3), 299–311. doi:10.1080/14616730500245963 PMID:16210241

Keltgen, J. (2016). *The impact of generational and gender effects on physician satisfaction in the US* (Doctoral dissertation). University of South Dakota.

Kessler, R. C., & Stipp, H. (1984). The impact of fictional television suicide stories on American fatalities. *American Journal of Sociology*, *90*, 151–167. doi:10.1086/228051

Keyder, Ç. (2007). Giriş. In Ç. Keyder (Ed.), *Avrupa'da ve Türkiye'de sağlık politikaları* (pp. 7–35). İstanbul: İletişim Yayınları.

Kiesler, S., Siegel, J., & McGuire, T. W. (1984). Social psychological aspects of computer-mediated communication. *The American Psychologist*, *39*(10), 1123–1134. doi:10.1037/0003-066X.39.10.1123

Kikuchi, T. (2013). Human-friendly mechatronics systems with functional fluids and elastomers. In J. Wu (Ed.), *Technological advancements in biomedicine for healthcare applications* (pp. 94–101). Hershey, PA: IGI Global. doi:10.4018/978-1-4666-2196-1.ch010

Kim, J., & Lee, J. E. (2011). The Facebook paths to happiness: Effects of the number of Facebook friends and self-presentation on subjective well-being. *Cyberpsychology, Behavior, and Social Networking*, *6*(6), 359–364. doi:10.1089/cyber.2010.0374 PMID:21117983

Kimura, T., Miura, T., Shinohara, K., & Doi, S. (2013). Visual attention in 3-D space while moving forward. In J. Wu (Ed.), *Biomedical engineering and cognitive neuroscience for healthcare: Interdisciplinary applications* (pp. 81–88). Hershey, PA: IGI Global. doi:10.4018/978-1-4666-2113-8.ch009

Kirk, S., & Milnes, L. (2015). An exploration of how young people and parents use online support in the context of living with cystic fibrosis. *Health Expectations*, *19*(2), 309–321. doi:10.1111/hex.12352 PMID:25691209

Kldiashvili, E. (2013). Implementation of telecytology in Georgia. In V. Gulla, A. Mori, F. Gabbrielli, & P. Lanzafame (Eds.), *Telehealth networks for hospital services: New methodologies* (pp. 341–361). Hershey, PA: IGI Global. doi:10.4018/978-1-4666-2979-0.ch022

Klein, J. D., & Wilson, K. M. (2002). Delivery quality care: Adolescents' discussion of health risks with their providers. *The Journal of Adolescent Health*, *30*(3), 190–195. doi:10.1016/S1054-139X(01)00342-1 PMID:11869926

Klemm, P., Bunnell, D., Cullen, M., Soneji, R., Gibbons, P., & Holecek, A. (2003). Online cancer support groups: a review of the research literature. CIN: Computers, Informatics. *Nursing*, *21*(3), 136–142. PMID:12792194

Klemm, P., Bunnell, D., Cullen, M., Soneji, R., Gibbons, P., & Holecek, A. (2003). Online cancer support groups: A review of the research literature. *CIN: Computers, Informatics. Nursing*, *21*(3), 136–142. PMID:12792194

Klemm, P., & Wheeler, E. (2005). Cancer caregivers online: Hope, emotional roller coaster, and physical/emotional/psychological responses. *CIN: Computers, Informatics. Nursing*, *23*(1), 38–45. PMID:15622203

Kolovou, L. T., & Lymberopoulos, D. K. (2013). The concept of interoperability for AAL systems. In I. Management Association (Ed.), User-driven healthcare: Concepts, methodologies, tools, and applications (pp. 1364-1385). Hershey, PA: IGI Global. doi:10.4018/978-1-4666-2770-3.ch068

Koppar, A. R., & Sridhar, V. (2013). Malaria parasite detection: Automated method using microscope color image. In J. Rodrigues (Ed.), *Digital advances in medicine, e-health, and communication technologies* (pp. 289–300). Hershey, PA: IGI Global. doi:10.4018/978-1-4666-2794-9.ch016

Kotsonis, E., & Eliakis, S. (2013). Information security standards for health information systems: The implementer's approach. In I. Management Association (Ed.), User-driven healthcare: Concepts, methodologies, tools, and applications (pp. 225-257). Hershey, PA: IGI Global. doi:10.4018/978-1-4666-2770-3.ch013

Koumpouros, Y., Toulias, T. L., & Koumpouros, N. (2015). The importance of patient engagement and the use of social media marketing in healthcare. *Technology and Health Care*, *23*(4), 495–507. doi:10.3233/THC-150918 PMID:26409912

Kraut, R., Olson, J., Banaji, M., Bruckman, A., Cohen, J., & Couper, M. (2004). Psychological research online: Report of Board of Scientific Affairs' Advisory Group on the Conduct of Research on the Internet. *The American Psychologist*, *59*(2), 105–117. doi:10.1037/0003-066X.59.2.105 PMID:14992637

Krishnaswamy, K., & Oates, T. (2014). Pathway to independence: Past, present, and beyond via robotics. In G. Kouroupetroglou (Ed.), *Disability informatics and web accessibility for motor limitations* (pp. 153–201). Hershey, PA: IGI Global. doi:10.4018/978-1-4666-4442-7.ch005

Kuehler, M., Schimke, N., & Hale, J. (2013). Privacy considerations for clectronic health records. In I. Management Association (Ed.), User-driven healthcare: Concepts, methodologies, tools, and applications (pp. 1387-1402). Hershey, PA: IGI Global. doi:10.4018/978-1-4666-2770-3.ch069

Kummervold, P., Chronaki, C., Lausen, B., Prokosch, H. U., Rasmussen, J., Santana, S., & Wangberg, S. et al. (2008). eHealth trends in Europe 2005-2007: A population-based survey. *Journal of Medical Internet Research*, *10*(4), e42. doi:10.2196/jmir.1023 PMID:19017584

Kurita, Y., Ikeda, A., Nagata, K., Okajima, M., & Ogasawara, T. (2013). Biomedical robotics for healthcare. In J. Wu (Ed.), *Technological advancements in biomedicine for healthcare applications* (pp. 160–169). Hershey, PA: IGI Global. doi:10.4018/978-1-4666-2196-1.ch017

Kuss, D. J., & Griffiths, M. D. (2011). Online social networking and addiction - A review of the psychological literature. *International Journal of Environmental Research and Public Health*, *8*(9), 3528–3552. doi:10.3390/ijerph8093528 PMID:22016701

Kyngäs, H., Hentinen, M., & Barlow, J. H. (1998). Adolescents' perceptions of physicians, nurses, parents and friends: Help or hindrance in compliance with diabetes self-care? *Journal of Advanced Nursing*, *27*(4), 760–769. doi:10.1046/j.1365-2648.1998.00608.x PMID:9578206

La Barbera, D., La Paglia, F., & Valsavoia, R. (2009). Social network and addiction. *Studies in Health Technology and Informatics*, *144*, 33–36. PMID:19592725

Labove, W. (n.d.). *Oral Narratives of Personal Experience*. Retrieved August 27, 2017, from http://www.ling.upenn.edu/~wlabov/Papers/FebOralNarPE.pdf

Labov, W., & Waletzky, J. (1967/1997). Narrative analysis. In J. Helm (Ed.), *Essays on the verbal and visual arts* (pp. 12–44). Seattle, WA: University of Washington Press.

Ladurantaye, S., & Robertson Krashinsky, S. (2013, February 13). "Let's Talk" campaign a boost for mental health and Bell. *The Globe and Mail.* Retrieved from: http://www.theglobeandmail.com/report-on-business/industry-news/marketing/lets-talk- campaign-a-boost-for-mental-health-and-bell/article8644553/

Lakkaraju, S., & Lakkaraju, S. (2013). Mobile device application in healthcare. In S. Sarnikar, D. Bennett, & M. Gaynor (Eds.), *Cases on healthcare information technology for patient care management* (pp. 276–307). Hershey, PA: IGI Global. doi:10.4018/978-1-4666-2671-3.ch016

Laskowski, M. (2013). A prototype agent based model and machine learning hybrid system for healthcare decision support. In J. Rodrigues (Ed.), *Digital advances in medicine, e-health, and communication technologies* (pp. 230–253). Hershey, PA: IGI Global. doi:10.4018/978-1-4666-2794-9.ch013

Lau, V. (2016, November 3). Ten things for pharma marketers to know about Facebook and Instagram. *Medical Marketing and Media*. Retrieved from http://www.mmm-online.com/technology/10-things-for-pharma-marketers-to-know-about-facebook-and-instagram/article/570439/

Lee, T. (2014). Mobile healthcare computing in the cloud. In J. Rodrigues, K. Lin, & J. Lloret (Eds.), *Mobile networks and cloud computing convergence for progressive services and applications* (pp. 275–294). Hershey, PA: IGI Global. doi:10.4018/978-1-4666-4781-7.ch015

Lelardeux, C., Alvarez, J., Montaut, T., Galaup, M., & Lagarrigue, P. (2013). Healthcare games and the metaphoric approach. In S. Arnab, I. Dunwell, & K. Debattista (Eds.), *Serious games for healthcare: Applications and implications* (pp. 23–49). Hershey, PA: IGI Global. doi:10.4018/978-1-4666-1903-6.ch002

Lemire, M., Paré, G., Sicotte, C., & Harvey, C. (2008). Determinants of Internet use as a preferred source of information on personal health. *International Journal of Medical Informatics*, *77*(11), 723–734. doi:10.1016/j.ijmedinf.2008.03.002 PMID:18434246

Lepping, P., Palmstierna, T., & Raveesh, B. N. (2016). Paternalism v. autonomy—Are we barking up the wrong tree? *The British Journal of Psychiatry*, *209*(2), 95–96. doi:10.1192/bjp.bp.116.181032 PMID:27482035

LeRouge, C., Van Slyke, C., Seale, D., & Wright, K. (2014). Baby boomers' adoption of consumer health technologies: Survey on readiness and barriers. *Journal of Medical Internet Research*, *16*(9), e200. doi:10.2196/jmir.3049 PMID:25199475

Leung, L. (2013). Generational differences in content generation in social media: The roles of the gratifications sought and of narcissism. *Computers in Human Behavior*, *29*(3), 997–1006. doi:10.1016/j.chb.2012.12.028

Lévy, P. (1997). *Collective Intelligence* (1st ed.). Basic Books.

Levy-Stein, R. (2009). Facebook suicide threat sparks massive manhunt in Eilat. *Haaretz*. Retrieved from: http://www.haaretz.com/news/facebook-suicide-threat-sparks-massive-manhunt-in-eilat-1.3436

Lewandowski, J., Rosenberg, B. D., Parks, M. J., & Siegel, J. T. (2011). The effect of informal social support: Face-to-face versus computer-mediated communication. *Computers in Human Behavior*, *27*(5), 1806–1814. doi:10.1016/j.chb.2011.03.008

Lewis, S., Thomas, S. L., Blood, R. W., Castle, D., Hyde, J., & Komesaroff, P. A. (2011). 'I'm searching for solutions': Why are obese individuals turning to the Internet for help and support with 'being fat'? *Health Expectations*, *14*(4), 339–350. doi:10.1111/j.1369-7625.2010.00644.x PMID:21199200

Ley, B. L. (2007). Vive les roses!: The architecture of commitment in an online pregnancy and mothering group. *Journal of Computer-Mediated Communication*, *12*(4), 1388–1408. doi:10.1111/j.1083-6101.2007.00378.x

Lhotska, L., Bursa, M., Huptych, M., Chudacek, V., & Havlik, J. (2013). Interoperability of medical devices and information systems. In M. Cruz-Cunha, I. Miranda, & P. Gonçalves (Eds.), *Handbook of research on ICTs for human-centered healthcare and social care services* (pp. 749–762). Hershey, PA: IGI Global. doi:10.4018/978-1-4666-3986-7.ch039

Liao, H. (2013). Biomedical information processing and visualization for minimally invasive neurosurgery. In J. Wu (Ed.), *Technological advancements in biomedicine for healthcare applications* (pp. 36–46). Hershey, PA: IGI Global. doi:10.4018/978-1-4666-2196-1.ch005

Libreri, C., & Graffigna, G. (2014). How web 2.0 shapes patient knowledge sharing: The case of diabetes in Italy. In C. El Morr (Ed.), *Research perspectives on the role of informatics in health policy and management* (pp. 238–260). Hershey, PA: IGI Global. doi:10.4018/978-1-4666-4321-5.ch014

Lieberman, M. A., & Goldstein, B. A. (2006). Not all negative emotions are equal: The role of emotional expression in online support groups for women with breast cancer. *Psycho-Oncology*, *15*(2), 160–168. doi:10.1002/pon.932 PMID:15880627

Lin, C., Huang, Y., Li, C., & Jalleh, G. (2013). Key health information systems outsourcing issues from six hospital cases. In I. Management Association (Ed.), User-driven healthcare: Concepts, methodologies, tools, and applications (pp. 824-837). Hershey, PA: IGI Global. doi:10.4018/978-1-4666-2770-3.ch041

Linde, C. (1993). *Life stories: The creation of coherence*. New York, NY: Oxford University Press.

Lin, L., Chen, Y., Wu, J., & Tennyson, R. D. (2013). What skill/knowledge is important to a nursing professional? In P. Ordóñez de Pablos (Ed.), *Business, technology, and knowledge management in Asia: Trends and innovations* (pp. 234–249). Hershey, PA: IGI Global. doi:10.4018/978-1-4666-2652-2.ch018

Litt, J. S. (2000). *Medicalized Motherhood: Perspectives from the Lives of African-American and Jewish Women*. New Brunswick, NJ: Rutgers University Press.

Littlejohn, S. W. (1992). Theories of human communication. Belmont, CA: Wadsworth Pub. Co.

Liu, G. (2014). Using case costing data and case mix for funding and benchmarking in rehabilitation hospitals. In C. El Morr (Ed.), *Research perspectives on the role of informatics in health policy and management* (pp. 62–78). Hershey, PA: IGI Global. doi:10.4018/978-1-4666-4321-5.ch005

Li, X., Lin, Z., & Wu, J. (2013). Language processing in the human brain of literate and illiterate subjects. In J. Wu (Ed.), *Biomedical engineering and cognitive neuroscience for healthcare: Interdisciplinary applications* (pp. 201–209). Hershey, PA: IGI Global. doi:10.4018/978-1-4666-2113-8.ch021

Lixun, Z., Dapeng, B., & Lei, Y. (2013). Design of and experimentation with a walking assistance robot. In J. Wu (Ed.), *Technological advancements in biomedicine for healthcare applications* (pp. 123–127). Hershey, PA: IGI Global. doi:10.4018/978-1-4666-2196-1.ch013

Lloyd, T., Shaffer, M. L., Christy, S., Widome, M. D., Repke, J., Weitekamp, M. R., & Paul, I. M. et al. (2013). Health knowledge among the millennial generation. *Journal of Public Health Research*, *2*(1), 38. doi:10.4081/jphr.2013.e8 PMID:25170479

Loeb, H. (2015). *The mindset of the millennial: Disruptive & committed for the long run. Huffington Post.*

Lui, K. (2013). The health informatics professional. In I. Management Association (Ed.), User-driven healthcare: Concepts, methodologies, tools, and applications (pp. 120-141). Hershey, PA: IGI Global. doi:10.4018/978-1-4666-2770-3.ch007

Luthans, F., & Avolio, B. (2003). Authentic leadership development. In K. S. Cameron, J. E. Dutton, & R. E. Quinn (Eds.), *Positive organizational scholarship: Foundations of a new discipline* (pp. 241–258). San Francisco, CA: Berrett-Koehler.

Luxton, D. D., McCann, R. A., Bush, N. E., Mishkind, M. C., & Reger, G. M. (2011). mHealth for mental health: Integrating smartphone technology in behavioral healthcare. *Professional Psychology, Research and Practice*, *42*(6), 505–512. doi:10.1037/a0024485

Madge, C., & O'Connor, H. (2002). On-line with e-mums: Exploring the internet as a medium for research. *Area*, *34*(1), 92–102. doi:10.1111/1475-4762.00060

Madge, C., & O'Connor, H. (2004). Online methods in geography educational research. *Journal of Geography in Higher Education*, *28*(1), 143–152. doi:10.1080/0309826042000198710

Makikawa, M., Okada, S., Fujiwara, Y., & Esaki, M. (2013). Sleep monitoring system equipped with a flexible non-contact ECG, respiration, and body motion sensor. In J. Wu (Ed.), *Technological advancements in biomedicine for healthcare applications* (pp. 287–297). Hershey, PA: IGI Global. doi:10.4018/978-1-4666-2196-1.ch030

Malik, S. H., & Coulson, N. S. (2008). Computer-mediated infertility support groups: An exploratory study of online experiences. *Patient Education and Counseling*, *73*(1), 105–113. doi:10.1016/j.pec.2008.05.024 PMID:18639409

Malindretos, G. (2013). Distribution and logistics outsourcing in the pharmaceutical sector. In D. Folinas (Ed.), *Outsourcing management for supply chain operations and logistics service* (pp. 202–222). Hershey, PA: IGI Global. doi:10.4018/978-1-4666-2008-7.ch012

Mann, C., & Stewart, F. (2000). Internet communication and qualitative research: A handbook for researching online. *Sage (Atlanta, Ga.).*

Manvi, S. S., & B., M. R. (2013). A survey on health care services using wireless sensor networks. In M. Cruz-Cunha, I. Miranda, & P. Gonçalves (Eds.), *Handbook of research on ICTs for human-centered healthcare and social care services* (pp. 587-606). Hershey, PA: IGI Global. doi:10.4018/978-1-4666-3986-7.ch031

Maples, M. F., & Han, S. (2008). Cybercounseling in the United States and South Korea: Implications for counseling college students of the millennial generation and the networked generation. *Journal of Counseling and Development*, *86*(2), 178–183. doi:10.1002/j.1556-6678.2008.tb00495.x

Marshall, S., & Hogan, J. (2013). The use of medical simulation to improve patient safety. In A. Moumtzoglou & A. Kastania (Eds.), *E-health technologies and improving patient safety: Exploring organizational factors* (pp. 155–172). Hershey, PA: IGI Global. doi:10.4018/978-1-4666-2657-7.ch011

Martin, V. (2013). Developing a library collection in bioinformatics: Support for an evolving profession. In I. Management Association (Ed.), Bioinformatics: Concepts, methodologies, tools, and applications (pp. 130-150). Hershey, PA: IGI Global. doi:10.4018/978-1-4666-3604-0.ch007

Martin, J., & McKay, E. (2013). Mental health, post-secondary education, and information communications technology. In J. Lannon & E. Halpin (Eds.), *Human rights and information communication technologies: Trends and consequences of use* (pp. 196–213). Hershey, PA: IGI Global. doi:10.4018/978-1-4666-1918-0.ch012

Martin, J., & McKay, E. (2014). Mental health, post-secondary education, and information communications technology. In *Assistive technologies: Concepts, methodologies, tools, and applications* (pp. 1209–1226). Hershey, PA: IGI Global. doi:10.4018/978-1-4666-4422-9.ch063

Masayuki, K., Eiji, K., Tetsuo, T., & Nozomu, M. (2013). Evaluation of olfactory impairment in Parkinson's disease using near-infrared spectroscopy. In J. Wu (Ed.), *Biomedical engineering and cognitive neuroscience for healthcare: Interdisciplinary applications* (pp. 293–302). Hershey, PA: IGI Global. doi:10.4018/978-1-4666-2113-8.ch030

Massanari, A. L. (2016). Contested Play. *Socialbots and Their Friends: Digital Media and the Automation of Sociality*, 110.

Ma, X., Chen, G., & Xiao, J. (2013). Understanding weight change behaviors through online social networks. In A. Gangopadhyay (Ed.), *Methods, models, and computation for medical informatics* (pp. 189–214). Hershey, PA: IGI Global. doi:10.4018/978-1-4666-2653-9.ch012

Maynard, E. G. [emilygmaynard]. (2016, August 6). Post [Instagram page]. Retrieved from https://www.instagram.com/p/BIpVQd_Ag4N/?taken-by=emilygmaynard

Mazzanti, I., Maolo, A., & Antonicelli, R. (2013). E-health and telemedicine in the elderly: State of the art. In V. Gulla, A. Mori, F. Gabbrielli, & P. Lanzafame (Eds.), *Telehealth Networks for Hospital Services: New Methodologies* (pp. 33–43). Hershey, PA: IGI Global. doi:10.4018/978-1-4666-2979-0.ch003

Mazzanti, I., Maolo, A., & Antonicelli, R. (2014). E-health and telemedicine in the elderly: State of the art. In *Assistive technologies: Concepts, methodologies, tools, and applications* (pp. 693–704). Hershey, PA: IGI Global. doi:10.4018/978-1-4666-4422-9.ch034

Mazzoni, D., & Cicognani, E. (2014). Sharing experiences and social support requests in an Internet forum for patients with systemic lupus erythematosus. *Journal of Health Psychology, 19*(5), 689–696. doi:10.1177/1359105313477674 PMID:23479300

McAlexander, A. [@alicemcalex]. (2017, February 6). Tweet [Twitter page]. Retrieved from https://twitter.com/alicemcalex/status/828600176344461312

McCormick, A. (2010). Supermothers on Film, or Maternal Melodrama in the 21st Century. In A. O'Reilly (Ed.), *Twenty-first-century motherhood: Experience, identity, policy, agency* (pp. 140–157). New York, NY: Columbia University Press.

McCrossan, B. A., & Casey, F. A. (2013). The role of telemedicine in paediatric cardiology. In V. Gulla, A. Mori, F. Gabbrielli, & P. Lanzafame (Eds.), *Telehealth networks for hospital services: New methodologies* (pp. 44–88). Hershey, PA: IGI Global. doi:10.4018/978-1-4666-2979-0.ch004

McDaniel, B. T., Coyne, S. M., & Holmes, E. K. (2012). New mothers and media use: Associations between blogging, social networking, and maternal well-being. *Maternal and Child Health Journal, 16*(7), 1509–1517. doi:10.1007/s10995-011-0918-2 PMID:22094592

McGaha, J. (2013). Implementation issues on a national electronic health record network. In I. Management Association (Ed.), User-driven healthcare: Concepts, methodologies, tools, and applications (pp. 1236-1251). Hershey, PA: IGI Global. doi:10.4018/978-1-4666-2770-3.ch062

McGinnes, S., & Burke, M. (2013). Hoping for the best: A qualitative study of information technology in primary care. In M. Cruz-Cunha, I. Miranda, & P. Gonçalves (Eds.), *Handbook of research on ICTs and management systems for improving efficiency in healthcare and social care* (pp. 1088–1108). Hershey, PA: IGI Global. doi:10.4018/978-1-4666-3990-4.ch057

McGrew, M. (2013). What's a baby boomer parent to do with a millennial? *Baltimore Sun.*

McKeever, R., & McKeever, B. W. (2017). Moms and Media: Exploring the Effects of Online Communication on Infant Feeding Practices. *Health Communication, 32*(9), 1059–1065. doi:10.1080/10410236.2016.1196638 PMID:27484216

Medhekar, A., Wong, H. Y., & Hall, J. (2014). Innovation in medical tourism service marketing: A case of India. In A. Goyal (Ed.), *Innovations in services marketing and management: Strategies for emerging economies* (pp. 49–66). Hershey, PA: IGI Global. doi:10.4018/978-1-4666-4671-1.ch003

Medhekar, A., Wong, H. Y., & Hall, J. (2014). Medical tourism: A conceptual framework for an innovation in global healthcare provision. In A. Goyal (Ed.), *Innovations in services marketing and management: Strategies for emerging economies* (pp. 148–169). Hershey, PA: IGI Global. doi:10.4018/978-1-4666-4671-1.ch009

Medimagazin. (2015, October 26). *Hastalar muayene sürelerinin kısalığından şikayetçi*. Retrieved from http://www.medimagazin.com.tr/ana-sayfa/guncel/tr-hastalar-muayene-surelerinin-kisaligindan-sikayetci-1-11-67485.html

Mehdizadeh, S. (2010). Self-presentation 2.0L Narcissism and self-esteem on Facebook. *Cyberpsychology, Behavior, and Social Networking*, *13*(4), 357–364. doi:10.1089/cyber.2009.0257 PMID:20712493

Meier, A., Lyons, E. J., Frydman, G., Forlenza, M., Rimer, B. K., & Winefield, H. (2007). How cancer survivors provide support on cancer-related Internet mailing lists. *Journal of Medical Internet Research*, *9*(2), e12. doi:10.2196/jmir.9.2.e12 PMID:17513283

Meltzer, D. (1967) *The Psycho-Analytical Process*. Perthshire, UK: Clunie.

Menciassi, A., & Laschi, C. (2014). Biorobotics. In I. Management Association (Ed.), Robotics: Concepts, methodologies, tools, and applications (pp. 1613-1643). Hershey, PA: IGI Global. doi:10.4018/978-1-4666-4607-0.ch079

Mendes, D., & Rodrigues, I. P. (2013). A semantic web pragmatic approach to develop clinical ontologies, and thus semantic interoperability, based in HL7 v2.xml messaging. In R. Martinho, R. Rijo, M. Cruz-Cunha, & J. Varajão (Eds.), *Information systems and technologies for enhancing health and social care* (pp. 205–214). Hershey, PA: IGI Global. doi:10.4018/978-1-4666-3667-5.ch014

Mendoza-González, R., Martin, M. V., & Rodríguez-Martínez, L. C. (2013). Identifying the essential design requirements for usable e-health communities in mobile devices. In I. Management Association (Ed.), User-driven healthcare: Concepts, methodologies, tools, and applications (pp. 533-552). Hershey, PA: IGI Global. doi:10.4018/978-1-4666-2770-3.ch027

Menzies, D., & Ellis, H. (1990). Intestinal obstruction from adhesions--how big is the problem? *Annals of the Royal College of Surgeons of England*, *72*(1), 60. PMID:2301905

Mettler, T. (2013). Transformation of the hospital supply chain: How to measure the maturity of supplier relationship management systems in hospitals? In J. Tan (Ed.), *Healthcare information technology innovation and sustainability: Frontiers and adoption* (pp. 180–192). Hershey, PA: IGI Global. doi:10.4018/978-1-4666-2797-0.ch011

Meyer, A., Coroiu, A., & Korner, A. (2015). One-to-one peer support in cancer care: A review of scholarship published between 2007 and 2014. *European Journal of Cancer Care*, *24*(3), 299–312. doi:10.1111/ecc.12273 PMID:25512107

Miesenberger, K., Nussbaum, G., & Ossmann, R. (2014). AsTeRICS: A framework for including sensor technology into AT solutions for people with motor disabilities. In G. Kouroupetroglou (Ed.), *Assistive technologies and computer access for motor disabilities* (pp. 154–179). Hershey, PA: IGI Global. doi:10.4018/978-1-4666-4438-0.ch006

Miller, K., & Sankaranarayanan, S. (2013). Applications of policy based agents in wireless body sensor mesh networks for patient health monitoring. In J. Rodrigues (Ed.), *Digital advances in medicine, e-health, and communication technologies* (pp. 85–101). Hershey, PA: IGI Global. doi:10.4018/978-1-4666-2794-9.ch005

Mills, E., Airey, C., & Yee, K. C. (2006). Generation Y in healthcare: The need for new socio-technical consideration for future technology design in healthcare. *Studies in Health Technology and Informatics*, *130*, 169–179. PMID:17917191

Mishra, S. I., Lucksted, A., Gioia, D., Barnet, B., & Baquet, C. R. (2009, January 01). Needs and preferences for receiving mental health information in an African American focus group sample. *Community Mental Health Journal*, *45*(2), 117–126. doi:10.1007/s10597-008-9157-4 PMID:18633704

Mitchell, M. (2016, December 31). Authentic leadership in illness blogs: What we can learn from jaw surgery bloggers. *Cogent Social Sciences*, *2*, 1.

Mohammadian, M., & Jentzsch, R. (2013). User and data classification for a secure and practical approach for patient-doctor profiling using an RFID framework in hospital. In S. Sarnikar, D. Bennett, & M. Gaynor (Eds.), *Cases on healthcare information technology for patient care management* (pp. 224–253). Hershey, PA: IGI Global. doi:10.4018/978-1-4666-2671-3.ch014

Monguet, J. M., Huerta, E., Fernández, J., Ferruzca, M., & Badillo, S. (2013). E-health business models prototyping by incremental design. In I. Management Association (Ed.), User-driven healthcare: Concepts, methodologies, tools, and applications (pp. 776-790). Hershey, PA: IGI Global. doi:10.4018/978-1-4666-2770-3.ch038

Monk, B. J., Berman, M. L., & Montz, F. J. (1994). Adhesions after extensive gynecologic surgery: Clinical significance, etiology, and prevention. *American Journal of Obstetrics and Gynecology*, *170*(5), 1396–1403. doi:10.1016/S0002-9378(13)90479-8 PMID:8178880

Montazemi, A. R., Pittaway, J. J., & Keshavjee, K. (2013). State of IS integration in the context of patient-centered care: A network analysis and research directions. In J. Tan (Ed.), *Healthcare information technology innovation and sustainability: Frontiers and adoption* (pp. 127–144). Hershey, PA: IGI Global. doi:10.4018/978-1-4666-2797-0.ch008

Montigny, F. D., Lacharité, C., & Amyot, É. (2006). The transition to fatherhood: The role of formal and informal support structures during the post-partum period. *Texto & Contexto Enfermagem*, *15*(4), 601–609. doi:10.1590/S0104-07072006000400008

Moorhead, S. A., Hazlett, D. E., Harrison, L., Carroll, J. K., Irwin, A., & Hoving, C. (2013). A new dimension of health care: Systematic review of the uses, benefits, and limitations of social media for health communication. *Journal of Medical Internet Research*, *15*(4), 85–100. doi:10.2196/jmir.1933 PMID:23615206

Mo, P. K. H., Malik, S. H., & Coulson, N. S. (2009). Gender differences in computer-mediated communication: A systematic literature review of online health-related support groups. *Patient Education and Counseling*, *75*(1), 16–24. doi:10.1016/j.pec.2008.08.029 PMID:19233586

Mo, P. K., & Coulson, N. S. (2013). Online support group use and psychological health for individuals living with HIV/AIDS. *Patient Education and Counseling, 93*(3), 426–432. doi:10.1016/j.pec.2013.04.004 PMID:23669152

Mori, A. R., Contenti, M., & Verbicaro, R. (2013). Policies on telemedicine-enhanced hospital services: Prioritization criteria for the interventions at regional level. In V. Gulla, A. Mori, F. Gabbrielli, & P. Lanzafame (Eds.), *Telehealth networks for hospital services: New methodologies* (pp. 1–14). Hershey, PA: IGI Global. doi:10.4018/978-1-4666-2979-0.ch001

Morita, A. (2013). The quantitative EEG change in Parkinson's disease. In J. Wu (Ed.), *Biomedical engineering and cognitive neuroscience for healthcare: Interdisciplinary applications* (pp. 225–234). Hershey, PA: IGI Global. doi:10.4018/978-1-4666-2113-8.ch023

Moromugi, S., & Ishimatsu, T. (2013). A strength training machine with a dynamic resistance control function based on muscle activity level. In J. Wu (Ed.), *Technological advancements in biomedicine for healthcare applications* (pp. 102–110). Hershey, PA: IGI Global. doi:10.4018/978-1-4666-2196-1.ch011

Morris, M. R. (2014). Social networking site use by mothers of young children. In K. P. O'Hara, M. Massimi, R. Harper, S. Rubens, & J. Morris (Eds.), *Proceedings of the 17th ACM conference on Computer supported cooperative work & social computing* (pp. 1272-1282). ACM. doi:10.1145/2531602.2531603

Morrow, D., & Chin, J. (2013). Technology as a bridge between health care systems and older adults. In I. Management Association (Ed.), User-driven healthcare: Concepts, methodologies, tools, and applications (pp. 99-119). Hershey, PA: IGI Global. doi:10.4018/978-1-4666-2770-3.ch006

Morrow, D., & Chin, J. (2013). Technology as a bridge between health care systems and older adults. In R. Zheng, R. Hill, & M. Gardner (Eds.), *Engaging older adults with modern technology: Internet use and information access needs* (pp. 59–79). Hershey, PA: IGI Global. doi:10.4018/978-1-4666-1966-1.ch004

Mostafa, R., Hasan, G. M., Kabir, A. A., & Rahman, M. A. (2013). Proposed framework for the deployment of telemedicine centers in rural Bangladesh. In J. Rodrigues (Ed.), *Digital advances in medicine, e-health, and communication technologies* (pp. 254–270). Hershey, PA: IGI Global. doi:10.4018/978-1-4666-2794-9.ch014

Motoi, K., Ogawa, M., Yamakoshi, T., & Yamakoshi, K. (2013). Fusion physiological sensing system for healthcare. In J. Wu (Ed.), *Technological advancements in biomedicine for healthcare applications* (pp. 298–313). Hershey, PA: IGI Global. doi:10.4018/978-1-4666-2196-1.ch031

Motorny, S. P. (2013). Big information technology bet of a small community hospital. In S. Sarnikar, D. Bennett, & M. Gaynor (Eds.), *Cases on healthcare information technology for patient care management* (pp. 70–94). Hershey, PA: IGI Global. doi:10.4018/978-1-4666-2671-3.ch004

Moumtzoglou, A. (2013). Health 2.0 and medicine 2.0: Safety, ownership and privacy issues. In I. Management Association (Ed.), User-driven healthcare: Concepts, methodologies, tools, and applications (pp. 1508-1522). Hershey, PA: IGI Global. doi:10.4018/978-1-4666-2770-3.ch075

Moumtzoglou, A. (2013). Risk perception as a patient safety dimension. In A. Moumtzoglou & A. Kastania (Eds.), *E-health technologies and improving patient safety: Exploring organizational factors* (pp. 285–299). Hershey, PA: IGI Global. doi:10.4018/978-1-4666-2657-7.ch017

Msanjila, S. S. (2013). Emerging ICT challenges on provision of online HIV/AIDS advisory services. In M. Cruz-Cunha, I. Miranda, & P. Gonçalves (Eds.), *Handbook of research on ICTs for human-centered healthcare and social care services* (pp. 248–269). Hershey, PA: IGI Global. doi:10.4018/978-1-4666-3986-7.ch013

Müller, A. (2013). Improving the identification of medication names by increasing phonological awareness via a language-teaching computer game (medicina). In S. Arnab, I. Dunwell, & K. Debattista (Eds.), *Serious games for healthcare: Applications and implications* (pp. 283–295). Hershey, PA: IGI Global. doi:10.4018/978-1-4666-1903-6.ch014

Mungham, S., & Lazard, L. (2011). Virtually experts: Exploring constructions of mothers' advice-seeking in online parenting communities. *Radical Psychology*, *9*(2).

Murakami, S., Kim, H., Tan, J. K., Ishikawa, S., & Aoki, T. (2013). The development of a quantitative method for the detection of periarticular osteoporosis using density features within ROIs from computed radiography images of the hand. In J. Wu (Ed.), *Technological advancements in biomedicine for healthcare applications* (pp. 55–67). Hershey, PA: IGI Global. doi:10.4018/978-1-4666-2196-1.ch007

Murry, V. M. B., Heflinger, C. A., Suiter, S. V., & Brody, G. H. (2011, January 01). Examining Perceptions About Mental Health Care and Help-Seeking Among Rural African American Families of Adolescents. *Journal of Youth and Adolescence*, *40*(9), 1118–1131. doi:10.1007/s10964-010-9627-1 PMID:21259067

Myrick, J. G., Holton, A. E., Himelboim, I., & Love, B. (2016). # Stupidcancer: Exploring a typology of social support and the role of emotional expression in a social media community. *Health Communication*, *31*(5), 596–605. doi:10.1080/10410236.2014.981664 PMID:26453480

Nadathur, S. G., & Warren, J. R. (2013). Formal-transfer in and out of stroke care units: An analysis using Bayesian networks. In J. Tan (Ed.), *Healthcare information technology innovation and sustainability: Frontiers and adoption* (pp. 193–207). Hershey, PA: IGI Global. doi:10.4018/978-1-4666-2797-0.ch012

Naidoo, V., & Naidoo, Y. (2014). Home telecare, medical implant, and mobile technology: Evolutions in geriatric care. In C. El Morr (Ed.), *Research perspectives on the role of informatics in health policy and management* (pp. 222–237). Hershey, PA: IGI Global. doi:10.4018/978-1-4666-4321-5.ch013

Nakagawa, S. (2013). Bone-conducted ultrasonic perception: An elucidation of perception mechanisms and the development of a novel hearing aid for the profoundly deaf. In J. Wu (Ed.), *Technological advancements in biomedicine for healthcare applications* (pp. 148–159). Hershey, PA: IGI Global. doi:10.4018/978-1-4666-2196-1.ch016

Nakai, M., & Niinomi, M. (2013). Recent progress in mechanically biocompatible titanium-based materials. In J. Wu (Ed.), *Technological advancements in biomedicine for healthcare applications* (pp. 206–212). Hershey, PA: IGI Global. doi:10.4018/978-1-4666-2196-1.ch022

Nakakuki, T., & Okada-Hatakeyama, M. (2013). Methods for the analysis of intracellular signal transduction systems. In J. Wu (Ed.), *Technological advancements in biomedicine for healthcare applications* (pp. 347–353). Hershey, PA: IGI Global. doi:10.4018/978-1-4666-2196-1.ch034

Nakku, J., Okello, E., Kizza, D., Honikman, S., Ssebunnya, J., Ndyanabangi, S., ... Kigozi, F. (2016). *Perinatal mental health care in a rural African district, Uganda: A qualitative study of barriers, facilitators and needs*. BioMed Central Ltd.

Nalin, M., Verga, M., Sanna, A., & Saranummi, N. (2013). Directions for ICT research in disease prevention. In M. Cruz-Cunha, I. Miranda, & P. Gonçalves (Eds.), *Handbook of research on ICTs for human-centered healthcare and social care services* (pp. 229–247). Hershey, PA: IGI Global. doi:10.4018/978-1-4666-3986-7.ch012

Nap, H. H., & Diaz-Orueta, U. (2013). Rehabilitation gaming. In S. Arnab, I. Dunwell, & K. Debattista (Eds.), *Serious games for healthcare: Applications and implications* (pp. 50–75). Hershey, PA: IGI Global. doi:10.4018/978-1-4666-1903-6.ch003

Narushima, T., & Ueda, K. (2013). Calcium phosphate coating on titanium by RF magnetron sputtering. In J. Wu (Ed.), *Technological advancements in biomedicine for healthcare applications* (pp. 223–233). Hershey, PA: IGI Global. doi:10.4018/978-1-4666-2196-1.ch024

Naslund, J. A., Aschbrenner, K. A., Marsch, L. A., & Bartels, S. J. (2016). The future of mental health care: Peer-to-peer support and social media. *Epidemiology and Psychiatric Sciences*, *25*(2), 113–122. doi:10.1017/S2045796015001067 PMID:26744309

National Cancer Institute. (2013). *Health Information National Trends Survey*. Retrieved from http://hints.cancer.gov

National Institutes of Health. (2014, October 17). *Using social media to better understand, prevent and treat substance abuse*. Retrieved from: https://www.nih.gov/news- events/news-releases/using-social-media-better-understand-prevent-treat-substance-use

Nava-Muñoz, S., & Morán, A. L. (2013). A review of notifications systems in elder care environments: Challenges and opportunities. In M. Cruz-Cunha, I. Miranda, & P. Gonçalves (Eds.), *Handbook of research on ICTs for human-centered healthcare and social care services* (pp. 407–429). Hershey, PA: IGI Global. doi:10.4018/978-1-4666-3986-7.ch022

Nganji, J. T., & Nggada, S. H. (2014). Adoption of blended learning technologies in selected secondary schools in Cameroon and Nigeria: Challenges in disability inclusion. In N. Ololube (Ed.), *Advancing technology and educational development through blended learning in emerging economies* (pp. 159–173). Hershey, PA: IGI Global. doi:10.4018/978-1-4666-4574-5.ch009

Niela-Vilén, H., Axelin, A., Salanterä, S., & Melender, H. L. (2014). Internet-based peer support for parents: A systematic integrative review. *International Journal of Nursing Studies*, *51*(11), 1524–1537. doi:10.1016/j.ijnurstu.2014.06.009 PMID:24998788

Nieuwboer, C. C., Fukkink, R. G., & Hermanns, J. M. (2013). Peer and professional parenting support on the Internet: A systematic review. *Cyberpsychology, Behavior, and Social Networking*, *16*(7), 518–528. doi:10.1089/cyber.2012.0547 PMID:23659725

Nikolov, S., Vera, J., & Wolkenhauer, O. (2013). Bifurcation analysis of a model accounting for the 14-3-3s signalling compartmentalisation. In I. Management Association (Ed.), Bioinformatics: Concepts, methodologies, tools, and applications (pp. 851-859). Hershey, PA: IGI Global. doi:10.4018/978-1-4666-3604-0.ch046

Nishiguchi, H. (2013). Description of and applications for a motion analysis method for upper limbs. In J. Wu (Ed.), *Technological advancements in biomedicine for healthcare applications* (pp. 1–10). Hershey, PA: IGI Global. doi:10.4018/978-1-4666-2196-1.ch001

Nokata, M. (2013). Small medical robot. In J. Wu (Ed.), *Technological advancements in biomedicine for healthcare applications* (pp. 170–179). Hershey, PA: IGI Global. doi:10.4018/978-1-4666-2196-1.ch018

Noritsugu, T. (2013). Wearable power assist robot driven with pneumatic rubber artificial muscles. In J. Wu (Ed.), *Technological advancements in biomedicine for healthcare applications* (pp. 139–147). Hershey, PA: IGI Global. doi:10.4018/978-1-4666-2196-1.ch015

Noteboom, C. (2013). Physician interaction with EHR: The importance of stakeholder identification and change management. In S. Sarnikar, D. Bennett, & M. Gaynor (Eds.), *Cases on healthcare information technology for patient care management* (pp. 95–112). Hershey, PA: IGI Global. doi:10.4018/978-1-4666-2671-3.ch005

Nutbeam, D. (2000). Health literacy as a public health goal: A challenge for contemporary health education and communication strategies into the 21st century. *Health Promotion International*, *15*(3), 259–267. doi:10.1093/heapro/15.3.259

O'Connor, H., & Madge, C. (2001). Cyber-mothers: Online synchronous interviewing using conferencing software. *Sociological Research Online*, *5*(4). doi:10.5153/sro.543

O'Hanlon, S. (2013). Avoiding adverse consequences of e-health. In A. Moumtzoglou & A. Kastania (Eds.), *E-health technologies and improving patient safety: Exploring organizational factors* (pp. 13–26). Hershey, PA: IGI Global. doi:10.4018/978-1-4666-2657-7.ch002

Oakley, A., & Roberts, H. (1981). Interviewing women: A contradiction in terms. In C. Seale (Ed.), *Social Research Methods: A reader* (pp. 261–268). London: Routledge.

Oeldorf-Hirsch, A., & Sundar, S. S. (2016). Social and technological motivations for online photo sharing. *Journal of Broadcasting & Electronic Media*, *60*(4), 624–642. doi:10.1080/08838151.2016.1234478

Ogawa, K., Nishio, S., Minato, T., & Ishiguro, H. (2013). Android robots as telepresence media. In J. Wu (Ed.), *Biomedical engineering and cognitive neuroscience for healthcare: Interdisciplinary applications* (pp. 54–63). Hershey, PA: IGI Global. doi:10.4018/978-1-4666-2113-8.ch006

Ohashi, M., Sakimura, N., Fujimoto, M., Hori, M., & Kurata, N. (2013). Technical perspective of authentication policy extension for the adaptive social services and e-health care management. In M. Cruz-Cunha, I. Miranda, & P. Gonçalves (Eds.), *Handbook of research on ICTs for human-centered healthcare and social care services* (pp. 719–726). Hershey, PA: IGI Global. doi:10.4018/978-1-4666-3986-7.ch037

Oh, H. J., & Lee, B. (2012). The effect of computer-mediated social support in online communities on patient empowerment and doctor–patient communication. *Health Communication*, *27*(1), 30–41. doi:10.1080/10410236.2011.567449 PMID:21797714

Oh, H. J., Ozkaya, E., & LaRose, R. (2014). How does online social networking enhance life satisfaction? The relationships among online supportive interaction, affect, perceived social support, sense of community, and life satisfaction. *Computers in Human Behavior*, *30*, 69–78. doi:10.1016/j.chb.2013.07.053

Ohta, Y., & Uchida, M. (2013). Non-contact pulse monitoring using live imaging. In J. Wu (Ed.), *Technological advancements in biomedicine for healthcare applications* (pp. 240–246). Hershey, PA: IGI Global. doi:10.4018/978-1-4666-2196-1.ch026

Oikonomou, D., Moulianitis, V., Lekkas, D., & Koutsabasis, P. (2013). DSS for health emergency response: A contextual, user-centred approach. In R. Biswas (Ed.), *Clinical solutions and medical progress through user-driven healthcare* (pp. 51–69). Hershey, PA: IGI Global. doi:10.4018/978-1-4666-1876-3.ch006

Ojelade, I. I., McCray, K., Ashby, J. S., & Meyers, J. (2011). Use of Ifá as a Means of Addressing Mental Health Concerns Among African American Clients. *Journal of Counseling and Development*, *89*(4), 406–412. doi:10.1002/j.1556-6676.2011.tb02837.x

Okamoto, S., Hirotomi, T., Aoki, K., & Hosomi, Y. (2013). Evaluation of walking motions with the aid of walkers using acceleration sensors. In J. Wu (Ed.), *Biomedical engineering and cognitive neuroscience for healthcare: Interdisciplinary applications* (pp. 346–354). Hershey, PA: IGI Global. doi:10.4018/978-1-4666-2113-8.ch036

Okamura, H. (2013). Rehabilitation of elderly people with dementia. In J. Wu (Ed.), *Biomedical engineering and cognitive neuroscience for healthcare: Interdisciplinary applications* (pp. 235–242). Hershey, PA: IGI Global. doi:10.4018/978-1-4666-2113-8.ch024

Ola, B., Crabb, J., Adewuya, A., Olugbile, F., & Abosede, O. A. (2014). The State of Readiness of Lagos State Primary Health Care Physicians to Embrace the Care of Depression in Nigeria. *Community Mental Health Journal*, *50*(2), 239–244. doi:10.1007/s10597-013-9648-9 PMID:23912148

Olson, V. D. (2011). Generational diversity: Implications for healthcare leaders. *Journal of Business & Economics Research*, *6*(11). doi:10.19030/jber.v6i11.2486

Olvera-Lobo, M., & Gutiérrez-Artacho, J. (2013). Searching health information in question-answering systems. In M. Cruz-Cunha, I. Miranda, & P. Gonçalves (Eds.), *Handbook of research on ICTs for human-centered healthcare and social care services* (pp. 474–490). Hershey, PA: IGI Global. doi:10.4018/978-1-4666-3986-7.ch025

Ordun, G., & Akun, A. (2016). Personality Characteristics and Emotional Intelligence Levels of Millenials: A Study in Turkish Context. *Journal of Economic and Social Studies*, *6*(1), 125. doi:10.14706/JECOSS16614

Öresland, S., Friberg, F., Määttä, S., & Öhlen, J. (2015). Disclosing discourses: Biomedical and hospitality discourses in patient education material. *Nursing Inquiry*, *22*(3), 240–248. doi:10.1111/nin.12097 PMID:25847051

Owen, J. E., Klapow, J. C., Roth, D. L., Nabell, L., & Tucker, D. C. (2004). Improving the effectiveness of adjuvant psychological treatment for women with breast cancer: The feasibility of providing online support. *Psycho-Oncology*, *13*(4), 281–292. doi:10.1002/pon.733 PMID:15054732

Owen, W. F. (1984). Interpretive themes in relational communication. *The Quarterly Journal of Speech*, *70*(3), 274–287. doi:10.1080/00335638409383697

Pace, S. (2014). *Millennials, Health, and the Doctor-Patient Relationship* (Thesis). Bard College.

Padovani, E., Orelli, R. L., Agnoletti, V., & Buccioli, M. (2013). Low cost and human-centered innovations in healthcare services: A case of excellence in Italy. In S. Saeed & C. Reddick (Eds.), *Human-centered system design for electronic governance* (pp. 239–252). Hershey, PA: IGI Global. doi:10.4018/978-1-4666-3640-8.ch014

Palfrey, J. S., Tonniges, T. F., Green, M., & Richmond, J. (2005). Introduction: Addressing the millennial morbidity—the context of community pediatrics. *Pediatrics*, *115*(4Supplement 3), 1121–1123. doi:10.1542/peds.2004-2825B PMID:15828080

Palmén, M., Korpela, M., & Saranto, K. (2012) Identifying health and wellbeing related information management activities and needs in families with young children. *Finnish Journal of eHealth and eWelfare, 4*(3), 165-176.

Paninchukunnath, A. (2014). Healthcare services delivery in India: special reference to mother and child health. In A. Goyal (Ed.), *Innovations in services marketing and management: Strategies for emerging economies* (pp. 170–189). Hershey, PA: IGI Global. doi:10.4018/978-1-4666-4671-1.ch010

Pantic, I., Damjanovic, A., & Todorovic, J. (2012). Association between online social networking and depression in high school students: Behavioral physiology viewpoint. *Psychiatria Danubina*, *24*, 90–93. PMID:22447092

Papacharissi, Z. (2002). The virtual sphere The internet as a public sphere. *New Media & Society*, *4*(1), 9–27. doi:10.1177/14614440222226244

Paparountas, T., Nikolaidou-Katsaridou, M. N., Rustici, G., & Aidinis, V. (2013). Data mining and meta-analysis on DNA microarray data. In I. Management Association (Ed.), Bioinformatics: Concepts, methodologies, tools, and applications (pp. 1196-1236). Hershey, PA: IGI Global. doi:10.4018/978-1-4666-3604-0.ch062

Parentela, G., Mancini, P., Naccarella, F., Feng, Z., & Rinaldi, G. (2013). Telemedicine, the European space agency, and the support to the african population for infectious disease problems: Potentiality and perspectives for Asia countries and China. In V. Gulla, A. Mori, F. Gabbrielli, & P. Lanzafame (Eds.), *Telehealth networks for hospital services: New methodologies* (pp. 89–96). Hershey, PA: IGI Global. doi:10.4018/978-1-4666-2979-0.ch005

Parker, M. C., Ellis, H., Moran, B. J., Thompson, J. N., Wilson, M. S., Menzies, D., & Buchan, S. (2001). Postoperative adhesions: Ten-year follow-up of 12,584 patients undergoing lower abdominal surgery. *Diseases of the Colon and Rectum*, *44*(6), 822–829. doi:10.1007/BF02234701 PMID:11391142

Parks, M. R. (2011). Social network sites as virtual communities. In Z. Papacharissi (Ed.), *A Networked Self. Identity, community, and culture on social network sites* (pp. 105–123). New York, NY: Routledge.

Parr, H. (2008). *Mental health and social space: Towards inclusionary geographies*. Malden, MA: Blackwell Publishing. doi:10.1002/9780470712924

Paterson, G. I., MacDonald, J. M., & Mensink, N. N. (2014). The administrative policy quandary in Canada's health service organizations. In C. El Morr (Ed.), *Research perspectives on the role of informatics in health policy and management* (pp. 116–134). Hershey, PA: IGI Global. doi:10.4018/978-1-4666-4321-5.ch008

Peek, H. (2015). Harnessing social media and mobile apps for mental health. *The Psychiatric Times*, *32*(3), 33.

Penchovsky, R. (2013). Engineering gene control circuits with allosteric ribozymes in human cells as a medicine of the future. In I. Management Association (Ed.), Bioinformatics: Concepts, methodologies, tools, and applications (pp. 860-883). Hershey, PA: IGI Global. doi:10.4018/978-1-4666-3604-0.ch047

Pereira, O. R., Caldeira, J. M., & Rodrigues, J. J. (2013). An advanced and secure symbian-based mobile approach for body sensor networks interaction. In J. Rodrigues (Ed.), *Digital advances in medicine, e-health, and communication technologies* (pp. 33–48). Hershey, PA: IGI Global. doi:10.4018/978-1-4666-2794-9.ch002

Petkovic, M., & Ibraimi, L. (2013). Privacy and security in e-health applications. In I. Management Association (Ed.), User-driven healthcare: Concepts, methodologies, tools, and applications (pp. 1141-1166). Hershey, PA: IGI Global. doi:10.4018/978-1-4666-2770-3.ch058

Petosa, R. L., & Smith, L. H. (2014). Peer mentoring for health behavior change: A systematic review. *American Journal of Health Education*, *45*(6), 351–357. doi:10.1080/19325037.2014.945670

Pew Research Centre. (2017). *Mobile fact sheet.* Retrieved from: http://www.pewinternet.org/fact-sheet/mobile/

Peyton, L., & Hu, J. (2013). Identity management and audit trail support for privacy protection in e-health networks. In I. Management Association (Ed.), User-driven healthcare: Concepts, methodologies, tools, and applications (pp. 1112-1125). Hershey, PA: IGI Global. doi:10.4018/978-1-4666-2770-3.ch056

Pham, D. V., Halgamuge, M. N., Nirmalathas, T., & Moran, B. (2013). A centralized real-time e-healthcare system for remote detection and prediction of epileptic seizures. In I. Management Association (Ed.), User-driven healthcare: Concepts, methodologies, tools, and applications (pp. 326-356). Hershey, PA: IGI Global. doi:10.4018/978-1-4666-2770-3.ch017

Phillips, D. P. (1974). The influence of suggestion on suicide: Substantive and theoretical implications of the Werther effect. *American Sociological Review*, *39*(3), 340–354. doi:10.2307/2094294 PMID:11630757

Phillips, D. P. (1979). Suicide, motor vehicle fatalities and the mass media: Evidence toward a theory of suggestion. *American Journal of Sociology*, *84*(5), 1150–1174. doi:10.1086/226904 PMID:507276

Phua, C., Roy, P. C., Aloulou, H., Biswas, J., Tolstikov, A., & Foo, V. S. … Xu, D. (2014). State-of-the-art assistive technology for people with dementia. In Assistive technologies: Concepts, methodologies, tools, and applications (pp. 1606-1625). Hershey, PA: IGI Global. doi:10.4018/978-1-4666-4422-9.ch085

Piette, J. D., Resnicow, K., Choi, H., & Heisler, M. (2013). A diabetes peer support intervention that improved glycemic control: Mediators and moderators of intervention effectiveness. *Chronic Illness*, *9*(4), 258–267. doi:10.1177/1742395313476522 PMID:23585636

Pink, , Horst, , Postill, , Hjorth, , & Lewis, , & Tacchi. (2016). *Digital Ethnography: Principles and Practices*. London: Sage.

Pino, A. (2014). Augmentative and alternative communication systems for the motor disabled. In G. Kouroupetroglou (Ed.), *Disability informatics and web accessibility for motor limitations* (pp. 105–152). Hershey, PA: IGI Global. doi:10.4018/978-1-4666-4442-7.ch004

Piper, L. E. (2012). Generation Y in healthcare: Leading millennials in an era of reform. *Frontiers of Health Services Management*, *29*(1), 16–28. PMID:23050334

Pirkis, J., & Blood, R. W. (2001). Suicide and the media: Reportage in nonfictional media. *Crisis*, *22*(4), 146–154. doi:10.1027//0227-5910.22.4.146 PMID:11848658

Pirkis, J., Francis, C., Blood, R. W., Burgess, P., Morley, B., & Stewart, A. et al.. (2002). Reporting of suicide in the Australian media. *The Australian and New Zealand Journal of Psychiatry*, *36*(2), 190–197. doi:10.1046/j.1440-1614.2002.01000.x PMID:11982539

Plantin, L., & Daneback, K. (2009). Parenthood, information and support on the internet. A literature review of research on parents and professionals online. *BioMed Center Family Practice*, *10*(1), 1–12. PMID:19450251

Poor, N. (2005). Mechanisms of an online public sphere: The website Slashdot. *Journal of Computer-Mediated Communication, 10*(2).

Popovic, K., Smith, C., & Hellebusch, S. J. (2013). Attitudes on the use of social media in healthcare communications. *Journal of Communication in Healthcare*, *6*(1), 22–28. doi:10.1179/1753807612Y.0000000029

Portela, F., Cabral, A., Abelha, A., Salazar, M., Quintas, C., Machado, J., & Santos, M. F. et al. (2013). Knowledge acquisition process for intelligent decision support in critical health care. In R. Martinho, R. Rijo, M. Cruz-Cunha, & J. Varajão (Eds.), *Information systems and technologies for enhancing health and social care* (pp. 55–68). Hershey, PA: IGI Global. doi:10.4018/978-1-4666-3667-5.ch004

Powell, J., Inglis, N., Ronnie, J., & Large, S. (2011). The characteristics and motivations of online health information seekers: Cross-selectional survey and qualitative interview study. *Journal of Medical Internet Research*, *13*(1), 1–11. doi:10.2196/jmir.1600 PMID:21345783

Previtali, P. (2013). Grid technology for archive solutions in health care organizations. In A. Moumtzoglou & A. Kastania (Eds.), *E-health technologies and improving patient safety: Exploring organizational factors* (pp. 148–154). Hershey, PA: IGI Global. doi:10.4018/978-1-4666-2657-7.ch010

Purkayastha, S. (2013). Design and implementation of mobile-based technology in strengthening health information system: Aligning mhealth solutions to infrastructures. In I. Management Association (Ed.), User-driven healthcare: Concepts, methodologies, tools, and applications (pp. 689-713). Hershey, PA: IGI Global. doi:10.4018/978-1-4666-2770-3.ch034

Qian, H., & Scott, C. R. (2007). Anonymity and self-disclosure on weblogs. *Journal of Computer-Mediated Communication*, *12*(4), 1428–1451. doi:10.1111/j.1083-6101.2007.00380.x

Qi, G., & Wu, J. (2013). Functional role of the left ventral occipito-temporal cortex in reading. In J. Wu (Ed.), *Biomedical engineering and cognitive neuroscience for healthcare: Interdisciplinary applications* (pp. 192–200). Hershey, PA: IGI Global. doi:10.4018/978-1-4666-2113-8.ch020

Queirós, A., Alvarelhão, J., Silva, A. G., Teixeira, A., & Pacheco da Rocha, N. (2013). A conceptual framework for the design and development of AAL services. In M. Cruz-Cunha, I. Miranda, & P. Gonçalves (Eds.), *Handbook of research on ICTs for human-centered healthcare and social care services* (pp. 568–586). Hershey, PA: IGI Global. doi:10.4018/978-1-4666-3986-7.ch030

Radulescu, V., & Cetina, I. (2011). The impact of health care consumer education on marketing strategies of health services organization. *Procedia: Social and Behavioral Sciences*, *15*, 388–393. doi:10.1016/j.sbspro.2011.03.109

Rains, S. A. (2014). The implications of stigma and anonymity for self-disclosure in health blogs. *Health Communication, 29*(1), 23–31. doi:10.1080/10410236.2012.714861 PMID:23356432

Rains, S. A., & Keating, D. M. (2011). The social dimension of blogging about health: Health blogging, social support, and well-being. *Communication Monographs, 78*(4), 511–534. doi:10.1080/03637751.2011.618142

Rains, S. A., Peterson, E. B., & Wright, K. B. (2015). Communicating social support in computer-mediated contexts: A meta-analytic review of content analyses examining support messages shared online among individuals coping with illness. *Communication Monographs, 82*(4), 403–430. doi:10.1080/03637751.2015.1019530

Rains, S. A., & Young, V. (2009). A meta-analysis of research on formal computer-mediated support groups: Examining group characteristics and health outcomes. *Human Communication Research, 35*(3), 309–336. doi:10.1111/j.1468-2958.2009.01353.x

Ransford, H. E., Carrillo, F. R., & Rivera, Y. (2010). Health care-seeking among Latino immigrants: Blocked access, use of traditional medicine, and the role of religion. *Journal of Health Care for the Poor and Underserved, 21*(3), 862–878. doi:10.1353/hpu.0.0348 PMID:20693732

Rao, D., Chen, W. T., Pearson, C. R., Simoni, J. M., Fredriksen-Goldsen, K., Nelson, K., & Zhang, F. et al. (2012). Social support mediates the relationship between HIV stigma and depression/quality of life among people living with HIV in Beijing, China. *International Journal of STD & AIDS, 23*(7), 481–484. doi:10.1258/ijsa.2009.009428 PMID:22844001

Rasmussen-Pennington, D. M., Richardson, G., Garinger, C., & Contursi, M. L. (2013). "I could be on Facebook by now": Insights from Canadian youth on online mental health information resources. *Canadian Journal of Information and Library Science, 37*(3), 183–200. doi:10.1353/ils.2013.0015

Ravka, N. (2014). Informatics and health services: The potential benefits and challenges of electronic health records and personal electronic health records in patient care, cost control, and health research – An overview. In C. El Morr (Ed.), *Research perspectives on the role of informatics in health policy and management* (pp. 89–114). Hershey, PA: IGI Global. doi:10.4018/978-1-4666-4321-5.ch007

Rawlings, B. (2015). Fashion bloggers, celebrities, and other influencers' endorsements and the FTC guidelines. *Entertainment and Sports Lawyer, 32*(2). Retrieved from http://www.americanbar.org/publications/entertainment-sports-lawyer/2015/firstedition/a-practitioner_s-column.html

Reblin, M., & Uchino, B. N. (2008). Social and emotional support and its implication for health. *Current Opinion in Psychiatry, 21*(2), 201–205. doi:10.1097/YCO.0b013e3282f3ad89 PMID:18332671

Reibling, N., & Wendt, C. (2013). Regulating patients' access to healthcare services. In M. Merviö (Ed.), *Healthcare management and economics: Perspectives on public and private administration* (pp. 53–68). Hershey, PA: IGI Global. doi:10.4018/978-1-4666-3982-9.ch005

Reichow, B., Halpern, J. I., Steinhoff, T. B., Letsinger, N., Naples, A., & Volkmar, F. R. (2012). Characteristics and quality of autism websites. *Journal of Autism and Developmental Disorders, 42*(6), 1263–1274. doi:10.1007/s10803-011-1342-6 PMID:21822761

Reis, C. I., Freire, C. S., Fernández, J., & Monguet, J. M. (2013). Patient centered design: Challenges and lessons learned from working with health professionals and schizophrenic patients in e-therapy contexts. In R. Martinho, R. Rijo, M. Cruz-Cunha, & J. Varajão (Eds.), *Information systems and technologies for enhancing health and social care* (pp. 120–135). Hershey, PA: IGI Global. doi:10.4018/978-1-4666-3667-5.ch008

Remmers, H., & Hülsken-Giesler, M. (2013). e-Health technologies in home care nursing: Recent survey results and subsequent ethical issues. In I. Management Association (Ed.), User-driven healthcare: Concepts, methodologies, tools, and applications (pp. 396-420). Hershey, PA: IGI Global. doi:10.4018/978-1-4666-2770-3.ch020

Repetti, R. L., & Wood, J. (1997). Effects of daily stress at work on mothers' interactions with preschoolers. *Journal of Family Psychology, 11*(1), 90–108. doi:10.1037/0893-3200.11.1.90

Ricketts, M. (2014). Making health information personal: How anecdotes bring concepts to life. In S. Hai-Jew (Ed.), *Packaging digital information for enhanced learning and analysis: Data visualization, spatialization, and multidimensionality* (pp. 1–36). Hershey, PA: IGI Global. doi:10.4018/978-1-4666-4462-5.ch001

Ridgeway, C. L., & Correll, S. J. (2004). Motherhood as a status characteristic. *The Journal of Social Issues, 60*(4), 683–700. doi:10.1111/j.0022-4537.2004.00380.x

Robehmed, N. (2016, July 26). Kim Kardashian West, mobile mogul: The Forbes cover story. *Forbes*. Retrieved from http://www.forbes.com/sites/natalierobehmed/2016/07/11/kim-kardashian-mobile-mogul-the-forbes-cover-story/#2c7a957d77ae

Robinson, J. D., Turner, J. W., Levine, B., & Tian, Y. (2011). Expanding the walls of the health care encounter: Support and outcomes for patients online. *Health Communication, 26*(2), 125–134. doi:10.1080/10410236.2010.541990 PMID:21294020

Roblin, D. W. (2011). The potential of cellular technology to mediate social networks for support of chronic disease self-management. *Journal of Health Communication, 16*(sup1), 59-76.

Rocha, Á. (2013). Evolution of information systems and technologies maturity in healthcare. In J. Tan (Ed.), *Healthcare information technology innovation and sustainability: Frontiers and adoption* (pp. 238–246). Hershey, PA: IGI Global. doi:10.4018/978-1-4666-2797-0.ch015

Rodgers, S., & Chen, Q. (2005). Internet community group participation: Psychosocial benefits for women with breast cancer. *Journal of Computer-Mediated Communication, 10*(4).

Rodríguez-Gómez, D., & Gairín, J. (2014). Communities of practice in the Catalan public administration: Promoting their improvement. In Y. Al-Bastaki & A. Shajera (Eds.), *Building a competitive public sector with knowledge management strategy* (pp. 383–402). Hershey, PA: IGI Global. doi:10.4018/978-1-4666-4434-2.ch018

Rodríguez-Solano, C., Lezcano, L., & Sicilia, M. (2013). Automated generation of SNOMED CT subsets from clinical guidelines. In R. Martinho, R. Rijo, M. Cruz-Cunha, & J. Varajão (Eds.), *Information systems and technologies for enhancing health and social care* (pp. 190–204). Hershey, PA: IGI Global. doi:10.4018/978-1-4666-3667-5.ch013

Rogers, E. M. (1962). *The Diffusion of Innovations*. Glencoe, IL: Free Press.

Rogers, E. M. (2003). *Diffusion of innovations* (5th ed.). New York: Free Press.

Rosland, A. M., Heisler, M., & Piette, J. D. (2012). The impact of family behaviors and communication patterns on chronic illness outcomes: A systematic review. *Journal of Behavioral Medicine*, *35*(2), 221–239. doi:10.1007/s10865-011-9354-4 PMID:21691845

Ross, C., Orr, E. S., Sisic, M., Arseneault, J. M., Simmering, M. G., & Orr, R. R. (2009). Personality and motivations associated with Facebook use. *Computers in Human Behavior*, *25*(2), 578–586. doi:10.1016/j.chb.2008.12.024

Rosu, S. M., & Dragoi, G. (2014). E-health sites development using open source software and OMT methodology as support for family doctors' activities: A Romanian case study. In M. Cruz-Cunha, F. Moreira, & J. Varajão (Eds.), *Handbook of research on enterprise 2.0: Technological, social, and organizational dimensions* (pp. 72–88). Hershey, PA: IGI Global. doi:10.4018/978-1-4666-4373-4.ch004

Roy, N., Das, S. K., & Julien, C. (2013). Resolving and mediating ambiguous contexts in pervasive environments. In I. Management Association (Ed.), User-driven healthcare: Concepts, methodologies, tools, and applications (pp. 630-654). Hershey, PA: IGI Global. doi:10.4018/978-1-4666-2770-3.ch031

Ruder, T. D., Hatch, G. M., Amponzi, G., Thali, M. J., & Fischer, N. (2011). Suicide announcement on Facebook. *Crisis: The Journal of Crisis Intervention and Suicide*, *32*(5), 280–282. doi:10.1027/0227-5910/a000086 PMID:21940257

Rushkoff, D. (2014). *Present shock: When everything happens now*. New York: Current.

Russo, M. R. (2014). Emergency management professional development: Linking information communication technology and social communication skills to enhance a sense of community and social justice in the 21st century. In I. Management Association (Ed.), Crisis management: Concepts, methodologies, tools and applications (pp. 651-665). Hershey, PA: IGI Global. doi:10.4018/978-1-4666-4707-7.ch031

Sabone, M. B., Mogobe, K. D., & Sabone, T. G. (2013). ICTS and their role in health promotion: A preliminary situation analysis in selected botswana rural communities. In I. Management Association (Ed.), User-driven healthcare: Concepts, methodologies, tools, and applications (pp. 211-224). Hershey, PA: IGI Global. doi:10.4018/978-1-4666-2770-3.ch012

Sağlık Bakanlığı (MOH). (2014). *Türkiye Kanser İstatistikleri.* Retrieved January 13, 2017, from http://kanser.gov.tr/Dosya/2017Haberler/2014-RAPOR._uzun.pdf

Saha, P. (2014). Systemic enterprise architecture as future: Tackling complexity in governments in the cusp of change. In P. Saha (Ed.), *A systemic perspective to managing complexity with enterprise architecture* (pp. 1–70). Hershey, PA: IGI Global. doi:10.4018/978-1-4666-4518-9.ch001

Saijo, Y. (2013). Biomedical application of multimodal ultrasound microscope. In J. Wu (Ed.), *Technological advancements in biomedicine for healthcare applications* (pp. 27–35). Hershey, PA: IGI Global. doi:10.4018/978-1-4666-2196-1.ch004

Santos, M. F., Portela, F., Miranda, M., Machado, J., Abelha, A., Silva, Á., & Rua, F. (2013). Grid data mining strategies for outcome prediction in distributed intensive care units. In R. Martinho, R. Rijo, M. Cruz-Cunha, & J. Varajão (Eds.), *Information systems and technologies for enhancing health and social care* (pp. 87–101). Hershey, PA: IGI Global. doi:10.4018/978-1-4666-3667-5.ch006

Santos, M., Bastião, L., Costa, C., Silva, A., & Rocha, N. (2013). Clinical data mining in small hospital PACS: Contributions for radiology department improvement. In R. Martinho, R. Rijo, M. Cruz-Cunha, & J. Varajão (Eds.), *Information systems and technologies for enhancing health and social care* (pp. 236–251). Hershey, PA: IGI Global. doi:10.4018/978-1-4666-3667-5.ch016

Santos, R. J., Bernardino, J., & Vieira, M. (2013). A hypotension surveillance and prediction system for critical care. In M. Cruz-Cunha, I. Miranda, & P. Gonçalves (Eds.), *Handbook of research on ICTs and management systems for improving efficiency in healthcare and social care* (pp. 341–355). Hershey, PA: IGI Global. doi:10.4018/978-1-4666-3990-4.ch017

Sanz, P. R., Mezcua, B. R., & Pena, J. M. (2013). ICTs for orientation and mobility for blind people: A state of the art. In M. Cruz-Cunha, I. Miranda, & P. Gonçalves (Eds.), *Handbook of research on ICTs for human-centered healthcare and social care services* (pp. 646–669). Hershey, PA: IGI Global. doi:10.4018/978-1-4666-3986-7.ch034

Sarabdeen, J. (2013). Legal issues in e-healthcare systems. In I. Management Association (Ed.), User-driven healthcare: Concepts, methodologies, tools, and applications (pp. 1194-1219). Hershey, PA: IGI Global. doi:10.4018/978-1-4666-2770-3.ch060

Saraceno, C. (2003). La conciliazione di responsabilità familiari e attività lavorative in Italia: Paradossi ed equilibri imperfetti. *Polis*, *17*(2), 199–228.

Sarasohn-Kahn, J. (2008). *The wisdom of patients: Healthcare meets online social media ihealth reports*. Accessed December 16, 2016 from http://www.chcf.org/topics/chronicdisease/index.cfm?itemID=133631

Sarbadhikari, S. N. (2013). Unlearning and relearning in online health education. In I. Management Association (Ed.), User-driven healthcare: Concepts, methodologies, tools, and applications (pp. 1348-1363). Hershey, PA: IGI Global. doi:10.4018/978-1-4666-2770-3.ch067

Sarringhaus, M. M. (2011). The great divide: Social media's role in bridging healthcare's generational shift. *Journal of Healthcare Management*, *56*(4), 235–244. PMID:21838022

Sasayama, T., Hamada, S., & Kobayashi, T. (2013). Application of prewhitening beamformer with linear constraints for correlated EEG signal source estimation. In J. Wu (Ed.), *Biomedical engineering and cognitive neuroscience for healthcare: Interdisciplinary applications* (pp. 243–254). Hershey, PA: IGI Global. doi:10.4018/978-1-4666-2113-8.ch025

Satoh, J. (2013). Molecular network analysis of target RNAs and interacting proteins of TDP-43, a causative gene for the neurodegenerative diseases ALS/FTLD. In I. Management Association (Ed.), Bioinformatics: Concepts, methodologies, tools, and applications (pp. 964-985). Hershey, PA: IGI Global. doi:10.4018/978-1-4666-3604-0.ch052

Satoh, J. (2013). Molecular network analysis of target RNAs and interacting proteins of TDP-43, a causative gene for the neurodegenerative diseases ALS/FTLD. In J. Wu (Ed.), *Technological advancements in biomedicine for healthcare applications* (pp. 314–335). Hershey, PA: IGI Global. doi:10.4018/978-1-4666-2196-1.ch032

Sato, T., & Minato, K. (2013). Differences in analysis methods of the human uncinate fasciculus using diffusion tensor MRI. In J. Wu (Ed.), *Biomedical engineering and cognitive neuroscience for healthcare: Interdisciplinary applications* (pp. 162–170). Hershey, PA: IGI Global. doi:10.4018/978-1-4666-2113-8.ch017

Scaioli, G., Bert, F., Galis, V., Brusaferro, S., De Vito, E., La Torre, G., & Siliquini, R. et al. (2015). Pregnancy and internet: Sociodemographic and geographic differences in e-health practice. Results from an Italian multicenter study. *Public Health*, *129*(9), 1258–1266. doi:10.1016/j.puhe.2015.06.012 PMID:26210071

Schafer, S. B. (2013). Fostering psychological coherence: With ICTs. In M. Cruz-Cunha, I. Miranda, & P. Gonçalves (Eds.), *Handbook of research on ICTs for human-centered healthcare and social care services* (pp. 29–47). Hershey, PA: IGI Global. doi:10.4018/978-1-4666-3986-7.ch002

Scharer, K. (2005). Internet social support for parents: The state of science. *Journal of Child and Adolescent Psychiatric Nursing*, *18*(1), 26–35. doi:10.1111/j.1744-6171.2005.00007.x PMID:15701096

Schmeida, M., & McNeal, R. (2013). Bridging the inequality gap to accessing medicare and medicaid information online: An empirical analysis of e-government success 2002 through 2010. In J. Gil-Garcia (Ed.), *E-government success around the world: Cases, empirical studies, and practical recommendations* (pp. 60–78). Hershey, PA: IGI Global. doi:10.4018/978-1-4666-4173-0.ch004

Scholl, J. C., & Olaniran, B. A. (2013). ICT use and multidisciplinary healthcare teams. In M. Cruz-Cunha, I. Miranda, & P. Gonçalves (Eds.), *Handbook of research on ICTs for human-centered healthcare and social care services* (pp. 627–645). Hershey, PA: IGI Global. doi:10.4018/978-1-4666-3986-7.ch033

Schulz, P. J., & Nakamoto, K. (2011). "Bad" Literacy, the Internet, and the Limits of Patinet Empowerment. *AI and Health Communication, Spring Symposium*, 65 – 69.

Seçkin, G. (2013). Satisfaction with health status among cyber patients: Testing a mediation model of electronic coping support. *Behaviour & Information Technology, 32*(1), 91–101. doi:10.1080/0144929X.2011.603359

Serenko, N. (2013). The impact of genetic testing and genetic information on ethical, legal and social issues in North America: The framework. In I. Management Association (Ed.), Bioinformatics: Concepts, methodologies, tools, and applications (pp. 1317-1333). Hershey, PA: IGI Global. doi:10.4018/978-1-4666-3604-0.ch067

Serrano, M., Elmisery, A., Foghlú, M. Ó., Donnelly, W., Storni, C., & Fernström, M. (2013). Pervasive computing support in the transition towards personalised health systems. In J. Rodrigues (Ed.), *Digital advances in medicine, e-health, and communication technologies* (pp. 49–64). Hershey, PA: IGI Global. doi:10.4018/978-1-4666-2794-9.ch003

Shapiro, J. (2009). *Patients turn to online community for help healing*. National Public Radio.

Sharf, B. F. (1997). Communicating breast cancer on-line: Support and empowerment on the Internet. *Women & Health, 26*(1), 65–84. doi:10.1300/J013v26n01_05 PMID:9311100

Shaw, V., & Braa, J. (2013). "Developed in the south": An evolutionary and prototyping approach to developing scalable and sustainable health information systems. In I. Management Association (Ed.), User-driven healthcare: Concepts, methodologies, tools, and applications (pp. 583-607). Hershey, PA: IGI Global. doi:10.4018/978-1-4666-2770-3.ch029

Shaw, R. B., Mctavish, F., Hawkins, R., Gustafson, D. H., & Pingree, S. (2000). Experiences of Women with Breast Cancer: Exchanging Social Support over the CHESS Computer Network. *Journal of Health Communication, 5*(2), 135–159. doi:10.1080/108107300406866 PMID:11010346

Shi, J., Upadhyaya, S., & Erdem, E. (2013). Health information exchange for improving the efficiency and quality of healthcare delivery. In I. Management Association (Ed.), User-driven healthcare: Concepts, methodologies, tools, and applications (pp. 714-736). Hershey, PA: IGI Global. doi:10.4018/978-1-4666-2770-3.ch035

Shibata, T. (2013). A human-like cognitive computer based on a psychologically inspired VLSI brain model. In J. Wu (Ed.), *Technological advancements in biomedicine for healthcare applications* (pp. 247–266). Hershey, PA: IGI Global. doi:10.4018/978-1-4666-2196-1.ch027

Shimada, S. (2013). Self-body recognition and its impairment. In J. Wu (Ed.), *Biomedical engineering and cognitive neuroscience for healthcare: Interdisciplinary applications* (pp. 156–161). Hershey, PA: IGI Global. doi:10.4018/978-1-4666-2113-8.ch016

Shimogonya, Y., Ishikawa, T., Yamaguchi, T., Kumamaru, H., & Itoh, K. (2013). Computational study of the hemodynamics of cerebral aneurysm initiation. In J. Wu (Ed.), *Technological advancements in biomedicine for healthcare applications* (pp. 267–277). Hershey, PA: IGI Global. doi:10.4018/978-1-4666-2196-1.ch028

Shimonomura, K. (2013). A neuromorphic robot vision system to predict the response of visual neurons. In J. Wu (Ed.), *Technological advancements in biomedicine for healthcare applications* (pp. 193–199). Hershey, PA: IGI Global. doi:10.4018/978-1-4666-2196-1.ch020

Shpigelman, C., & Gill, C. (2014). Facebook Use by Persons with Disabilities. *Journal of Computer-Mediated Communication*, *19*(3), 610–624. doi:10.1111/jcc4.12059

Shrestha, S. (2013). Clinical decision support system for diabetes prevention: An illustrative case. In S. Sarnikar, D. Bennett, & M. Gaynor (Eds.), *Cases on healthcare information technology for patient care management* (pp. 308–329). Hershey, PA: IGI Global. doi:10.4018/978-1-4666-2671-3.ch017

Siddiqui, Z. S., & Jonas-Dwyer, D. R. (2013). Mobile learning in health professions education: A systematic review. In J. Keengwe (Ed.), *Pedagogical applications and social effects of mobile technology integration* (pp. 193–205). Hershey, PA: IGI Global. doi:10.4018/978-1-4666-2985-1.ch011

Silva, J. M. (2014). Slight expectations: Making sense of the "Me me me" generation. *Sociology Compass*, *8*(12), 1388–1397. doi:10.1111/soc4.12227

Silvana de Rosa, A., Fino, E., & Bocci, E. (2014). Addressing healthcare on-line demand and supply relating to mental illness: Knowledge sharing about psychiatry and psychoanalysis through social networks in Italy and France. In A. Kapoor & C. Kulshrestha (Eds.), *Dynamics of competitive advantage and consumer perception in social marketing* (pp. 16–55). Hershey, PA: IGI Global. doi:10.4018/978-1-4666-4430-4.ch002

Singer, N. (2014, December 26). Risks in using social media to spot signs of distress. *The New York Times*. Retrieved from: https://www.nytimes.com/2014/12/27/technology/risks-in-using-social-posts-to-spot-signs-of-distress.html?_r=0

Singer, P., Flöck, F., Meinhart, C., Zeitfogel, E., & Strohmaier, M. (2014, April). Evolution of reddit: from the front page of the internet to a self-referential community? In *Proceedings of the 23rd International Conference on World Wide Web* (pp. 517-522). ACM. doi:10.1145/2567948.2576943

Sinnenberg, L., Buttenheim, A. M., Padrez, K., Mancheno, C., Ungar, L., & Merchant, R. M. (2017). Twitter as a tool for health research: A systematic review. *American Journal of Public Health*, *107*(1), e1–e8. doi:10.2105/AJPH.2016.303512 PMID:27854532

Siqueira, S. R., Rocha, E. C., & Nery, M. S. (2013). Brazilian occupational therapy perspective about digital games as an inclusive resource to disabled people in schools. In I. Management Association (Ed.), User-driven healthcare: Concepts, methodologies, tools, and applications (pp. 918-937). Hershey, PA: IGI Global. doi:10.4018/978-1-4666-2770-3.ch046

Slade, A., Cohen, L. J., Sadler, L. S., & Miller, M. (2009) The psychology and psychopathology of pregnancy. Handbook of infant mental health, 3, 22-39.

Sliedrecht, S., & Kotzé, E. (2013). Patients with a spinal cord injury inform and co-construct services at a spinal cord rehabilitation unit. In I. Management Association (Ed.), User-driven healthcare: Concepts, methodologies, tools, and applications (pp. 1054-1072). Hershey, PA: IGI Global. doi:10.4018/978-1-4666-2770-3.ch053

Smedberg, Å. (2013). E-health communities for learning healthy habits: How to consider quality and usability. In I. Management Association (Ed.), User-driven healthcare: Concepts, methodologies, tools, and applications (pp. 310-325). Hershey, PA: IGI Global. doi:10.4018/978-1-4666-2770-3.ch016

Smedberg, Å., & Sandmark, H. (2013). Dynamic stress management: Self-help through holistic system design. In I. Management Association (Ed.), User-driven healthcare: Concepts, methodologies, tools, and applications (pp. 1469-1486). Hershey, PA: IGI Global. doi:10.4018/978-1-4666-2770-3.ch073

Smith, A. (2014, February 3). 6 new facts about Facebook. *Facttank*. Retrieved from http://www.pewresearch.org/fact-tank/2014/02/03/6-new-facts-about-facebook/

Smith, D. W. (2016). Phenomenology. In E. N. Zalta (Ed.), *The Stanford Encyclopedia of Philosophy*. Retrieved from https://plato.stanford.edu/entries/phenomenology/

Smith, E. E., & Aaker, J. L. (2013). Millennial searchers. *New York Times*.

Sobol, M., & Prater, E. (2013). Adoption, usage and efficiency: Benchmarking healthcare IT in private practices. In J. Tan (Ed.), *Healthcare information technology innovation and sustainability: Frontiers and adoption* (pp. 145–159). Hershey, PA: IGI Global. doi:10.4018/978-1-4666-2797-0.ch009

Sobrinho, Á. A., Dias da Silva, L., Melo de Medeiros, L., & Pinheiro, M. E. (2013). A mobile assistant to aid early detection of chronic kidney disease. In R. Martinho, R. Rijo, M. Cruz-Cunha, & J. Varajão (Eds.), *Information systems and technologies for enhancing health and social care* (pp. 309–323). Hershey, PA: IGI Global. doi:10.4018/978-1-4666-3667-5.ch020

Soomlek, C., & Benedicenti, L. (2013). Agent-based wellness indicator. In V. Gulla, A. Mori, F. Gabbrielli, & P. Lanzafame (Eds.), *Telehealth networks for hospital services: New methodologies* (pp. 300–330). Hershey, PA: IGI Global. doi:10.4018/978-1-4666-2979-0.ch020

Sorkin, D., Rook, K. S., & Lu, J. L. (2002). Loneliness, lack of emotional support, lack of companionship, and the likelihood of having a heart condition in an elderly sample. *Annals of Behavioral Medicine*, *24*(4), 290–298. doi:10.1207/S15324796ABM2404_05 PMID:12434940

South African Depression and Anxiety Group. (2017). Retrieved from http://www.sadag.org/

Spadaro, L., Timpano, F., Marino, S., & Bramanti, P. (2013). Telemedicine and Alzheimer disease: ICT-based services for people with Alzheimer disease and their caregivers. In V. Gulla, A. Mori, F. Gabbrielli, & P. Lanzafame (Eds.), *Telehealth networks for hospital services: New methodologies* (pp. 191–206). Hershey, PA: IGI Global. doi:10.4018/978-1-4666-2979-0.ch013

Sparks, H., Collins, F. L., & Kearns, R. (2016). Reflecting on the risks and ethical dilemmas of digital research. *Geoforum, 77*, 40–46. doi:10.1016/j.geoforum.2016.09.019

Speed, E., Davison, C., & Gunnell, C. (2016). The anonymity paradox in patient engagement: Reputation, risk and web-based public feedback. *Medical Humanities, 42*(2), 135–140. doi:10.1136/medhum-2015-010823 PMID:26879526

Spinelli, M., Frigerio, A., Montali, L., Fasolo, M., Spada, M. S., & Mangili, G. (2016). 'I still have difficulties feeling like a mother': The transition to motherhood of preterm infants mothers. *Psychology & Health, 31*(2), 184–204. doi:10.1080/08870446.2015.1088015 PMID:26359768

Springer, J. A., Beever, J., Morar, N., Sprague, J. E., & Kane, M. D. (2013). Ethics, privacy, and the future of genetic information in healthcare information assurance and security. In I. Management Association (Ed.), Bioinformatics: Concepts, methodologies, tools, and applications (pp. 1405-1423). Hershey, PA: IGI Global. doi:10.4018/978-1-4666-3604-0.ch072

Stachura, M. E., Wood, J., Angjellari-Dajci, F., Grayson, J., Astapova, E. V., Tung, H., . . . Lawless, W. (2013). Representing organizational conservation of information: A review of telemedicine and e-health in Georgia. In I. Management Association (Ed.), User-driven healthcare: Concepts, methodologies, tools, and applications (pp. 1220-1235). Hershey, PA: IGI Global. doi:10.4018/978-1-4666-2770-3.ch061

Stack, S. (1996). The effect of media on suicide: Evidence from Japan, 1955-1985. *Suicide & Life-Threatening Behavior, 26*(2), 132–142. PMID:8840417

Stack, S. (2002). Media coverage as a risk factor in suicide. *Injury Prevention, 8*(90004Suppl IV), 30–32. doi:10.1136/ip.8.suppl_4.iv30 PMID:12460954

Stack, S. (2005). Suicide in the media: A quantitative review of studies based on non-fictional stories. *Suicide & Life-Threatening Behavior, 35*(2), 121–133. doi:10.1521/suli.35.2.121.62877 PMID:15843330

Stanton, A. L., Danoff-burg, S., & Huggins, M. E. (2002). The first year after breast cancer diagnosis: Hope and coping strategies as predictors of adjustment. *Psycho-Oncology, 11*(2), 93–102. doi:10.1002/pon.574 PMID:11921325

Stefaniak, J. E. (2013). Resuscitating team roles within wayburn health system. In A. Ritzhaupt & S. Kumar (Eds.), *Cases on educational technology implementation for facilitating learning* (pp. 130–145). Hershey, PA: IGI Global. doi:10.4018/978-1-4666-3676-7.ch008

Stein, J. (2013). Millennials: The me me me generation. *Time Magazine, 20*, 1-8.

Steinfield, C., Ellison, N. B., & Lampe, C. (2008). Social capital, self-esteem, and use of online social network sites: A longitudinal analysis. *Journal of Applied Developmental Psychology, 29*(6), 434–445. doi:10.1016/j.appdev.2008.07.002

Stern, D. N., & Bruschweiler-Stern, N. (1998). *The birth of a mother: How the motherhood experience changes you forever*. Basic Books.

Stone, R. A. (1996). *The war of desire and technology at the close of the mechanical age*. Cambridge, MA: MIT Press.

Strine, T. W., Chapman, D. P., Balluz, L., & Mokdad, A. H. (2008). Health-related quality of life and health behaviors by social and emotional support. *Social Psychiatry and Psychiatric Epidemiology*, *43*(2), 151–159. doi:10.1007/s00127-007-0277-x PMID:17962895

Stuart, J. (2007). Work and motherhood: Preliminary report of a psychoanalytic study. *The Psychoanalytic Quarterly*, *76*(2), 439–485. doi:10.1002/j.2167-4086.2007.tb00264.x PMID:17503624

Sugiura, M. (2013). A cognitive neuroscience approach to self and mental health. In J. Wu (Ed.), *Biomedical engineering and cognitive neuroscience for healthcare: Interdisciplinary applications* (pp. 1–10). Hershey, PA: IGI Global. doi:10.4018/978-1-4666-2113-8.ch001

Suler, J. R. (2002). Identity management in cyberspace. *Journal of Applied Psychoanalytic Studies*, *4*(4), 455–459. doi:10.1023/A:1020392231924

Suler, J. R. (2004). The online disinhibition effect. *Cyberpsychology & Behavior*, *7*(3), 321–326. doi:10.1089/1094931041291295 PMID:15257832

Sullivan, M. F. (2011). *Asthma Management In Millenial College Students: Attitudes and Perceptions of Resources* (Doctoral dissertation). The Ohio State University, Columbus, OH.

Sundstrom, B. (2016). Mothers "Google It Up:" Extending communication channel behavior in diffusion of innovations theory. *Health Communication*, *31*(1), 91–101. doi:10.1080/10410236.2014.936339 PMID:26075413

Supnithi, T., Buranarach, M., Thatphithakkul, N., Junsirimongkol, B., Wongrochananan, S., Kulnawan, N., & Jiamjarasrangsi, W. (2014). A self-management service framework to support chronic disease patients' self-management. In M. Kosaka & K. Shirahada (Eds.), *Progressive trends in knowledge and system-based science for service innovation* (pp. 425–450). Hershey, PA: IGI Global. doi:10.4018/978-1-4666-4663-6.ch023

Syed-Abdul, S., Fernandez-Luque, L., Jian, W. S., Li, Y. C., Crain, S., Hsu, M. H., & Liou, D. M. (2013). Misleading health-related information promoted through video-based social media: Anorexia on YouTube. *Journal of Medical Internet Research*, *15*(2), e30. doi:10.2196/jmir.2237 PMID:23406655

Takahashi, K., & Watanabe, K. (2013). Crossmodal interactions in visual competition. In J. Wu (Ed.), *Biomedical engineering and cognitive neuroscience for healthcare: Interdisciplinary applications* (pp. 64–72). Hershey, PA: IGI Global. doi:10.4018/978-1-4666-2113-8.ch007

Tamiya, T., Kawanishi, M., Miyake, K., Kawai, N., & Guo, S. (2013). Neurosurgical operations using navigation microscope integration system. In J. Wu (Ed.), *Technological advancements in biomedicine for healthcare applications* (pp. 128–138). Hershey, PA: IGI Global. doi:10.4018/978-1-4666-2196-1.ch014

Tanaka, H., & Furutani, M. (2013). Sleep management promotes healthy lifestyle, mental health, QOL, and a healthy brain. In J. Wu (Ed.), *Biomedical engineering and cognitive neuroscience for healthcare: Interdisciplinary applications* (pp. 211–224). Hershey, PA: IGI Global. doi:10.4018/978-1-4666-2113-8.ch022

Tang, C., & Carpendale, S. (2013). Human-centered design for health information technology: A qualitative approach. In I. Management Association (Ed.), User-driven healthcare: Concepts, methodologies, tools, and applications (pp. 158-179). Hershey, PA: IGI Global. doi:10.4018/978-1-4666-2770-3.ch009

Tangherlini, T. R., Roychowdhury, V., Glenn, B., Crespi, C. M., Bandari, R., Wadia, A., ... Bastani, R. (2016). "Mommy Blogs" and the Vaccination Exemption Narrative: Results From A Machine-Learning Approach for Story Aggregation on Parenting Social Media Sites. *JMIR public Health and Surveillance, 2*(2).

Tang, X., Gao, Y., Yang, W., Zhang, M., & Wu, J. (2013). Audiovisual integration of natural auditory and visual stimuli in the real-world situation. In J. Wu (Ed.), *Biomedical engineering and cognitive neuroscience for healthcare: Interdisciplinary applications* (pp. 337–344). Hershey, PA: IGI Global. doi:10.4018/978-1-4666-2113-8.ch035

Tanis, M. (2008). Health-related online forums: What's the big attraction. *Journal of Health Communication, 13*(7), 698–714. doi:10.1080/10810730802415316 PMID:18958781

Tan, R., Wang, S., Jiang, Y., Ishida, K., & Fujie, M. G. (2013). Motion control of an omni-directional walker for walking support. In J. Wu (Ed.), *Biomedical engineering and cognitive neuroscience for healthcare: Interdisciplinary applications* (pp. 20–28). Hershey, PA: IGI Global. doi:10.4018/978-1-4666-2113-8.ch003

Targowski, A. (2013). Well-being, wisdom, health, and IT: From the big-picture to the small-picture. In M. Cruz-Cunha, I. Miranda, & P. Gonçalves (Eds.), *Handbook of research on ICTs for human-centered healthcare and social care services* (pp. 1–28). Hershey, PA: IGI Global. doi:10.4018/978-1-4666-3986-7.ch001

Tayabali, S., & Martin, C. M. (2013). The need to transform the core values of medical care and health organizations. In R. Biswas (Ed.), *Clinical solutions and medical progress through user-driven healthcare* (pp. 85–92). Hershey, PA: IGI Global. doi:10.4018/978-1-4666-1876-3.ch009

Taylor, B. W. (2014). Decision-making and decision support in acute care. In C. El Morr (Ed.), *Research perspectives on the role of informatics in health policy and management* (pp. 1–18). Hershey, PA: IGI Global. doi:10.4018/978-1-4666-4321-5.ch001

Taylor, S. E., Klein, L. C., Gruenewald, T. L., Gurung, R. A. R., & Fernandes-Taylor, S. (2003). Affiliation, social support, and biobehavioral responses to stress. In J. Suls & K. A. Wallston (Eds.), *Social Psychological Foundations of Health and Illness* (pp. 314–331). doi:10.1002/9780470753552.ch12

Taylor, S. E., & Lobel, M. (1989). Social comparison activity under threat: Downward evaluation and upward contacts. *Psychological Review*, *96*(4), 569–575. doi:10.1037/0033-295X.96.4.569 PMID:2678204

Teixeira, C., Pinto, J. S., Ferreira, F., Oliveira, A., Teixeira, A., & Pereira, C. (2013). Cloud computing enhanced service development architecture for the living usability lab. In R. Martinho, R. Rijo, M. Cruz-Cunha, & J. Varajão (Eds.), *Information systems and technologies for enhancing health and social care* (pp. 33–53). Hershey, PA: IGI Global. doi:10.4018/978-1-4666-3667-5.ch003

Teixeira, L., Saavedra, V., Ferreira, C., & Santos, B. S. (2013). The role of ICTs in the management of rare chronic diseases: The case of hemophilia. In M. Cruz-Cunha, I. Miranda, & P. Gonçalves (Eds.), *Handbook of research on ICTs and management systems for improving efficiency in healthcare and social care* (pp. 635–649). Hershey, PA: IGI Global. doi:10.4018/978-1-4666-3990-4.ch033

Teoh, S. Y., Singh, M., & Chong, J. (2013). An overview of e-health development in Australia. In I. Management Association (Ed.), User-driven healthcare: Concepts, methodologies, tools, and applications (pp. 901-917). Hershey, PA: IGI Global. doi:10.4018/978-1-4666-2770-3.ch045

Terzioğlu, A. (2011). Küreselleşme, Kanser ve Hastalık Anlatıları. In C. Özbay, A. Terzioğlu, & Y. Yasin (Eds.), *Neoliberalizm ve Mahremiyet Türkiye'de Beden Sağlık ve Cinsellik* (pp. 111–132). İstanbul: Metis.

Thoits, P. A. (2011). Mechanisms linking social ties and support to physical and mental health. *Journal of Health and Social Behavior*, *52*(2), 145–161. doi:10.1177/0022146510395592 PMID:21673143

Thomson, R. (2011). *Making modern mothers*. Policy Press. doi:10.2307/j.ctt1t898c8

Tidwell, L. C., & Walther, J. B. (2002). Computer-mediated communication effects on disclosure, impression, and interpersonal evaluations: Getting to know one another a bit at a time. *Human Communication Research*, *28*(3), 317–348. doi:10.1111/j.1468-2958.2002.tb00811.x

Tiwari, S., & Srivastava, R. (2014). Research and developments in medical image reconstruction methods and its applications. In R. Srivastava, S. Singh, & K. Shukla (Eds.), *Research developments in computer vision and image processing: Methodologies and applications* (pp. 274–312). Hershey, PA: IGI Global. doi:10.4018/978-1-4666-4558-5.ch014

Tobolcea, I. (2013). The psychosocial impact of ICT efficiency on speech disorders-treatment. In M. Cruz-Cunha, I. Miranda, & P. Gonçalves (Eds.), *Handbook of research on ICTs for human-centered healthcare and social care services* (pp. 70–92). Hershey, PA: IGI Global. doi:10.4018/978-1-4666-3986-7.ch004

Toda, T., Chen, P., Ozaki, S., Fujita, K., & Ideguchi, N. (2013). A simple web-based image database system for facilitating medical care in dermatological clinics. In I. Management Association (Ed.), User-driven healthcare: Concepts, methodologies, tools, and applications (pp. 502-513). Hershey, PA: IGI Global. doi:10.4018/978-1-4666-2770-3.ch025

Toda, T., Chen, P., Ozaki, S., Fujita, K., & Ideguchi, N. (2013). A simple web-based image database system for facilitating medical care in dermatological clinics. In J. Wu (Ed.), *Technological advancements in biomedicine for healthcare applications* (pp. 385–397). Hershey, PA: IGI Global. doi:10.4018/978-1-4666-2196-1.ch038

Tong, S. T., Heinmann-LaFave, D., Jeon, J., Kolodziej-Smith, R., & Warshay, N. (2013). The use of pro-ana blogs for online social support. *Eating Disorders*, *21*(5), 408–422. doi:10.1080/10640266.2013.827538 PMID:24044597

Tozzi, A. E., Mingarelli, R., Gonfiantini, M., Pandolfi, E., Carloni, E., Gesualdo, F., & Dallapiccola, B. (2013). The internet user profile of Italian families of patients with rare diseases: A web survey. *Orphanet Journal of Rare Diseases*, *8*(1), 1–8. doi:10.1186/1750-1172-8-76 PMID:23680013

Trudeau, S. (2013). CoRDS registry: An HIT case study concerning setup and maintenance of a disease registry. In S. Sarnikar, D. Bennett, & M. Gaynor (Eds.), *Cases on healthcare information technology for patient care management* (pp. 197–207). Hershey, PA: IGI Global. doi:10.4018/978-1-4666-2671-3.ch012

Tseng, R., & Yi-Luen Do, E. (2013). The role of information and computer technology for children with autism spectrum disorder and the facial expression wonderland (FEW). In A. Gangopadhyay (Ed.), *Methods, models, and computation for medical informatics* (pp. 98–116). Hershey, PA: IGI Global. doi:10.4018/978-1-4666-2653-9.ch006

TUIK. (2011). *Hanehalkı Bilişim Teknolojileri Kullanım Araştırması, 2011*. Retrieved January 3, 2017, from http://www.tuik.gov.tr/PreHaberBultenleri.do?id=8572

TUIK. (2016). *Hanehalkı Bilişim Teknolojileri Kullanım Araştırması, 2016*. Retrieved January 3, 2017, from http://www.tuik.gov.tr/PreHaberBultenleri.do?id=21779

Turkle, S. (2011). *Alone together: Why we expect more from technology and less from each other*. Academic Press.

Turkle, S. (2011). *Alone, together: Why we expect more from technology and less from each other*. New York: Basic Books.

Turkle, S. (2012). *Alone together: Why we expect more from technology and less from each other*. New York: Basic Books.

Turner, J. W., Grube, J. A., & Meyers, J. (2001). Developing an optimal match within online communities: An exploration of CMC support communities and traditional support. *Journal of Communication*, *51*(2), 231–251. doi:10.1111/j.1460-2466.2001.tb02879.x

Uchino, B. N. (2004). *Social support and physical health: Understanding the health consequences of relationships*. Yale University Press. doi:10.12987/yale/9780300102185.001.0001

Uchino, B. N., Cacioppo, J. T., & Kiecolt-Glaser, J. K. (1996). The relationship between social support and physiological processes: A review with emphasis on underlying mechanisms and implications for health. *Psychological Bulletin*, *119*(3), 488–531. doi:10.1037/0033-2909.119.3.488 PMID:8668748

Uchitomi, H., Suzuki, K., Nishi, T., Hove, M. J., Miyake, Y., Orimo, S., & Wada, Y. (2013). Gait rhythm of Parkinson's disease patients and an interpersonal synchrony emulation system based on cooperative gait. In J. Wu (Ed.), *Biomedical engineering and cognitive neuroscience for healthcare: Interdisciplinary applications* (pp. 38–53). Hershey, PA: IGI Global. doi:10.4018/978-1-4666-2113-8.ch005

Usher, W., & San Too, L. (2013). E-health knowledge management by australian university students. In I. Management Association (Ed.), User-driven healthcare: Concepts, methodologies, tools, and applications (pp. 938-953). Hershey, PA: IGI Global. doi:10.4018/978-1-4666-2770-3.ch047

Ussher, J., Kirsten, L., Butow, P., & Sandoval, M. (2006). What do cancer support groups provide which other supportive relationships do not? The experience of peer support groups for people with cancer. *Social Science & Medicine*, *62*(10), 2565–2576. doi:10.1016/j.socscimed.2005.10.034 PMID:16303220

van Dam, H. A., van der Horst, F. G., Knoops, L., Ryckman, R. M., Crebolder, H. F., & van den Borne, B. H. (2005). Social support in diabetes: A systematic review of controlled intervention studies. *Patient Education and Counseling*, *59*(1), 1–12. doi:10.1016/j.pec.2004.11.001 PMID:16198213

Van Genderen, E. (2014). Intensive care. In V. Jham & S. Puri (Eds.), *Cases on consumer-centric marketing management* (pp. 53–67). Hershey, PA: IGI Global. doi:10.4018/978-1-4666-4357-4.ch006

Van Leuven, N., Newton, D., Leuenberger, D. Z., & Esteves, T. (2014). Reaching citizen 2.0: How government uses social media to send public messages during times of calm and times of crisis. In I. Management Association (Ed.), Crisis management: Concepts, methodologies, tools and applications (pp. 839-857). Hershey, PA: IGI Global. doi:10.4018/978-1-4666-4707-7.ch041

Van Tilburg, T. (1998). Losing and gaining in old age: Changes in personal network size and social support in a four-year longitudinal study. *The Journals of Gerontology. Series B, Psychological Sciences and Social Sciences*, *53*(6), S313–S323. doi:10.1093/geronb/53B.6.S313 PMID:9826973

Van Uden-Kraan, N. (2008). *Online Peer Support for Patients with Somatic Diseases* (Thesis). University of Twente. Retrieved January 12, 2017, from http://purl.utwente.nl/publications/60136

van Uden-Kraan, C. F., Drossaert, C. H., Taal, E., Shaw, B. R., Seydel, E. R., & van de Laar, M. A. (2008). Empowering processes and outcomes of participation in online support groups for patients with breast cancer, arthritis, or fibromyalgia. *Qualitative Health Research*, *18*(3), 405–417. doi:10.1177/1049732307313429 PMID:18235163

Vanable, P. A., Carey, M. P., Blair, D. C., & Littlewood, R. A. (2006). Impact of HIV-related stigma on health behaviors and psychological adjustment among HIV-positive men and women. *AIDS and Behavior*, *10*(5), 473–482. doi:10.1007/s10461-006-9099-1 PMID:16604295

Vasudevan, V., & Rao, H. (2013). E-discovery and health care IT: An investigation. In I. Management Association (Ed.), User-driven healthcare: Concepts, methodologies, tools, and applications (pp. 1622-1635). Hershey, PA: IGI Global. doi:10.4018/978-1-4666-2770-3.ch080

Vat, K. H. (2013). Conceiving community knowledge records as e-governance concerns in wired healthcare provision. In I. Management Association (Ed.), User-driven healthcare: Concepts, methodologies, tools, and applications (pp. 1093-1111). Hershey, PA: IGI Global. doi:10.4018/978-1-4666-2770-3.ch055

Venkatasubramanian, K. K., Nabar, S., Gupta, S. K., & Poovendran, R. (2013). Cyber physical security solutions for pervasive health monitoring systems. In I. Management Association (Ed.), User-driven healthcare: Concepts, methodologies, tools, and applications (pp. 447-465). Hershey, PA: IGI Global. doi:10.4018/978-1-4666-2770-3.ch022

Vevea, N., & Miller, A. (2010). Patient Narratives: Exploring the Fit of Uncertainty-Management Models of Health Care. *Review of Communication*, *10*(4), 276–289. doi:10.1080/15358593.2010.501907

Victan, H. (2013). Emerging trends in user-driven healthcare: Negotiating disclosure in online health community organizations. In I. Management Association (Ed.), User-driven healthcare: Concepts, methodologies, tools, and applications (pp. 1589-1606). Hershey, PA: IGI Global. doi:10.4018/978-1-4666-2770-3.ch078

Vidal, B., Pereira, J. M., & Santos, G. (2013). SimBody: An interactive simulator for health education. In S. Arnab, I. Dunwell, & K. Debattista (Eds.), *Serious games for healthcare: Applications and implications* (pp. 265–282). Hershey, PA: IGI Global. doi:10.4018/978-1-4666-1903-6.ch013

Vilhauer, R. P. (2009). Perceived benefits of online support groups for women with metastatic breast cancer. *Women & Health*, *49*(5), 381–404. doi:10.1080/03630240903238719 PMID:19851944

Vivekananda-Schmidt, P. (2013). Ethics in the design of serious games for healthcare and medicine. In S. Arnab, I. Dunwell, & K. Debattista (Eds.), *Serious games for healthcare: Applications and implications* (pp. 91–106). Hershey, PA: IGI Global. doi:10.4018/978-1-4666-1903-6.ch005

Von Muhlen, M., & Ohno-Machado, L. (2012). Reviewing social media use b clinicians. *Journal of the American Medical Informatics Association*, *19*(5), 777–781. doi:10.1136/amiajnl-2012-000990 PMID:22759618

Wahbeh, A. (2013). Application of handheld computing and mobile phones in diabetes self-care. In S. Sarnikar, D. Bennett, & M. Gaynor (Eds.), *Cases on healthcare information technology for patient care management* (pp. 254–275). Hershey, PA: IGI Global. doi:10.4018/978-1-4666-2671-3.ch015

Waidyanatha, N., & Dekker, S. (2013). The RTBP – Collective intelligence driving health for the user. In R. Biswas (Ed.), *Clinical solutions and medical progress through user-driven healthcare* (pp. 70–78). Hershey, PA: IGI Global. doi:10.4018/978-1-4666-1876-3.ch007

Waidyanatha, N., Dubrawski, A. M. G., & Gow, G. (2013). Affordable system for rapid detection and mitigation of emerging diseases. In J. Rodrigues (Ed.), *Digital advances in medicine, e-health, and communication technologies* (pp. 271–288). Hershey, PA: IGI Global. doi:10.4018/978-1-4666-2794-9.ch015

Walker, D. (2013). How would a ban on prescriber-identifying information impact pharmaceutical marketing? In M. Merviö (Ed.), *Healthcare management and economics: Perspectives on public and private administration* (pp. 141–153). Hershey, PA: IGI Global. doi:10.4018/978-1-4666-3982-9.ch011

Wallston, B. S., Alagna, S. W., DeVellis, B. M., & DeVellis, R. F. (1983). Social support and physical health. *Health Psychology*, *2*(4), 367–391. doi:10.1037/0278-6133.2.4.367

Walther, J. B., & Parks, M. R. (2002). Cues filtered out, cues filtered in. Handbook of interpersonal communication, 3, 529-563.

Walther, J. B. (1992). Interpersonal effects in computer-mediated interaction: A relational perspective. *Communication Research*, *19*(1), 52–90. doi:10.1177/009365092019001003

Walther, J. B. (1996). Computer-mediated communication: Impersonal, interpersonal, and hyperpersonal interaction. *Communication Research*, *23*(1), 3–43. doi:10.1177/009365096023001001

Walther, J. B. (2007). Selective self-presentation in computer-mediated communication: Hyperpersonal dimensions of technology, language, and cognition. *Computers in Human Behavior*, *23*(5), 2538–2557. doi:10.1016/j.chb.2006.05.002

Walther, J. B., & Boyd, S. (2002). Attraction to computer-mediated social support. In C. A. Lin & D. Atkin (Eds.), *Communication technology and society: Audience adoption and uses* (pp. 153–188). Cresskill, NJ: Hampton Press.

Walther, J. B., Slovacek, C., & Tidwell, L. C. (2001). Is a picture worth a thousand words? Photographic images in long term and short term virtual teams. *Communication Research*, *28*(1), 105–134. doi:10.1177/009365001028001004

Walumbwa, F. O., Avolio, B. J., Gardner, W. L., Wernsing, T. S., & Peterson, S. J. (2008). Authentic leadership: Development and validation of a theory-based measure. *Journal of Management*, *34*(1), 89–126. doi:10.1177/0149206307308913

Wang, B., Yan, T., & Wu, J. (2013). Neuronal function in the cortical face perception network. In J. Wu (Ed.), *Biomedical engineering and cognitive neuroscience for healthcare: Interdisciplinary applications* (pp. 171–182). Hershey, PA: IGI Global. doi:10.4018/978-1-4666-2113-8.ch018

Wang, Y., & Wang, Q. (2013). Evaluating the IEEE 802.15.6 2.4GHz WBAN proposal on medical multi-parameter monitoring under WiFi/bluetooth interference. In J. Rodrigues (Ed.), *Digital advances in medicine, e-health, and communication technologies* (pp. 312–325). Hershey, PA: IGI Global. doi:10.4018/978-1-4666-2794-9.ch018

Wang, Z., Walther, J. B., Pingree, S., & Hawkins, R. P. (2008). Health information, credibility, homophily, and influence via the Internet: Web sites versus discussion groups. *Health Communication*, *23*(4), 358–368. doi:10.1080/10410230802229738 PMID:18702000

Watanabe, T., & Miura, N. (2013). Functional electrical stimulation (FES) control for restoration and rehabilitation of motor function. In J. Wu (Ed.), *Technological advancements in biomedicine for healthcare applications* (pp. 80–93). Hershey, PA: IGI Global. doi:10.4018/978-1-4666-2196-1.ch009

Watanabe, Y., Tanaka, H., & Hirata, K. (2013). Evaluation of cognitive function in migraine patients: A study using event-related potentials. In J. Wu (Ed.), *Biomedical engineering and cognitive neuroscience for healthcare: Interdisciplinary applications* (pp. 303–310). Hershey, PA: IGI Global. doi:10.4018/978-1-4666-2113-8.ch031

Watfa, M. K., Kaur, M., & Daruwala, R. F. (2013). RFID applications in e-healthcare. In I. Management Association (Ed.), User-driven healthcare: Concepts, methodologies, tools, and applications (pp. 259-287). Hershey, PA: IGI Global. doi:10.4018/978-1-4666-2770-3.ch014

Weinert, C., & Hill, W. G. (2005). Rural women with chronic illness: Computer use and skill acquisition. *Women's Health Issues*, *15*(5), 230–236. doi:10.1016/j.whi.2005.06.002 PMID:16165009

Weldon, T. (2017, January 25). Grand Falls radio host says Bell Media fired her for mental health issues. *CBC News*. Retrieved from: http://www.cbc.ca/news/canada/new-brunswick/bell-media-host-mental-health-1.3950097

Wesorick, B. (2013). Essential steps for successful implementation of the EHR to achieve sustainable, safe, quality care. In A. Moumtzoglou & A. Kastania (Eds.), *E-health technologies and improving patient safety: Exploring organizational factors* (pp. 27–55). Hershey, PA: IGI Global. doi:10.4018/978-1-4666-2657-7.ch003

Whitaker, R. (2013). Securing health-effective medicine in practice: A critical perspective on user-driven healthcare. In R. Biswas (Ed.), *Clinical solutions and medical progress through user-driven healthcare* (pp. 35–50). Hershey, PA: IGI Global. doi:10.4018/978-1-4666-1876-3.ch005

White, M., & Dorman, S. M. (2001). Receiving social support online: Implications for health education. *Health Education Research*, *16*(6), 693–707. doi:10.1093/her/16.6.693 PMID:11780708

Wickramasinghe, N., Troshani, I., Hill, S. R., Hague, W., & Goldberg, S. (2013). A transaction cost assessment of a pervasive technology solution for gestational diabetes. In J. Tan (Ed.), *Healthcare information technology innovation and sustainability: Frontiers and adoption* (pp. 109–126). Hershey, PA: IGI Global. doi:10.4018/978-1-4666-2797-0.ch007

Widarsson, M., Kerstis, B., Sundquist, K., Engström, G., & Sarkadi, A. (2012). Support needs of expectant mothers and fathers: A qualitative study. *Journal of Perinatal Education*, *21*(1), 36–44. doi:10.1891/1058-1243.21.1.36 PMID:23277729

Wilkowska, W., & Ziefle, M. (2013). User diversity as a challenge for the integration of medical technology into future smart home environments. In I. Management Association (Ed.), User-driven healthcare: Concepts, methodologies, tools, and applications (pp. 553-582). Hershey, PA: IGI Global. doi:10.4018/978-1-4666-2770-3.ch028

Williams, J. C., & Segal, N. (2003). Beyond the maternal wall: Relief for family caregivers who are discriminated against on the job. *Harvard Women's Law Journal, 26*, 77–162.

Willis, E., Wang, Y., & Rodgers, S. (2013). Online health communities and health literacy: Applying a framework for understanding domains of health literacy. In I. Management Association (Ed.), User-driven healthcare: Concepts, methodologies, tools, and applications (pp. 180-196). Hershey, PA: IGI Global. doi:10.4018/978-1-4666-2770-3.ch010

Willson, M. A. (2006). *Technically together: Rethinking community within techno-society*. New York, NY: Peter Lang.

Winefield, H. R. (2006). Support provision and emotional work in an Internet support group for cancer patients. *Patient Education and Counseling, 62*(2), 193–197. doi:10.1016/j.pec.2005.07.002 PMID:16139466

Winnicott, D. W. (1951). Transitional Objects and Transitional Phenomena: A Study of the First Not-Me. *The International Journal of Psycho-Analysis, 34*(2), 89–97. PMID:13061115

Wolburg, J. M., & Pokrywczynski, J. (2001). A psychographic analysis of Generation Y college students. *Journal of Advertising Research, 41*(5), 33–52. doi:10.2501/JAR-41-5-33-52

Wolitski, R. J., Pals, S. L., Kidder, D. P., Courtenay-Quick, C., & Holtgrave, D. R. (2008). The effects of HIV stigma on health, disclosure of HIV status, and risk behavior of homeless and unstably housed persons living with HIV. *AIDS and Behavior, 13*(6), 1222–1232. doi:10.1007/s10461-008-9455-4 PMID:18770023

Wright, K. B. (2005). Researching Internet-based popu0lations: Advantages and disadvantages of online survey research, online questionnaire authoring software packages, and web survey services. *Journal of Computer-Mediated Communication, 10*(3), article 11. Available: http://jcmc.indiana.edu/vol10/issue3/wright.html

Wright, K. B. (1999). Computer-mediated support groups: An examination of relationships among social support, perceived stress, and coping strategies. *Communication Quarterly, 47*(4), 402–414. doi:10.1080/01463379909385570

Wright, K. B. (2000). Perceptions of online support providers: An examination of perceived homophily, source credibility, communication and social support within online support groups. *Communication Quarterly, 48*(1), 44–59. doi:10.1080/01463370009385579

Wright, K. B. (2002). Social support within an online cancer community: An assessment of emotional support, perceptions of advantages and disadvantages, and motives for using the community. *Journal of Applied Communication Research, 30*, 195–209. doi:10.1080/00909880216586

Wright, K. B. (2012). Emotional support and perceived stress among college students using Facebook.com: An exploration of the relationship between source perceptions and emotional support. *Communication Research Reports, 29*(3), 1–10. doi:10.1080/08824096.2012.695957

Wright, K. B., Bell, S. B., Wright, K. B., & Bell, S. B. (2003). Health-related support groups on the Internet: Linking empirical findings to social support and computer-mediated communication theory. *Journal of Health Psychology*, *8*(1), 37–52. doi:10.1177/1359105303008001429 PMID:22113899

Wright, K. B., Johnson, A. J., Bernard, D. R., & Averbeck, J. (2011). Computer-mediated social support: Promises and pitfalls for individuals coping with health concerns. In T. L. Thompson, R. Parrott, & J. F. Nussbaum (Eds.), *The Routledge handbook of health communication* (2nd ed.; pp. 349–362). New York: Routledge.

Wright, K. B., & Miller, C. H. (2010). A measure of weak tie/strong tie support network preference. *Communication Monographs*, *77*(4), 502–520. doi:10.1080/03637751.2010.502538

Wright, K. B., & Rains, S. A. (2014). Weak tie support preference and preferred coping styles as predictors of perceived credibility within health-related computer-mediated support groups. *Health Communication*, *29*(3), 281–287. doi:10.1080/10410236.2012.751084 PMID:23790220

Wright, K. B., Rains, S., & Banas, J. (2010). Weak tie support network preference and perceived life stress among participants in health-related, computer-mediated support groups. *Journal of Computer-Mediated Communication*, *15*(4), 606–624. doi:10.1111/j.1083-6101.2009.01505.x

Wright, K. B., Rosenberg, J., Egbert, N., Ploeger, N., Bernard, D. R., & King, S. (2013). Communication competence, social support, and depression among college students. A model of Facebook and face-to-face support network influence. *Journal of Health Communication*, *18*(1), 41–47. doi:10.1080/10810730.2012.688250 PMID:23030518

Wu, Q., Li, C., Takahashi, S., & Wu, J. (2013). Visual-tactile bottom-up and top-down attention. In J. Wu (Ed.), *Biomedical engineering and cognitive neuroscience for healthcare: Interdisciplinary applications* (pp. 183–191). Hershey, PA: IGI Global. doi:10.4018/978-1-4666-2113-8.ch019

Yamaguchi, S., Onoda, K., & Abe, S. (2013). Feedback-related negativity and its clinical implications. In J. Wu (Ed.), *Biomedical engineering and cognitive neuroscience for healthcare: Interdisciplinary applications* (pp. 283–292). Hershey, PA: IGI Global. doi:10.4018/978-1-4666-2113-8.ch029

Yan, B., Lei, Y., Tong, L., & Chen, K. (2013). Functional neuroimaging of acupuncture: A systematic review. In J. Wu (Ed.), *Biomedical engineering and cognitive neuroscience for healthcare: Interdisciplinary applications* (pp. 142–155). Hershey, PA: IGI Global. doi:10.4018/978-1-4666-2113-8.ch015

Yang, J. (2014). Towards healthy public policy: GIS and food systems analysis. In C. El Morr (Ed.), *Research perspectives on the role of informatics in health policy and management* (pp. 135–152). Hershey, PA: IGI Global. doi:10.4018/978-1-4666-4321-5.ch009

Yang, J. J., Liu, J. F., Kurokawa, T., Kitamura, N., Yasuda, K., & Gong, J. P. (2013). Tough double-network hydrogels as scaffolds for tissue engineering: Cell behavior in vitro and in vivo test. In J. Wu (Ed.), *Technological advancements in biomedicine for healthcare applications* (pp. 213–222). Hershey, PA: IGI Global. doi:10.4018/978-1-4666-2196-1.ch023

Yang, J., Li, Q., Gao, Y., & Wu, J. (2013). Temporal dependency of multisensory audiovisual integration. In J. Wu (Ed.), *Biomedical engineering and cognitive neuroscience for healthcare: Interdisciplinary applications* (pp. 320–326). Hershey, PA: IGI Global. doi:10.4018/978-1-4666-2113-8.ch033

Yang, W., Gao, Y., & Wu, J. (2013). Effects of selective and divided attention on audiovisual interaction. In J. Wu (Ed.), *Biomedical engineering and cognitive neuroscience for healthcare: Interdisciplinary applications* (pp. 311–319). Hershey, PA: IGI Global. doi:10.4018/978-1-4666-2113-8.ch032

Yano, Y. (2013). An EMG control system for an ultrasonic motor using a PSoC microcomputer. In J. Wu (Ed.), *Technological advancements in biomedicine for healthcare applications* (pp. 11–17). Hershey, PA: IGI Global. doi:10.4018/978-1-4666-2196-1.ch002

Yap, K. Y. (2013). The evolving role of pharmacoinformatics in targeting drug-related problems in clinical oncology practice. In I. Management Association (Ed.), User-driven healthcare: Concepts, methodologies, tools, and applications (pp. 1541-1588). Hershey, PA: IGI Global. doi:10.4018/978-1-4666-2770-3.ch077

Yardi, S., Romero, D., Schoenebeck, G., & Boyd, D. (2009). Detecting spam in a twitter network. *First Monday, 15*(1). doi:10.5210/fm.v15i1.2793

Yokoi, H., Kato, R., Mori, T., Yamamura, O., & Kubota, M. (2013). Functional electrical stimulation based on interference-driven PWM signals for neuro-rehabilitation. In J. Wu (Ed.), *Technological advancements in biomedicine for healthcare applications* (pp. 180–192). Hershey, PA: IGI Global. doi:10.4018/978-1-4666-2196-1.ch019

York, A. M., & Nordengren, F. R. (2013). E-learning and web 2.0 case study: The role of gender in contemporary models of health care leadership. In H. Yang & S. Wang (Eds.), *Cases on formal and informal e-learning environments: Opportunities and practices* (pp. 292–313). Hershey, PA: IGI Global. doi:10.4018/978-1-4666-1930-2.ch016

Yu, W. D., & Bhagwat, R. (2013). Modeling emergency and telemedicine health support system: A service oriented architecture approach using cloud computing. In J. Rodrigues (Ed.), *Digital advances in medicine, e-health, and communication technologies* (pp. 187–213). Hershey, PA: IGI Global. doi:10.4018/978-1-4666-2794-9.ch011

Yu, Y., Yang, J., & Wu, J. (2013). Cognitive functions and neuronal mechanisms of tactile working memory. In J. Wu (Ed.), *Biomedical engineering and cognitive neuroscience for healthcare: Interdisciplinary applications* (pp. 89–98). Hershey, PA: IGI Global. doi:10.4018/978-1-4666-2113-8.ch010

Zaheer, S. (2014). Implementation of evidence-based practice and the PARIHS framework. In C. El Morr (Ed.), *Research perspectives on the role of informatics in health policy and management* (pp. 19–36). Hershey, PA: IGI Global. doi:10.4018/978-1-4666-4321-5.ch002

Zalzala, A., Chia, S., Zalzala, L., Sahu, S., Vaghasiya, S., & Karimi, A. (2013). Rural e-health infrastructure development. In I. Management Association (Ed.), User-driven healthcare: Concepts, methodologies, tools, and applications (pp. 870-900). Hershey, PA: IGI Global. doi:10.4018/978-1-4666-2770-3.ch044

Zapirain, B. G., & Zorrilla, A. M. (2013). Independent living support for disabled and elderly people using cell phones. In M. Cruz-Cunha, I. Miranda, & P. Gonçalves (Eds.), *Handbook of research on ICTs for human-centered healthcare and social care services* (pp. 379–397). Hershey, PA: IGI Global. doi:10.4018/978-1-4666-3986-7.ch020

Zgodavová, K., & Bourek, A. (2013). Potential of web based learning in managing for the sustained success of a healthcare organization based on IMPROHEALTH® project. In I. Management Association (Ed.), User-driven healthcare: Concepts, methodologies, tools, and applications (pp. 1523-1540). Hershey, PA: IGI Global. doi:10.4018/978-1-4666-2770-3.ch076

Zhao, X., Zuo, M. J., & Moghaddass, R. (2013). Generating indicators for diagnosis of fault levels by integrating information from two or more sensors. In I. Management Association (Ed.), User-driven healthcare: Concepts, methodologies, tools, and applications (pp. 288-309). Hershey, PA: IGI Global. doi:10.4018/978-1-4666-2770-3.ch015

Zhou, X., & Ren, X. (2013). Speed-accuracy tradeoff models of target-based and trajectory-based movements. In J. Wu (Ed.), *Biomedical engineering and cognitive neuroscience for healthcare: Interdisciplinary applications* (pp. 355–368). Hershey, PA: IGI Global. doi:10.4018/978-1-4666-2113-8.ch037

Zouag, N., & Driouchi, A. (2014). Trends and prospects of the Moroccan health system: 2010-2030. In A. Driouchi (Ed.), *Labor and health economics in the mediterranean region: Migration and mobility of medical doctors* (pp. 314–336). Hershey, PA: IGI Global. doi:10.4018/978-1-4666-4723-7.ch013

Zvikhachevskaya, A., & Mihaylova, L. (2013). Advanced video distribution for wireless e-healthcare systems. In I. Management Association (Ed.), User-driven healthcare: Concepts, methodologies, tools, and applications (pp. 421-446). Hershey, PA: IGI Global. doi:10.4018/978-1-4666-2770-3.ch021

About the Contributors

Aslıhan Ardıç Çobaner is a asistant professor at Mersin University. She graduated from Ankara University, Faculty of Communication Departmant of Journalism in 2000. She has received her PhD degree with the thesis about "Media Framing of Tobacco control News in the Context of Right-Based Health Aproach" from Ankara University in 2013. Her studies focus on the health communication, media and health literacy, media studies and news analysis.

Mine Gencel Bek is currently Georg Bollenbeck fellow at the University of Siegen. She completed her Ph.D at Loughborough University in 1999. She was a visiting lecturer at MIT Comparative Media Studies, Open Documentary Lab and Civic Media Lab in 2013 and 2014. Her current research and teaching are focused on immigration and exile cultures; memory; journalism, peace and trauma; changing media forms, technological innovations and the use of participatory tools in civic advocacy.

Valentina Boursier graduated in Clinical Psychology, PhD in Gender Studies, Researcher at Naples University "Federico II", Psychotherapist for Children and Adolescents, Member of the Winnicott's Institute (iW) and of the Italian Psychoanalytical Psychotherapy Society for Children and Adolescents (SIPsIA). Her occupational fields and research areas are Clinical Psychology and Development Psychoanalysis, Gender Studies, Feminine Identity, Maternity and motherhood, Mother-Infant interactions, Children's psychopathology prevention, Direct observation for training, intervention and clinical research tools. One specific study direction focus on the web use and misuse among parents as e-health users and adolescents, underlying related risks and opportunities.

Federica Coppola graduated in Clinical, Dynamic, and Social Psychology at University of Naples Federico II, Psychologist. Her occupational fields and research areas are Clinical and Dynamic Psychology, Gender Studies, adolescence, Cyberpsychology, and Internet Addiction, parenthood, and children with special needs.

Francesca Gioia graduated in Clinical, Dynamic and Social Psychology, PhD student in Mind, Gender and Language at University of Naples Federico II, Psychologist. Her occupational fields and research areas are Clinical and Dynamic Psychology, Gender Studies, Feminine Identity, Maternity and Motherhood, Parenthood, Children with Special Needs and Cyberpsychology. One specific direction focus on the web use and misuse among parents as e-health users and adolescents, underlying related risks and opportunities.

Kristin Maki is currently a PhD candidate at the University at Buffalo, The State University of New York. Her research is in health communication, with a focus on persuasion, social support, and adherence.

Valentina Manna, PhD, post-doctoral fellow at Naples University, is clinical psychologist and post-graduate student in Psychoanalytic Psychotherapy of the child, adolescent and parents. She mostly works with schoolers/preschoolers, also being engaged as educator at a nursery school. She collaborated, as project manager, in several national/international projects about prevention of risk in childhood and adolescence, equal opportunities and gender issues. She has been awarded (2015) by the Italian Order of Psychologists for the project Dear Sibling, addressed to young siblings of children with Down Syndrome. She has been enrolled in home-visiting programs for at-risk-children, and currently runs help-desks for parents. She is vice-president of Roots in Action Association. Her research interests include sibling relationships in disabilities, psychodynamic observation, videobservation/videofeedback, identity processes and technologies in adolescence, infant psychoanalysis and maternity

Claudia Lisa Moeller was born in 1992, in Milano. She studied Philosophy during her BA and MA. She focused her studies particularly on Kierkegaard and Bioethics.

Liza Ngenye is a PhD student of Health Communication at George Mason University.

Brandon Niezgoda is a graduating PhD student, and Adjunct Professor at Drexel University. Originally from upstate New York he received a Master's in Humanities with a concentration in film from the University at Buffalo, and a BA in Cinema and Screen Studies from SUNY Oswego. His dissertation focused on the pragmatics of micro-budget film collectives across the United States.

Aisha K. O'Mally is a PhD candidate at the State University of New York at Buffalo. Her area of research is health communication with an interest in patient-provider communication, self-efficacy, and adherence.

Gemma Richardson is a professor in the degree programs in the School of Media Studies and Information at Humber College in Toronto, Canada and is the program coordinator of the Bachelor of Digital Communications program. She has a PhD in Media Studies from the University of Western Ontario. Her dissertation provided the first ever historical analysis of Canadian newspaper coverage of suicide and explored the ethical norms around reporting on suicide.

Noemi Venosa graduated in Clinical, Dynamic and Social Psychology, Psychologist. Her occupational fields and research areas are Clinical and Dynamic Psychology, Narcisism and Identity, Gender Studies, Maternity and Motherhood, Parenthood, and Cyberpsychology. One specific direction focus on the construction of identity among the web use.

Kevin Wright is a professor at George Mason University. He has focused much of his research on social support processes and health outcomes in both face-to-face and computer-mediated contexts. He is the author of five books, including Health Communication in the 21st Century and Computer-Mediated Communication in Personal Relationships. He has published over 70 articles and book chapters, and his research appears in numerous journals such as Communication Monographs, Journal of Computer-Mediated Communication, Journal of Communication, Health Communication, Journal of Health Communication, Journal of Applied Communication Research, Journal of Personal and Social Relationships, Communication Quarterly, Communication Studies, and several other publications. Dr. Wright served from 2007 to 2010 as editor of the Journal of Computer-Mediated Communication published by the International Communication Association. He also serves on numerous editorial boards of various communication journals and is a frequent presenter at regional, national, and international communication conferences.

Index

A

Africa 107, 109, 111
algorithm 216, 223
alternative treatments 93, 98, 106
Asynchronous/ Computer Mediated Communication 27
authentic leadership 108, 110-111, 126-127, 130

B

Baby Boomers 164, 166, 183
Bell Canada 217
breast cancer patients 86, 88-89, 101-102, 104

C

caregivers 1-2, 59-60, 63-64, 84
chronic illness 14, 60, 63, 68, 76-79, 84, 171
clinical anxiety 107-109, 112-114, 116-117, 125-127, 130
clinical anxiety and depression 107, 126-127, 130
comparison 7, 30, 32, 34, 38, 41, 48-49, 57, 66, 69, 78, 89
cyber 57, 89, 96-97

D

Deconstruction 206
depression 4-5, 9, 12-14, 34, 59, 87, 107-109, 111-121, 123, 125-127, 130-131, 135-138, 141-148, 150-156, 158-159, 173, 176, 212-214, 224

E

e-group 29, 39, 41, 44-45, 47-49, 57
emoji reactions 71, 73, 84
Emotional Empathy 85, 106
emotional support 4, 7, 27, 61-63, 67, 73-74, 78, 84, 88-89, 106
e-parents 30, 34, 45, 47
ethnographic analysis 90

F

Facebook 63-66, 68-69, 71, 73-74, 76-79, 84-87, 89-91, 104, 108-109, 163-164, 168, 173, 188, 207, 210-211, 213-218
FDA 167, 185-187, 189-193, 195, 199-201, 206
framing 168-169, 171, 173, 175, 183
Framing Theory 183
FTC 191-193, 206

G

Gaslighting 171-172, 184
gender 37, 45, 47, 64, 86, 89, 91, 96-97, 101, 104, 175
generation Y 162, 164, 166-168, 170
Group Think 174, 184

H

hashtag 64-66, 77-79, 191-192, 195, 200, 211, 217-218, 223
health system 95, 102, 104

I

Immanuel Kant 188, 196
informational support 2, 27, 59, 61-62, 64, 74, 77-79, 84, 106
instrumental support 27, 33-34, 61

K

Kim Kardashian 185, 187, 193-194

M

maternity 36, 42-43, 48-49, 57
mental health 4, 14, 60, 108-110, 120, 127, 137, 148, 171, 210-219
mental illness 109, 170, 173, 177, 210-214, 216-219, 224
Morgellons 174, 176, 184
motherhood 29, 31-34, 46, 57

O

Obama-Care 184
online community 2, 7, 11, 27, 48, 62, 77
online social support 1, 3, 13-14, 59, 62-64, 79, 87-88, 101, 108
online support 1-15, 27, 33, 57, 62-63, 85-86, 88-89
online support community 2, 6, 8, 27
Owen's Thematic Analytical Framework 130

P

patient empowerment 185, 190, 202, 206
peer-to-peer 3, 212, 219, 224
Phenomenology 206
pregnancy 30-31, 36, 41-42, 44, 57, 186

Q

qualitative analysis 29

R

retweet 69, 73-74, 84

S

SADAG 107, 109, 112-114, 118, 125-126, 130, 150, 153
Self-Fulfilling Prophecy 177, 184
Slippery Slope Argument 207
social media 14, 27, 57, 59-60, 62-66, 69, 71, 76-79, 84-86, 101, 109, 164-168, 173, 176, 186, 188, 191-192, 198, 201, 207, 210-214, 216-219, 223-224
Social Networks 2-3, 8, 12-13, 15, 27, 33, 46, 48, 63-64, 77-78, 87, 89, 164, 167, 187, 189, 199, 215, 217
Social Security 164, 184
social support 1-14, 27, 30, 32, 59-69, 71, 75-79, 84-91, 99-102, 108
stigma 9, 107-109, 210-211, 213-219, 224
Stigmatization 87, 106
Story-Arc 113, 130
Sub-Saharan Africa 107
suicide prevention 210-211, 213-216, 218, 224

T

tech-moms 29, 39, 46, 48, 57
transition to parenthood 30, 32
Turkey 85-87, 91, 97, 101-102, 104, 157
tweet 84, 218
Twitter 64-66, 68-69, 71, 73-79, 84, 86, 108, 168, 193, 207, 211-213, 216-217
Type 1 Diabetes (T1D) 59-60, 84, 108

U

Uses and Gratifications 165

W

Web 2.0 63, 174, 213, 219
Web Forum 57
website 32, 57, 107, 109, 112-114, 118, 125-126

Purchase Print, E-Book, or Print + E-Book

IGI Global books can now be purchased from three unique pricing formats: Print Only, E-Book Only, or Print + E-Book. Shipping fees apply.

www.igi-global.com

Recommended Reference Books

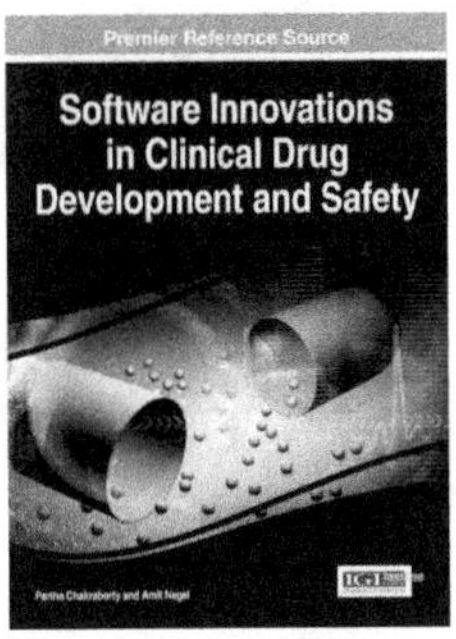

ISBN: 978-1-4666-8726-4
© 2016; 305 pp.
List Price: $225

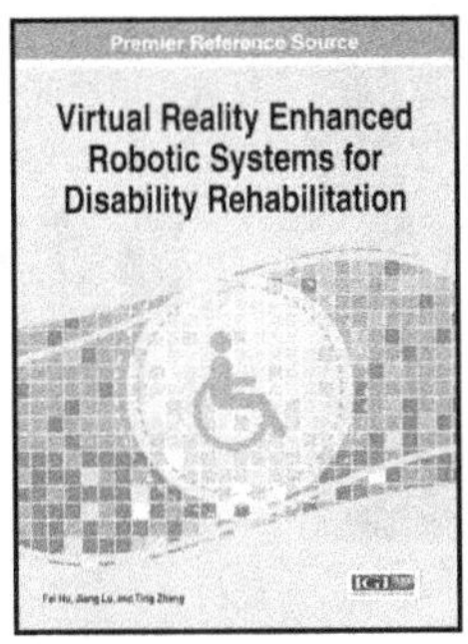

ISBN: 978-1-4666-9740-9
© 2016; 383 pp.
List Price: $210

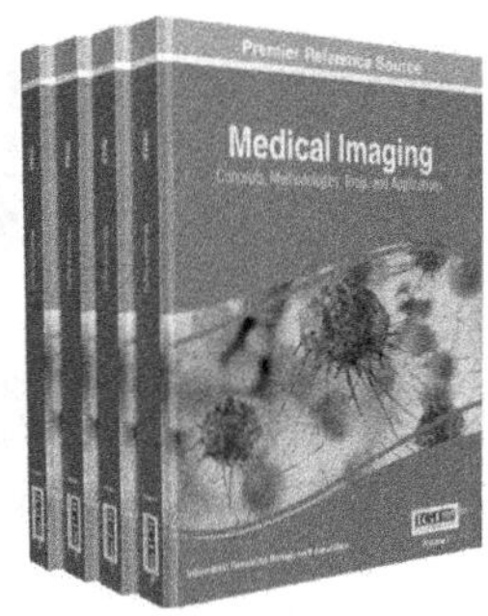

ISBN: 978-1-5225-0571-6
© 2017; 2,081 pp.
List Price: $2,150

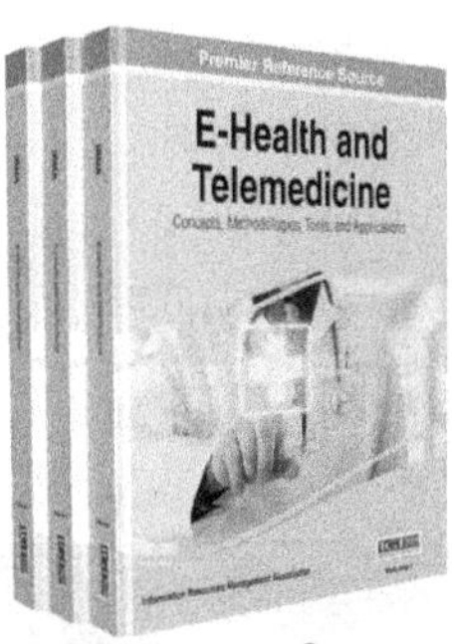

ISBN: 978-1-4666-8756-1
© 2016; 1,759 pp.
List Price: $2,435

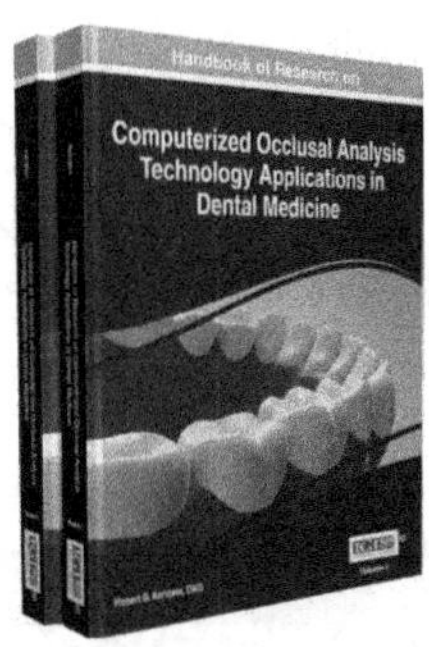

ISBN: 978-1-4666-6587-3
© 2015; 973 pp.
List Price: $475

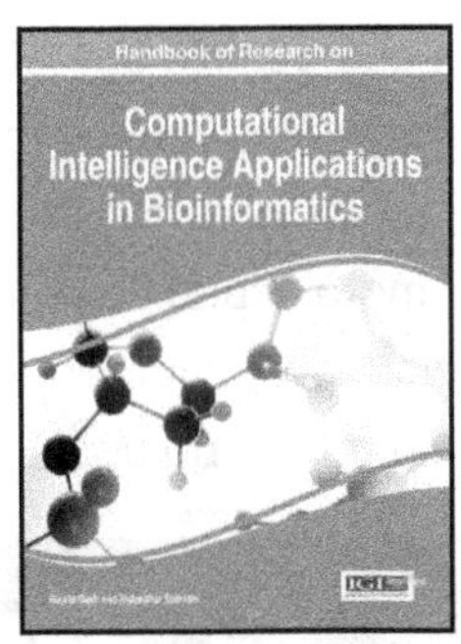

ISBN: 978-1-5225-0427-6
© 2016; 514 pp.
List Price: $230

Looking for free content, product updates, news, and special offers?
Join IGI Global's mailing list today and start enjoying exclusive perks sent only to IGI Global members.
Add your name to the list at **www.igi-global.com/newsletters.**

Publishing Information Science and Technology Research Since 1988

IGI Global
DISSEMINATOR OF KNOWLEDGE

www.igi-global.com Sign up at www.igi-global.com/newsletters facebook.com/igiglobal twitter.com/igiglobal

Stay Current on the Latest Emerging Research Developments

Become an IGI Global Reviewer for Authored Book Projects

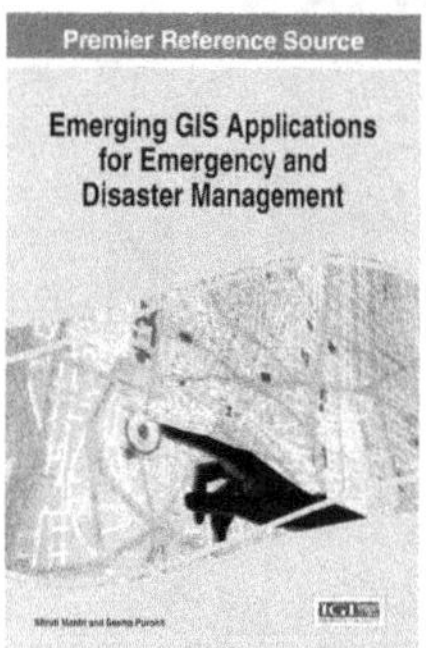

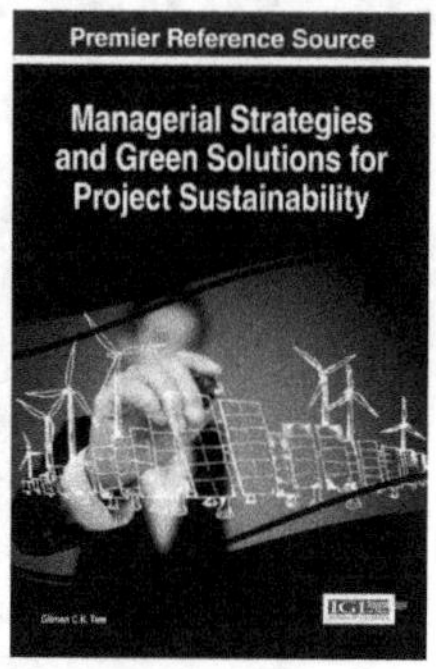

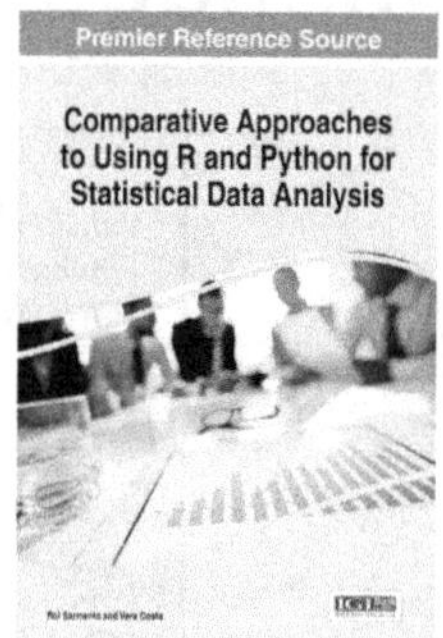

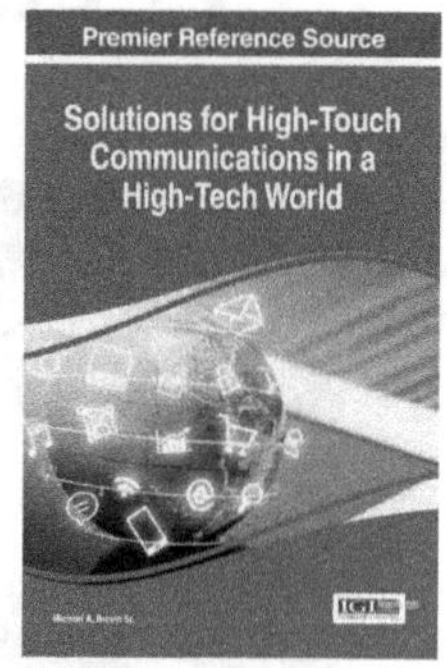

The overall success of an authored book project is dependent on quality and timely reviews.

In this competitive age of scholarly publishing, constructive and timely feedback significantly decreases the turnaround time of manuscripts from submission to acceptance, allowing the publication and discovery of progressive research at a much more expeditious rate. Several IGI Global authored book projects are currently seeking highly qualified experts in the field to fill vacancies on their respective editorial review boards:

Applications may be sent to:
development@igi-global.com

Applicants must have a doctorate (or an equivalent degree) as well as publishing and reviewing experience. Reviewers are asked to write reviews in a timely, collegial, and constructive manner. All reviewers will begin their role on an ad-hoc basis for a period of one year, and upon successful completion of this term can be considered for full editorial review board status, with the potential for a subsequent promotion to Associate Editor.

If you have a colleague that may be interested in this opportunity, we encourage you to share this information with them.

www.igi-global.com

InfoSci®-Books

A Database for Information Science and Technology Research

Maximize Your Library's Book Collection!

Invest in IGI Global's InfoSci®-Books database and gain access to hundreds of reference books at a fraction of their individual list price.

The InfoSci®-Books database offers unlimited simultaneous users the ability to precisely return search results through more than 80,000 full-text chapters from nearly 3,900 reference books in the following academic research areas:

Business & Management Information Science & Technology • Computer Science & Information Technology
Educational Science & Technology • Engineering Science & Technology • Environmental Science & Technology
Government Science & Technology • Library Information Science & Technology • Media & Communication Science & Technology
Medical, Healthcare & Life Science & Technology • Security & Forensic Science & Technology • Social Sciences & Online Behavior

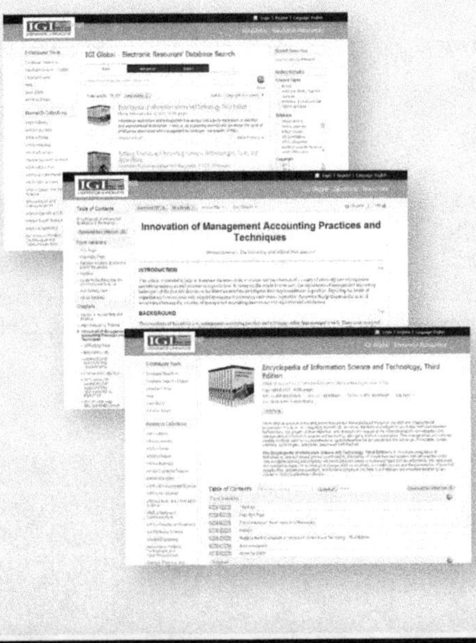

Peer-Reviewed Content:
- Cutting-edge research
- No embargoes
- Scholarly and professional
- Interdisciplinary

Award-Winning Platform:
- Unlimited simultaneous users
- Full-text in XML and PDF
- Advanced search engine
- No DRM

Librarian-Friendly:
- Free MARC records
- Discovery services
- COUNTER4/SUSHI compliant
- Training available

To find out more or request a free trial, visit: www.igi-global.com/eresources

IGI Global
DISSEMINATOR OF KNOWLEDGE
www.igi-global.com

IGI Global
DISSEMINATOR OF KNOWLEDGE
www.igi-global.com

IGI Global Proudly Partners with

eContent Pro International

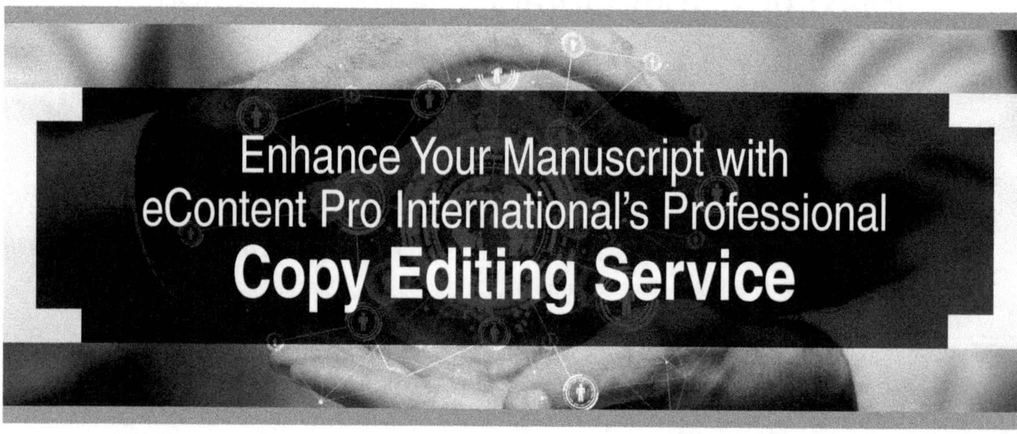

Expert Copy Editing

eContent Pro International copy editors, with over 70 years of combined experience, will provide complete and comprehensive care for your document by resolving all issues with spelling, punctuation, grammar, terminology, jargon, semantics, syntax, consistency, flow, and more. In addition, they will format your document to the style you specify (APA, Chicago, etc.). All edits will be performed using Microsoft Word's Track Changes feature, which allows for fast and simple review and management of edits.

Additional Services

eContent Pro International also offers fast and affordable proofreading to enhance the readability of your document, professional translation in over 100 languages, and market localization services to help businesses and organizations localize their content and grow into new markets around the globe.

IGI Global Authors Save 25% on eContent Pro International's Services!

Scan the QR Code to Receive Your 25% Discount

The 25% discount is applied directly to your eContent Pro International shopping cart when placing an order through IGI Global's referral link. Use the QR code to access this referral link. eContent Pro International has the right to end or modify any promotion at any time.

Email: customerservice@econtentpro.com **econtentpro.com**

Information Resources Management Association

Advancing the Concepts & Practices of Information Resources Management in Modern Organizations

Become an IRMA Member

Members of the **Information Resources Management Association (IRMA)** understand the importance of community within their field of study. The Information Resources Management Association is an ideal venue through which professionals, students, and academicians can convene and share the latest industry innovations and scholarly research that is changing the field of information science and technology. Become a member today and enjoy the benefits of membership as well as the opportunity to collaborate and network with fellow experts in the field.

IRMA Membership Benefits:

- **One FREE Journal Subscription**
- **30% Off Additional Journal Subscriptions**
- **20% Off Book Purchases**
- Updates on the latest events and research on Information Resources Management through the IRMA-L listserv.
- Updates on new open access and downloadable content added to Research IRM.
- A copy of the Information Technology Management Newsletter twice a year.
- A certificate of membership.

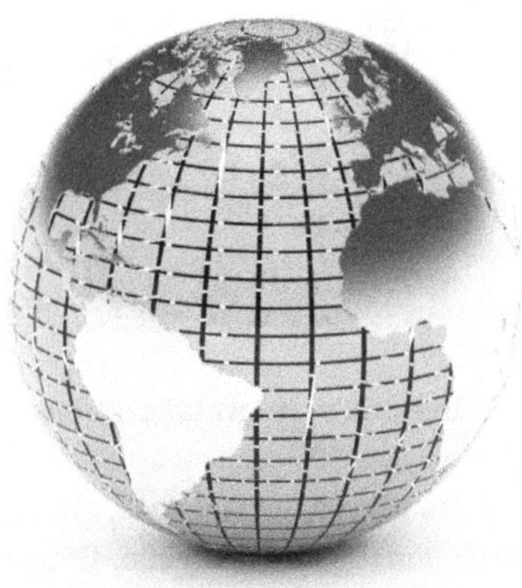

IRMA Membership $195

Scan code or visit **irma-international.org** and begin by selecting your free journal subscription.

Membership is good for one full year.

www.irma-international.org

IGI Global
DISSEMINATOR OF KNOWLEDGE
www.igi-global.com

Available to Order Now

Order through www.igi-global.com with Free Standard Shipping.*

The Premier Reference for Information Science & Information Technology

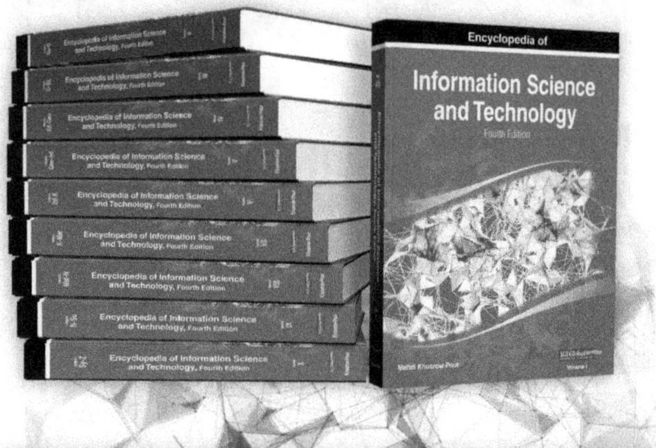

100% Original Content
Contains 705 new, peer-reviewed articles with color figures covering over 80 categories in 11 subject areas

Diverse Contributions
More than 1,100 experts from 74 unique countries contributed their specialized knowledge

Easy Navigation
Includes two tables of content and a comprehensive index in each volume for the user's convenience

Highly-Cited
Embraces a complete list of references and additional reading sections to allow for further research

Included in:
InfoSci®-Books

Encyclopedia of Information Science and Technology Fourth Edition

A Comprehensive 10-Volume Set

Mehdi Khosrow-Pour, D.B.A. (Information Resources Management Association, USA)
ISBN: 978-1-5225-2255-3; © 2018; Pg: 8,104; Release Date: July 31, 2017

The **Encyclopedia of Information Science and Technology, Fourth Edition** is a 10-volume set which includes 705 original and previously unpublished research articles covering a full range of perspectives, applications, and techniques contributed by thousands of experts and researchers from around the globe. This authoritative encyclopedia is an all-encompassing, well-established reference source that is ideally designed to disseminate the most forward-thinking and diverse research findings. With critical perspectives on the impact of information science management and new technologies in modern settings, including but not limited to computer science, education, healthcare, government, engineering, business, and natural and physical sciences, it is a pivotal and relevant source of knowledge that will benefit every professional within the field of information science and technology and is an invaluable addition to every academic and corporate library.

Scan for Online Bookstore

Pricing Information

Hardcover: **$5,695** E-Book: **$5,695** Hardcover + E-Book: **$6,895**

Recommend this Title to Your Institution's Library: www.igi-global.com/books

www.igi-global.com/infosci-ondemand

InfoSci®-OnDemand

Continuously updated with new material on a weekly basis, InfoSci®-OnDemand offers the ability to search through thousands of quality full-text research papers. Users can narrow each search by identifying key topic areas of interest, then display a complete listing of relevant papers, and purchase materials specific to their research needs.

Comprehensive Service

- Over 81,600+ journal articles, book chapters, and case studies.
- All content is downloadable in PDF format and can be stored locally for future use.

No Subscription Fees

- One time fee of $37.50 per PDF download.

Instant Access

- Receive a download link immediately after order completion!

Database Platform Features:

- Comprehensive Pay-Per-View Service
- Written by Prominent International Experts/Scholars
- Precise Search and Retrieval
- Updated With New Material on a Weekly Basis
- Immediate Access to Full-Text PDFs
- No Subscription Needed
- Purchased Research Can Be Stored Locally for Future Use

"It really provides an excellent entry into the research literature of the field. It presents a manageable number of highly relevant sources on topics of interest to a wide range of researchers. The sources are scholarly, but also accessible to 'practitioners'."

- Lisa Stimatz, MLS, University of North Carolina at Chapel Hill, USA

"It is an excellent and well designed database which will facilitate research, publication and teaching. It is a very very useful tool to have."

- George Ditsa, PhD, University of Wollongong, Australia

"I have accessed the database and find it to be a valuable tool to the IT/IS community. I found valuable articles meeting my search criteria 95% of the time."

- Lynda Louis, Xavier University of Louisiana, USA

Recommended for use by researchers who wish to immediately download PDFs of individual chapters or articles.
www.igi-global.com/e-resources/infosci-ondemand

IGI Global
DISSEMINATOR OF KNOWLEDGE
www.igi-global.com

www.ingramcontent.com/pod-product-compliance
Lightning Source LLC
LaVergne TN
LVHW081347300926
849161LV00008B/2088

* 9 7 8 1 5 2 2 5 3 7 1 6 8 *